The Clinical Encounter

A Guide to the Medical Interview and Case Presentation

The Clinical Encounter

A Guide to the Medical Interview and Case Presentation

J. ANDREW BILLINGS, MD

Assistant Clinical Professor, Harvard Medical School
Director of the Palliative Care Service and
Physician, Massachusetts General Hospital
Boston, Massachusetts

JOHN D. STOECKLE, MD

Professor of Medicine, Emeritus, Harvard Medical School
Physician, Massachusetts General Hospital
Boston, Massachusetts

SECOND EDITION

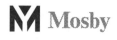

An Affiliate of Elsevier

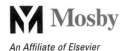
An Affiliate of Elsevier

SECOND EDITION

Printed in the United States of America

Mosby, Inc.
11830 Westline Industrial Drive
St. Louis, Missouri 63146

Library of Congress Cataloging-in-Publication Data

Billings, J. Andrew.
    The clinical encounter: a guide to the medical interview and case
presentation / J. Andrew Billings, John D. Stoeckle.—2nd ed.
        p.   cm.
    Includes bibliographical references and index.
    ISBN-13: 978-0-8151-1374-4   ISBN-10: 0-8151-1374-9
    1. Medical history taking.   I. Stoeckle, John D.   II. Title.
    [DNLM: 1. Medical History Taking—methods.   2. Physician–Patient
Relations.   3. Patient Education.   WB 290 B598c 1998]
RC65.B55 1998
616.07'51—dc21
DNLM/DLC   98–21886
ISBN-13: 978-0-8151-1374-4
ISBN-10: 0-8151-1374-9
  05 06 07 08 / 9 8 7 6

To

S.D.B., J.H.B., and especially **Gabriel**

J.A.B.

To

A.Y.S.

J.D.S.

FOREWORD

The patient-doctor relationship is arguably the most extraordinary social contract in human history. Two strangers meet in a confidential, unobserved setting that emphasizes their differences: the pain and subjective needs of one contrasted with the professionally defined availability of the other; the scientific naiveté and personal orientation of the one contrasted with the highly trained and fiduciary role of the other. Yet within minutes and precisely because one is there as a healer, an incredible evolution occurs. The physician is granted an access, an intimacy, and a candor that the patient would not extend to another human being. A remarkably intense bond is forged, within which information is obtained, analyzed, and exploited for therapeutic advantage.

What allows this to happen? At the social level, tradition and experience institutionalize a role that the doctor is allowed to occupy on the basis of designated training and continued technical competence. But at the personal level, the physician's role is expressed in empathic and deeply caring behavior dedicated to achieving the best possible outcome for the patient. In other words, the effective physician must continually improve skills that foster the remarkable connectedness within which a healing role can be exercised. Similarly, all medical students have to learn this behavior, and almost all need help in doing so. Now they need look no further, because Andy Billings and John Stoeckle have provided exactly the guidance needed.

The Clinical Encounter: A Guide to the Medical Interview and Case Presentation is a primer, at once electively naive and disarmingly sophisticated. It begins where a student book ought to—at the beginning. What is the basis of the student's presence in the patient's room? How to introduce oneself . . . how to ask the initial question . . . how to cover an awkward silence (and when not to) . . . how to know the individual behind the symptom and yet track the symptom to the disease . . . how to recognize the difference between the vulnerable dependence of the inpatient and the negotiative equality of the ambulatory. The beginner is led through all of these and many other challenges by a felicitous combination of simple exposition and beautifully chosen examples. Almost every page includes quotations and suggested wordings that both neophyte and expert can use not as absolutes but as models for individualized variation.

Billings and Stoeckle have much to say to the experienced clinician as well. An accurate but sensitive history of sexual practice and drug use is a critical step in modern clinical practice. Recognizing covert alcoholism can be the most valuable outcome of an encounter initiated by a sore throat.

Understanding the patient well enough is crucial in developing preventive health behavior for the person. Teaching effectively is a requisite in eliciting patient participation in therapeutic strategies. Yet all this must often be done across great cultural and linguistic gaps. Almost half of *The Clinical Encounter* is specifically addressed to these advanced challenges. Continuing reference to its lessons will thus be useful for both maturing student and seasoned clinician.

The greatest accomplishment of this book, however, is behind—rather than in—its pages. It would be easy for the authors' recommendations to be seen as a rote set of tactics for negotiating an uncertain field. Quite the contrary: every page implicitly displays the respect, affection, and dedication that justify the physician's presence in the service of the sick.

Daniel D. Federman
Dean for Medical Education
Carl W. Walter Professor of
Medicine and
Medical Education
Harvard Medical School
Boston, Massachusetts

PREFACE

Interview [from entrevoir *to have a glimpse of,* s'entrevoir *to see each other]: A meeting of persons face to face, esp. one sought or arranged for the purpose of formal conference on some point.*

OXFORD ENGLISH DICTIONARY

With modern medicine proclaiming its intricacy and dazzling high technology, why write about a simple, old fashioned theme—interviewing patients?

First, we have the notion that words and communicative behaviors still count. They may seem familiar and commonplace, but they are complex, requiring earnest study to be appreciated as well as careful practice to be effective. In everyday medical work, the physician's words and behavior convey and elicit meanings, emotions, and values not to be found in technologies alone. Moreover, when properly applied, words and behavior provide relief. The machines and medications that are the applications and commodities of modern medicine complement, but cannot substitute for, communicative acts.

A second notion drives the authors: namely, that the interview is not simply an interpersonal communication skill or technique, but a meeting of persons full of emotions, attachments, ideologies, values, rights, duties, politics, and conflicts—a relationship that is central to the physician's therapeutic and moral responsibility to patients. Attention to these dimensions of the relationship is diminished with the promotion of medical technologies alone and with the notion of interviewing as "interpersonal skills," as defined by increasingly commercialized and competitive medical practices. "We care" advertisements and those training programs in interviewing that are aimed at "avoiding malpractice" and "satisfying the customer" may trivialize the relationship, so we strive to reassert its importance and centrality.

A third idea moves the writers: namely, that the interview—the relationship—has new importance. The traditional uses of the interview and the customary focus of clinical instruction has been on "history-taking"—eliciting information for the task of diagnosis. But information gathering is essential not only for diagnosis but also for effective clinical management of many patients with known chronic disease, while information sharing and other reciprocal acts between patient and doctor—questioning, explaining, persuading each other—are central to today's notions of good care, including psychological, ethical, and preventive care. Thus attention has recently been directed to "patient education"—transmitting information about diagnosis

ix

and management—and to "motivational interviewing" for "behavioral change."

A still newer use of the interview is for patients' participation in shared decision-making—the expression of patient preferences, particularly after diagnosis and treatment have been explained. The doctor and patient now must explore new themes to individualize care: What are the patient's choices among the many options for diagnosis and treatment? For instance, why do patients request diagnostic studies, and how necessary and effective are these tests? As patients search for "quality of life" and live longer lives with impairment, disability, and disease, what is their own assessment of their function and of the meaning of their illness, and what are their preferences for interventions?

The rhetoric, relationship, and functions of interviewing for diagnosis, management, health education, and patients' decision-making complement the advances of modern medicine and can continue the tradition of personal care in the use of biomedical interventions. In a world of more technological medicine and more commercialized medical practice, the importance of words and behavior and of comprehensive therapeutic responsibility in the care of patients seems worthy of fresh exploration.

J. Andrew Billings
John D. Stoeckle

ACKNOWLEDGMENTS

The authors are medical practitioners who have trained in internal medicine, but are grateful to have collaborated with and studied the writings of teachers from a variety of disciplines. Diverse interprofessional exchanges have stimulated this text in which we synthesize old and new interview functions, content, and techniques. Colleagues from medicine, psychiatry, psychology, and the social sciences, some as co-instructors, have shown us how they teach and practice interviewing, while others have informed us from their studies of doctor-patient encounters in the teaching group practices of the Massachusetts General Hospital—the Medical Clinic (now Internal Medicine Associates)—and the Chelsea Memorial Health Center, and now the Palliative Care Service. Still others shared their insights on clinical communication by presenting their research at our continuing doctor-patient relationship seminar.

We acknowledge our particular indebtedness to Aaron Lazare (University of Massachusetts), Robert Coles, Arthur Kleinman, Gerald Adler, Jerome Schwartz, Ned Cassem, Arthur Barsky, Bernard Levy, Jerome Weinberger, Susan Block, and Bruce Fischberg (all at Harvard), as well as Michael McGuire (UCLA) and Harrison Sadler (UCSF)—all psychiatrists; Sherman Eisenthal (Harvard)—clinical and social psychology; Howard Waitskin (UC Irvine)—medicine and sociology; Irving K. Zola (Brandeis, deceased), Mark Field and John B. McKinlay (Boston University)—medical sociology; George Abbot White—lay therapist; David Barnard (Hershey Medical Center) and Stanley Reiser (University of Texas, Houston)—medical humanities; and Patricia McArdle (Harvard) and LuAnn Wilkerson (UCLA)—education consultants. Outside our practice, we have been invigorated by experiences with the "New Pathway" curricular reform at the Harvard Medical School, where we worked with Gordon Moore, Bob Lawrence, Arthur Keinman, Byron Good, Mary Jo Delvecchio, Leon Eisenberg, and many others, and with the Interviewing Workshops, Society for General Internal Medicine, organized by Mack Lipkin (NYU), Dennis Novack (Hahneman), Bill Clark (Midcoast Hospital, Bath, ME), Sam Putnam (Boston University), and William Branch (Emory University).

The text originally grew out of a 1981 publication entitled *Introduction to the Clinical Interview—A Handbook for Optometry Students* by David Greenberg, Stanley Reiser, and the present authors. The first version of Part I was prepared in 1982 for "Introduction to Clinical Medicine," a major course for second-year Harvard medical students, given at Massachusetts General Hospital under the direction of Allan Goroll. Recent revisions, as well as chapters from Part II: Advanced Topics, have been used for students in the "New Pathway" Patient/Doctor Curriculum under the direction of Gordon Moore, Susan Block, Allan Goroll, J. Andrew Billings, William Branch, Beverly Woo, and Ron Arky.

Dr. Billings's recent work has been supported by the Open Society Institute Project on Death in America. He is grateful for the collegiality shared with the project's board and his fellow faculty scholars. A National Cancer Institute grant allowed Dr. Billings, along with Dr. Susan Block, to develop a new Harvard Medical School course, "Living with Life-Threatening Illness." In this course he has benefited enormously from working with the students and from shared teaching and curricular design with Lynn Peterson, Anne Hallward, Joshua Hauser, Loring Conant, Ruth Fischback, Dan Goodenough, Susan MacDonald, Marshall Forstein, and others.

Dr. Stoeckle's recent interests have focused on doctor-doctor relationships, interprofessional manners and communication, and their effects on patient care and the doctor-patient relationship. He is grateful for his association with colleagues in the Cabot Group Primary Care Program, including Drs. Lawrence Ronan, Linda Emanuel, and Carol Ehrlich.

Andrea Cousins provided valuable editorial advice for earlier versions of Part I. We are also grateful for comments from Skip Atkins, Robin Barnes, Michael Bierer, Allan Brandt, Tom Glick, Byron Good, John Goodson, Eleanor Hanna, Charles Hatem, Ralph Minear, Ted Stern, Eliza Sutton, and William Zinn. Robert Coope's anthology, *The Quiet Art,* republished by the University of Alabama School of Medicine through the initiative of its dean, James A. Pittman, Jr., was a source of favorite quotations.

Sarah Bollinger has been a tireless and loyal typist. Additional valued technical assistance was provided by Joanne Perry, Karen Natsios, Guy Pugh, Nan Lawless, and Harrison Schreppel.

To our families, for their sacrifices and support in getting this book out, we are deeply grateful.

Finally, the authors thank our students and patients who have been a continuing and wonderful stimulus to examine the medical interview. Many of them have inadvertently contributed to this text in the course of daily clinical activities—by having their unique encounters videotaped and by participating in numerous teaching exercises, seminars, lectures, and studies on interviewing and the doctor-patient relationship—while some (L.D., W.H., E.S., and E.B.S.), also as friends, generously support our work.

CONTENTS

GUIDE TO THE INTERVIEW

CHAPTER 1

OVERVIEW

The relationship between physician and patient, if it were literally followed, would give us a world of extraordinary fertility of the imagination which we can hardly afford. There's no use trying to multiply cases, it is there, it is magnificent, it fills my thoughts, it reaches to the farthest limits of our lives.

WILLIAM CARLOS WILLIAMS
The Autobiography (1967)

This book is about essential skills for clinical medicine. It introduces you to the medical interview and to the problems that may arise in communication between doctors and patients.

The text is addressed to medical students and is structured to facilitate their learning, though the material has proven useful for graduate physicians, other physicians-in-training, and teachers of interviewing. For the student, the book will guide initial encounters with patients, especially those seen in ambulatory settings. Rather than merely exhorting you to be kind, sensitive, informative, or persuasive, it describes specific actions you can take to achieve these and other clinical goals. Numerous samples of the dialogue between doctors and patients let you "hear" and learn about clinical discourse away from the bedside and then adapt the examples to your own encounters with patients. The text shows you how to organize and present your findings. Finally, the text aims to promote analytic skills and self-awareness in interviewing, thus helping you throughout your medical career to develop greater facility in talking with and listening to patients.

Interviewing is unlike everyday conversation. You will now be undertaking the physician's tasks in providing personal care, which include:
- Making your patient comfortable
- Establishing a helping relationship—a therapeutic alliance
- Eliciting the information necessary to diagnose and manage your patient's medical and psychosocial problems
- Informing your patient about the diagnosis, negotiating a plan, and advising on management
- Counseling about health concerns, the prevention of disease and disability, and the distress of your patient's everyday life

Of the many ways to carry out these tasks, some approaches are better than others; some are appropriate for one patient but not for another; some will come easily to you, while others will not. This book suggests tactics for making the clinical process efficient, effective, humane, and gratifying.

HOW TO USE THIS BOOK

Part I (Chapters 1 to 9) of this text guides you through the initial process of becoming confident and comfortable in interviewing patients. It covers the basics of the medical interview, including oral and written case presentations. We suggest reading the brief overview (Chapter 1) for an introduction to the clinical encounter and to the organization of the text. Then focus on the opening phases of the interview by reviewing Chapter 2 (Beginning the Interview and Establishing a Relationship) and Chapter 3 (Eliciting Information for Diagnosis and Management I: The Interviewing Process). These chapters cover most of the skills you initially need to begin talking with patients, and they form the basis for excellence in more advanced tasks. Chapters 2 and 3 describe the essential competencies to be achieved in our first-year required course for medical students on the doctor-patient relationship and deserve repeated study both early and late in your introductory interviewing training.

As you extend the range of your basic interview and strive for greater completeness, review parts of Chapter 4 (Eliciting Information for Diagnosis and Management II: The Content of the Medical Interview) on the standard data base and Chapter 5 (More Interviewing Techniques). Chapter 4 includes detailed instructions for performing a "complete" interview. This extremely detailed, idealized interview may be quite intimidating initially, but you can learn it gradually and will also recognize that data collection is abbreviated in many clinical encounters or accomplished over multiple visits.

At some early phase of your training in interviewing, you may begin presenting your findings orally or in writing. Chapter 6 describes the process of consulting with your preceptor and making an oral presentation about the interview. Chapter 8 (Recording) explains how to make a written case presentation. Eventually, you will have the opportunity to discuss the diagnosis and proposed management with your patients. These tasks are described in Chapter 7 (The Exposition Phase: Informing and Counseling the Patient).

Interviewing requires highly complex and demanding skills. Indeed, even well-trained and experienced doctors are constantly challenged by many of the principles set forth in this text. Moreover, while your study of written material on how to talk with patients can be extremely valuable, it will not be sufficient for learning good interviewing. You need lots of practice—talking with simulated or real patients—as well as opportunities to see model interviews and to reflect on your own encounters (either through videotape review, role-playing, or direct supervision by your preceptor) and to learn from watching your fellow students. In the office, sit with other doctors or watch your supervisor repeating portions of the interview with your patient. In the hospital, look for "bedside teaching." Seek out model physicians who are good at talking *with* patients, as well as those who are good at talking *about* patients.

We encourage you to learn from your patients. As you become familiar with the varied problems for which people seek medical help, and as you become acquainted with how different persons experience sickness, health, and medical care, you continually have the opportunity to improve your skills in relating to patients. Ask yourself:

How can I make my patient comfortable?

How can I establish a helping relationship?

How can I best acquire the information I need to understand and manage this patient's problems?

How can I explain to this patient the nature of the problem and its management and negotiate a mutually satisfactory plan?

How can I help the patient promote his or her health?

How can I help the patient reduce risks, prevent illness, manage current problems, and rehabilitate disablements?

These concerns now become your responsibility and will remain so throughout your professional life as a doctor. We wish you success.

Part II (Chapters 10 to 19) addresses selected advanced topics in interviewing and related clinical skills. We have not attempted a comprehensive review of interviewing, but rather have chosen to address a number of crucial areas and representative issues that will challenge you in your ongoing work with patients. Some chapters reinforce or elaborate on difficult fundamentals presented in Part I, whereas others introduce key clinical skills (e.g., the mental status examination and psychosocial assessment) or some of the problems that students and physicians regularly encounter in their daily work (e.g., talking about sexuality or substance abuse, breaking bad news, finding patients difficult). We have also addressed a number of critical topics for which good teaching material is not readily available. Part II may be read consecutively, but you may want to study separate chapters in conjunction with other training exercises or when questions arise in the course of learning and practicing clinical skills. Suggestions for further reading are included at the end of most chapters.

THE SIX TASKS OF THE MEDICAL ENCOUNTER

Your supervised encounters with patients involve six broad tasks. Part I of this text is divided accordingly into sections for each task:

I. **Beginning the interview and establishing a relationship** (Chapter 2). Start by introducing yourself, making the patient comfortable, and describing your general plan for the visit. In this first section of the text, we examine the setting of the interview and discuss ways of establishing a helping relationship and putting the patient at ease.

II. **Eliciting information for diagnosis and management** (Chapters 3 and 4). Three kinds of information are obtained: (1) the medical history (the patient's report about present and past health, as well as reports from other sources, such as the family, previous doctors, or records, (2) the physical examination, and (3) laboratory tests.

A. The medical history. The history can be conceptualized as consisting of two distinct parts: (1) the present illness, which deals with the patient's major immediate concerns (or "problems" or "complaints"), and (2) the standard data base, which deals with old problems, background health information, and coexisting minor problems.

1. **The present illness,** including the reason(s) for the visit and the request(s). A detailed account of the patient's major concerns is obtained. You begin by asking why he or she came to you and thus identify the reason for the visit, also termed the chief complaint.

   > My left shoulder has been aching for 2 days.
   >
   > I've been feeling run-down for the past few months.
   >
   > I haven't seen a doctor in 6 years, so my wife scheduled me for a checkup.

   The patient may also have requests, as distinct from "problems" or "complaints." The requests describe what the patient wants from the visit.

   > I want my blood checked for anemia.
   >
   > I think I need an x-ray.
   >
   > I'm seeing spots before my left eye and want to be sure it's nothing serious.
   >
   > I want a letter to my employer saying that I can't work this week.

   You obtain a full account of the present illness (or "present problems"), including the time of onset, precipitating factors, what the patient thinks is causing the problem, attempts at self-treatment, and the effect of symptoms on the patient's life. You seek out the data that will help you decide among various possible diagnoses.

2. **The standard data base.** This includes the patient's past medical history, social history, family history, and review of systems. You acquire a standard set of background data on the patient's health. Facts about previous illnesses and treatments and about various health-related practices make up the past medical history. The inquiry into the patient's life and background—the social history—places the illness in a biographical and socioeconomic perspective, and allows you to plan for personal care. The family history identifies health problems of relatives. A standard set of questions about symptoms—the review of systems—may provide further

information about the present illness and also identify unrelated problems.

   B. The physical examination. Here, the text offers suggestions for putting your patient at ease during the physical examination.

   C. Laboratory tests (not discussed).

III. Consulting with your preceptor (Chapter 6). On completion of the history and physical examination, you present and review your findings with your preceptor. The corresponding section of the book suggests a format for the consultation.

IV. Assessment and plan (Chapters 6 and 8). You and your preceptor formulate your diagnostic conclusions—the assessment, impression, or differential diagnosis. You then make initial plans for management, including further diagnostic studies, treatment, and patient education.

V. The exposition phase: informing and counseling the patient (Chapter 7). In the closing portion of the interview, you may:

- Inform the patient of your opinions about the illness (its diagnosis, treatment, and prognosis), offer reassurance where appropriate, and propose a plan for management
- Encourage the patient to ask questions and express concerns
- Negotiate a mutually satisfactory plan
- Review the specific information required to carry out the plan, ask the patient for feedback on the communication, and counsel the patient on behavioral change
- Counsel the patient on health promotion and disease prevention, using motivational interviewing
- Offer advice on further use of medical services, including arrangements for follow-up visits and telephone calls
- Say goodbye

VI. Recording (Chapter 8). You now prepare a written case presentation, or "write-up," that records the information you have gathered and documents other clinical acts that were performed in the medical encounter. The format of this write-up is described in the sections on recording and in the case write-up example in the Appendix.

GROUND RULES OF STUDENT-PATIENT ENCOUNTERS

During your clinical training, you have the privilege, under supervision, to be the patient's primary doctor or a member of the medical team responsible for the patient. You may be the first person to take the patient's history and to organize diagnostic studies and treatments, perhaps aided by data collected on a printed questionnaire or a computer. On follow-up visits, you will have the opportunity to evaluate these efforts. As trust and familiarity develop, you may also see changes in your relationship with the patient.

While patients know that you are a student, you will also be viewed as a doctor, though perhaps as a relatively young, inexperienced one. Some patients enjoy taking part in your training and seem to have a parental interest in your professional development. For years afterward, patients may ask fondly about their student-doctors. Your comprehensive write-up for the medical record becomes a landmark in the patient's continuing care.

A few ground rules about the ambulatory encounter need to be made explicit. Patients should be asked beforehand—generally by your preceptor—whether they are willing to see a student, and, of course, they may refuse at any time. The patient should have been advised on roughly how long the visit will last. Patients should also be told that you will be working with a staff physician who will supervise their care. Your preceptor's involvement assures you and the patient that proper care is provided and may also allow the patient to begin an ongoing relationship with a physician. A visit with you may offer the patient the advantage of getting an unusually complete evaluation and perhaps of being seen sooner than if he or she had waited for an appointment with the physician alone. For a returning "old" patient, your review of chronic disablements allows for a fresh accounting of distress and discomfort. In many settings, the fee for the patient is based on the time your preceptor spends or would have spent handling a similar visit, so there is no extra cost for the added attention.

BOUNDARIES AND ETHICAL PROFESSIONAL BEHAVIOR

In a professional relationship the physician's actions are governed by what is best for the patient. The patient, who almost inevitably feels some dependence on the physician and senses a disparity in power in the relationship, should be able to trust physicians to act in a manner that, first and foremost, promotes the patient's welfare. Any conduct that exploits or distorts the doctor-patient relationship for the benefit of the physician or others, or that similarly undermines the patient's basic trust, is a violation of professional duty and may be labeled a boundary violation. Such unethical activities are immediately harmful to a patient and may undermine future professional relationships.

Boundary violations are most obvious and egregious when they involve sexual misconduct. In general, any physical contact or intimate involvement with a patient that is not part of usual clinical activities, regardless of whether it occurs outside of a clinical setting or after a professional relationship has terminated, may be interpreted as inappropriate and, in some states, illegal. Whenever aspects of a routine physical examination might be construed as sexual contact, the physician, whether male or female, should clearly explain the purpose of the examination and have a chaperone present.

Drawing a clear line between a close, meaningful professional relationship and a more intimate personal relationship—one that serves needs of the student or physician while at least initially bringing pleasure to the patient—may be difficult. Patients may particularly have difficulty understanding or recognizing the importance of boundaries; the responsibility falls on the professional to maintain appropriate behavior and avoid any likelihood of appearing or acting in an unethical fashion.

A variety of other boundary transgressions deserve note: writing prescriptions, particularly for controlled substances, for friends or relatives, business transactions with patients, accepting expensive gifts, disclosing confidential information about one patient to another, inappropriate self-disclosure, providing special favors to a particular patient, and seeing a patient at unusual times or locations. Instances of physicians receiving remuneration or similar benefits for enrolling patients in a research protocol, using particular drugs, or reducing the cost of care can also be viewed as unprincipled acts or boundary violations unless the patient is properly informed.

HOW OFFICE CARE DIFFERS FROM INPATIENT MEDICINE

This text focuses on care in the office, a setting that is congenial to learning about interviewing and other basic clinical skills. With the current reorganization of medical practice and teaching, hospitals have assumed an increasingly narrow role in the care of sick persons, often as sites for managing complex technologies. Patients are spending less time in hospitals, and students are finding fewer opportunities to get to know their inpatients well. The important process of talking with patients, including essential steps in diagnosis and treatment, must increasingly be carried out in ambulatory settings. You should be aware of ways in which ambulatory care differs from inpatient care, and thus of how the two settings place different demands on the interviewer.

Inpatient care generally is directed toward acute, severe medical disorders. A single major problem is usually evident, perhaps superimposed on or aggravating a host of chronic problems. All the energy and expertise of the staff and all the technology of the modern hospital are directed toward rapidly discovering the diagnosis of the acute illness and managing the immediate problem so that patients can be quickly discharged when they no longer require acute care. Hospitalizations tend to be brief, and the relationship between the patient and the hospital staff, while often intense, is time-limited and may be focused on technical diagnosis and treatment.

Outpatients, more often than not, have chronic disorders. Eighty percent of office encounters are return visits, initiated by the doctor and patient for ongoing problems. Outpatients in the United States visit a doctor an average of 4.8 times each year. Unlike hospitalized patients, ambulatory patients monitor their own symptoms and signs, take their own medicines, set a level of exercise, prepare a diet, and administer other treatments. Rather than lying in bed, constantly surveyed by the hospital staff, waiting to be visited on rounds, these "walking patients" will sometimes decide to seek out lay or professional medical advice. Most of the time, outpatients know their diagnosis and are their own doctor.

In helping patients care for themselves, rather than being cared for by the hospital staff, the outpatient physician must be particularly aware of the patient's perspective on his or her illness and its management and of the environment—social, psychological, economic, and so on—in which the patient lives. In your study of ambulatory patients, you will be introduced to the concept of "illness behavior," a characterization of patients' actions and rationales in managing their health. While the nature and severity of patients' physical complaints play a role in this behavior, psychological and social factors prove to be important "triggers" in the decision to see a doctor. The patients' attributions, expectations, and requests characterize their perceptions about the illness, their reasons for seeking help, and their attitude toward medical advice and treatment and toward changing their behaviors. Your ability to elicit and respond to these elements of the patient's perspective will influence, in turn, patient satisfaction, understanding, adherence to treatment, and prevention—important aspects of personal care.

Patients "comply" with or "adhere" to medical advice in varying degrees. Patient conduct often falls short of the doctor's recommendations. In office practice, the physician develops strategies for assessing and improving compliance. Moreover, to promote optimal treatment and provide support, the physician may enlist the patient's family, social network, and community resources.

Accessibility and continuity of care are important functions of primary care practice. These organizational goals reflect a concern with how patients gain entry to medical care and with how to maintain an ongoing doctor-patient relationship. A single physician who is familiar with the patient's background should supervise and coordinate care, yet many health care providers, such as nurse practitioners, physician assistants, and various specialists, may provide services and, at times, assume major responsibility. When the primary physician is unavailable (e.g., temporarily away for the evening, weekend, sick leave, or vacation or permanently leaving the practice), arrangements are made to ensure availability of care.

The picture of illness in the office—its nature, severity, and stage—is different from that in the hospital. Primary care practitioners may have a special interest in studying minor or self-limited disorders, chronic illness, convalescence, rehabilitation, and health promotion/disease prevention. Alexander Pope's phrase, "This long disease, my life," points to the burden of chronic illness that patients bring to the ambulatory setting. A visit, rather than being triggered by a major new disease, often turns out to be an episode, both in the course of a person's health and in the long-term relationship between doctor and patient. In contrast to the "complete" hospital workup that is carried out as rapidly as possible, the appropriate tactics of diagnosis and management in the office setting may be a carefully sequenced evaluation and treatment trial. A leisurely yet systematic approach may allow for problems to be sorted out, not all at once, but over time, and may avoid the personal and financial costs of unnecessary testing. During this orderly, measured process, both the patient and the doctor may be faced with the prospect of tolerating considerable uncertainty about the diagnosis and prognosis.

BEGINNING THE INTERVIEW AND ESTABLISHING A RELATIONSHIP

Most patients long for someone to whom they can confide their troubles. For this they look to the doctor, and it makes little difference whether he is clerk, interne or practitioner so long as he is the right sort. It may only be necessary for students to have recourse to a simple conversation; to show real interest in this man or that woman, as an individual, in order to let loose a flood of startling confidences. At other times, the way is not so clear; suspicions and fears must be allayed before the friendly relation can be established. And then there comes, little by little, or sometimes in torrents, a more or less disjointed story, which, when pieced together, gives the record of a human life surprisingly valuable, at times, in disclosing an explanation for the actual physical ailment. You thus increase your knowledge of human nature, often learn a way to help the patient in his distress, and in addition gain a friend.

WARFIELD T. LONGCOPE
Methods and Medicine (1932)

This section presents introductory approaches to the interview, emphasizing what everyone knows as common courtesy or good manners—but may easily forget.

INTRODUCING YOURSELF

The interview, like other social encounters, begins with a greeting and an introduction:

> Mrs. O'Connor, [seeking her out in the waiting room]. Hi, [shaking hands] I'm Jane Miller. Welcome to the Medical Clinic. I'm a student from University Medical School, and I will be talking to you this morning about your health and then giving you a thorough examination. Dr. O'Malley is my instructor, and he will also be seeing you in about 2 hours. Have you ever been here before? . . . Let me escort you to the office.

This is an effective introduction: it identifies the interviewer and her plans and gives the patient some notion of what to anticipate. A welcoming handshake can ease a person's initial apprehension. Consider the difference between this introduction and one in which the patient is simply led into a room after being greeted with "Mrs. O'Connor, come this way."

Here is another greeting:

> Mr. Kafka, I'm Fred Smith, a second-year medical student, and I will be giving you a good general checkup today. Let's go into my room. We have about an hour to talk

about what brings you here. Dr. Serrell and I are working together. She is going to join us later and will be your doctor at the Health Center after I leave next month.

For patients who are new to you but familiar with your preceptor, your instructor may introduce you after having obtained the patient's permission for your examination:

Mrs. Woolf, this is Derek Brown. He is our medical student-assistant who is helping out and learning in the practice. He's going to check you, and then I'll be in.

Greet your patients by their last names, preceded by conventional titles—Mr., Ms., Mrs., or Miss—unless they are adolescents or younger. Initially, avoid informal address, such as first names or those often demeaning endearments like "honey" or "dear." Patients, especially older ones, may interpret such presumed intimacy or egalitarianism as frankly disrespectful rather than as a sign of friendliness.

Your patient, of course, may suggest that you use a first name or nickname. As you and your patient get to know each other better, you may sense that titles are no longer called for, in which case you can negotiate a less formal address:

Examiner: Should I call you Jacob or Mr. Jones?
Patient: Actually, I prefer my nickname, Jake.

Even when you are using informal address in the office, formal titles are generally appropriate in public spaces, such as the waiting room, as well as for referring to patients in communications among physicians or other health care personnel. When you are not sure about pronunciation of the patient's name, ask the patient to repeat his or her name and to verify that you are saying it correctly.

SHOWING PERSONAL INTEREST

The village doctor was a great success. His success was due to his sympathy with his patients, each of whom he treated as an individual with an idiosyncrasy of his own and worthy of special and separate consideration. It was as if, instead of giving every one mass-produced medicine, he had moulded the portrait of each on his pill. He specialized in his patients ... in contradistinction to the town specialists who are identified with certain diseases or disasters ...

Oliver St. John Gogarty
Going Native (1940)

On the whole, you must remember, when associating with the sick, that these require kindness most of all, and that they first and foremost wish and hope to find a comprehending and sympathetic friend in their physician; and when treated in this manner will, in a few moments, give you their fullest confidence.

Thorkild Rovsing
Clinical Lectures on Abdominal Surgery

As an interview begins, patients quickly notice whether you seem friendly, warm, and personally interested in them. Immediate clues include your greeting, handshake, and attentiveness to the patient's comfort, as well as a host of additional nonverbal cues: appearance (particularly dress and grooming), tone of voice and other speech qualities, facial expression, quality of eye contact, gestures, posture and body orientation, how closely you position yourself in relation to the patient, congruence of your nonverbal communication with your verbal statements, and how your various features remind the patient of other people. Multiple clues are registered rapidly and may profoundly affect how you are perceived, though the patient may have little conscious awareness of this process. Conversely, you instantly judge the patient on similar evidence and may also be unaware of how you have been strongly influenced by such impressions.

Students can establish excellent rapport with their patients. As a novice interviewer, you naturally may feel anxious and uncertain about your skills and role, but your patients will appreciate your eagerness to understand and to help, your unhurried and concerned manner, your thoroughness and nonjudgmental stance. Many will be grateful for the hours of attention at an initial examination: the careful review of their history and meticulous physical examination, followed by a full explanation of the illness and its management.

Make an effort to connect with the patient. Know your patient, not just his or her medical problems (see Quick Tips: Establishing Rapport with Your Patient). At some phase in the interview, despite the pressure to do a complete workup in a limited time, briefly put aside your diagnostic pursuit and take a few minutes to learn about and enjoy the person you are interviewing—to "gossip." We usually go directly from the greeting to a standard medical inquiry (e.g., "What brings you in today?") but pick up on engaging features of the patient's background. Examples include:

You grew up in the North End! What was it like back then?

How do you move those big pipes on that kind of job?

QUICK TIPS

Establishing Rapport with Your Patient

- Begin the interview with a personal inquiry, for example:
  Ask about something in the patient's background that catches your fancy
  Identify a shared interest
  Engage in "small talk"
- Ask about basic demographic data, such as name, age, occupation, and marital status
- Ask about the patient's general health before asking the reason for the visit
- Find something you like about each patient

What's your recipe?

Tell me more about your work [or hobby, special interests, or use of free time].

Illness threatens and transforms many people's identity. New patients, in turning to you or other unfamiliar persons for help, will particularly be anxious about depending on a stranger. Show your patients that you recognize and value them for who they are. By demonstrating a personal interest in each patient, you will develop a more comfortable and effective relationship. In turn, you can draw great sustenance from your daily encounters, as you discover the marvelous variety of human experiences and personalities, and as you learn how people cope with illness and adversity.

Furthermore, by finding aspects of patients that particularly excite your curiosity or admiration, you also will be better able to remember them as unique persons. You can use this special knowledge to reconnect quickly with patients on subsequent visits.

THE OFFICE SETTING

A proper interview requires privacy (visual and auditory), absence of distractions or interruptions, and comfort. Arrange the furniture to put the patient at ease and to facilitate conversation. You will want neither to crowd the patient nor sit so far away as to seem distant. Large desks imposed between doctor and patient tend to define the relationship as distanced, authoritarian, or dominant-submissive. Close arrangements that foster constant eye contact may feel intrusive or too intimate.

Eye contact is an essential ingredient for establishing a personal relationship and for conveying your interest in the patient and his or her story. Establish a position that permits but does not force eye contact. Eye level for yourself and the patient should be about the same. Also, don't let note-taking or your attention to a written medical record or a computer screen prevent crucial visual engagement with the patient.

If such spatial details (or "proxemics") seem trivial, you can remind yourself of the profound effects of physical arrangements by having a casual conversation with a friend when your noses are 6 inches apart or while you are sitting 10 feet away. Compare how it feels to talk when your head is 1 foot higher or lower than that of the other person or when one person is lying down, as when a doctor stands above a patient who is in bed.

It is generally comfortable to be seated about 3 feet from the patient and to be positioned nearly face-to-face. With this arrangement, the doctor and patient can gaze directly at each other but are also able to distance themselves by looking away (Fig. 2-1).

Show your patient where to sit. The office is your territory. Also, help with personal belongings as you would with a visitor in your home. Don't let the patient go through an interview wearing a street coat or holding a pocketbook or hat for lack of your offering a place to put them down.

1. Dyadic Interaction

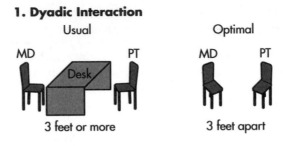

2. Interpreter (I) in Three-Way Interaction

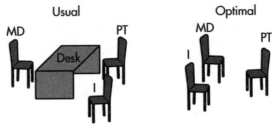

Fig. 2-1   Seating arrangements.

THE HOSPITAL SETTING

Hospitalized patients are generally interviewed in the emergency ward or a hospital room. Patients often find such settings unfamiliar and frightening. Patients may experience helplessness and a loss of identity as they relinquish their clothes and belongings, don a standard hospital gown, have a name tag placed on their wrist, lie down on a stretcher or hospital bed, and become "the patient in 309." Patients wait in bed, worrying about their health, sparsely clothed in a hospital "johnny"—attire generally reserved for the privacy of the home—while numerous fully clothed and mobile strangers walk in and out, stand over them, examine and test their bodies, feed them, and otherwise tell them what to do. The setting is not conducive to a relaxed, intimate interview, and requires extra effort on your part to assure privacy and comfort. An interview held while the patient is lying on his or her back is decidedly unnatural and uncomfortable, though sometimes necessitated by the patient's condition. For suggestions, see Quick Tips: Conducting a Bedside Interview.

ESCORTS, FAMILY, AND INTERPRETERS

Relatives or friends who accompany the patient, as well as interpreters who are called in, pose new challenges and possibilities. If you and the patient desire a confidential relationship, you may exclude the others from the room during parts or all of the interview. If you merely wish to get the initial story directly from the patient, you may seat the escorts off to the side, focusing your attention on the patient. If you and the patient prefer to include escorts and to seek their participation throughout the interview, you might arrange seats in a circle. The optimal arrangement for you, the patient, and the escorts may evolve with the initial interview:

To the patient: Would you like to talk alone? Who's going to start telling the story?

To the spouse: I'd like to talk to you after I've chatted with your husband. Let's let him tell the story in his own words. Then I'd be interested in hearing anything you would like to add.

To a family member or friend: Let's spend a few minutes hearing your view of the problem. Then I'll want to talk privately with Mr. Williams.

If you are using an escort as an interpreter, a triangular seating arrangement can be awkward. You can often maximize face-to-face conversation with the patient (who "comes to *see* the doctor") by sitting alongside the interpreter; let the patient's gaze encompass both of you, while directing your gaze to the patient, not the translator.

QUICK TIPS

Conducting a Bedside Interview

- If possible, raise the head of the bed or ask the patient to sit up so that your head and the patient's are at the same level. Try not to stand over the patient.
- Let the patient sit in a bedside chair, if possible, wearing a bathrobe or other clothes brought from home. Bring your seat close to the patient.
- Lower the bed rail so that it does not act as a barrier between you and the patient (but remember to put it up again if the patient is liable to fall out of bed).
- Minimize distractions. Turn off the television. Close the door to the room. Draw a curtain around you and your patient for at least visual privacy.
- If possible, ask other health care workers not to interrupt you.
- If the patient's room does not allow privacy and quiet, and the patient can be moved, consider moving to a nearby, more suitable location.

THE PROCESS OF THE VISIT

At the beginning of the interview, sketch your intentions for the visit, as in the previous introductory examples. Scheduled outpatient appointments and most inpatient visits should allow you ample time for a thorough history and physical examination. Rarely, acutely uncomfortable or anxious patients require abbreviated interviews and prompt intervention. Check with your preceptor if you think such immediate attention might be advisable.

Note-Taking

When you write during the interview, the patient will wonder what you are doing. Remove some of the mystery by acknowledging and explaining the process.

> I'll be jotting down some notes about what I learn from you so that I can put an accurate account in your record.

> Let me make a note on that so that I don't forget it.

Try not to pay more attention to your clipboard or the paper on your desktop than to the patient. When an interviewer becomes absorbed with note-taking, patients may feel uncomfortable because of a lack of frequent eye contact and the interruption of the normal flow of questions and answers. Conversely, you can quickly make your patient feel welcomed and can encourage him or her to talk freely by using nonverbal behaviors: maintaining good eye contact, leaning slightly forward to indicate your interest and involvement in the conversation, and listening carefully with an attentive, friendly facial expression.

Dress

According to a Russian proverb, "At meeting you're judged by your clothes; at parting you're judged by your wits." Clothing styles and grooming habits are important signals of social status and role. First impressions may set the tone of the encounter. Rather than dressing solely according to your own inclinations, consider the effect on your patient. There are no hard-and-fast rules. Remember that informal dress, although it may signify friendly, nonauthoritarian behavior to you, may suggest professional sloppiness and incompetence to others. Many patients dress carefully for their appointments, sometimes in their best "Sunday clothes." Your casual attire—perhaps intended to resemble the patient's ordinary appearance—may inadvertently demean the patient: it may signify condescension or presumptuousness, or even suggest indifference toward the patient and your own professional skill.

In the settings where you first meet patients, white coats or other formal attire may constitute the standard of professional dress. Patients often expect such formality and may feel more comfortable with familiar physician apparel and manners. Try to meet your patients' expectations and those of your instructor for the appropriate dress and conduct for a doctor, treating everyone in a manner that communicates respect.

A badge, name tag, or article of clothing that identifies you as a physician-in-training also assures patients that you have a legitimate basis for participating in their care.

CHAPTER 3

ELICITING INFORMATION FOR DIAGNOSIS AND MANAGEMENT I: THE INTERVIEWING PROCESS

...my "medicine" was the thing which gained me entrance to these secret gardens of the self. It lay there, another world, in the self. I was permitted by my medical badge to follow the poor, defeated body into those gulfs and grottos. And the astonishing thing is that at such times and in such places—foul as they may be with the stinking ischio-rectal abscesses of our comings and goings—just there, the thing, in all its greatest beauty, may for a moment be freed to fly for a moment guiltily about the room.

The physician enjoys a wonderful opportunity actually to witness the words being born. Their actual colors and shapes are laid before him carrying their tiny burdens which he is privileged to take into his care with their unspoiled newness. He may see the difficulty with which they have been born and what they are destined to do. No one else is present but the speaker and ourselves, we have been the words' very parents. Nothing is more moving.

WILLIAM CARLOS WILLIAMS
The Autobiography (1951)

QUESTIONING

Questions are the clinical interviewer's special tool. Well-chosen questions let the patient's story be told fully, quickly, precisely, and intelligibly (see Quick Tips: Questioning Techniques).

Open-Ended Questions

An accurate account of the patient's problems and perspectives can generally be best obtained by providing only minimal direction in the opening of the interview. Begin your inquiry with broad, open-ended questions (also called *nondirective* questions) that allow the patient latitude in describing complaints and only minimally specify what topics should be addressed:

How would you like us to help you?

What's on your mind in coming in today?

Could you tell me what is bothering you?

Let the patient tell the story; allow time for the history to emerge. Follow the patient's associations. By listening carefully and not interrupting, you encourage the patient to give his or her personal narrative of the illness and

> **QUICK TIPS**
>
> **Questioning Techniques**
> - Begin with open-ended (nondirective) questions
>   Beware of interrupting the patient
> - Facilitate the patient's report
>   Promote elaboration
>   Use silence to encourage amplification
> - Later, after surveying the patient's story, clarify the account
>   Repeat, rephrase, and summarize the patient's narrative to demonstrate
>   your grasp of the report and to invite correction and amplification
>   Use directive questions
>   Consider asking the patient to outline the chronological course of the
>   illness
> - Redirect the patient when he or she is wandering, repetitious, or having
>   difficulty focusing
>   Suggest answers only to clarify vague responses

of the experience of being sick. Typically, a patient will give a burst of information that includes the major elements of the history, setting the stage for the remainder of the interview.

Facilitation and Silence

Facilitate the patient's report by nodding or by saying "Yes" or "Uh-huh" or "What else?" Simply looking attentively at the patient will also encourage elaboration. For the patient who is shy or apologetic, you might say, "You're doing fine. Go on." Other phrases that encourage patients to speak freely and yet do not direct them to a specific topic might be:

> What is it like?
>
> Tell me more of the story of this illness.
>
> What happened?

You can foster elaboration by repeating or echoing a few words of the patient's last sentence:

> Chest pain?
>
> You were worried?

You can also briefly summarize what the patient has said and then encourage comment:

> So, if I understand you correctly, you have been having aching and stiffness in your shoulders for about 3 weeks now, and you have generally been feeling more tired than usual.
>
> Let me see if I have the story straight . . . Does that sound right to you?

Summary statements demonstrate to patients that you grasp their story, while inviting correction and elaboration. When patients seem to be wandering, a summary may direct them back to the main topic. These statements also give you a chance to gather your thoughts and catch your breath before going on to new questions.

Learn to use silence. If the patient pauses, don't feel you have to jump in with a question. If you wait attentively, your silence will usually prompt the patient to continue to elaborate about the complaint. In first learning to interview, long pauses may make you uneasy; practice using silence so that you become comfortable with this important technique.

You can often elicit the bulk of the information about the present illness simply by asking a few open-ended questions and by using facilitation, repetition, silence, and summarization. While some clinicians fear that such an approach gives the patient a license to ramble, this technique for opening the interview is both efficient and the best method for assuring that you get a complete picture of the illness. By encouraging the patient to tell the story as he or she sees it, you can recognize the full range of problems that bear on the illness and can appreciate essential relationships between events. You are unlikely to get this broad view by relying on your own ability to ask specific questions. Additionally, the quality of your information will be better because nondirective questions do not bias the patient's report. Moreover, patients will be appreciative of having the opportunity to tell their story fully.

Clarification and Directive Questions

Later in the interview, you may become more directive. Encourage the patient to expand on important topics:

> You said you were having pain?
>
> You also mentioned headaches. Tell me more about them.

Clarification is invariably necessary:

> I'm not sure I understand. Would you explain that again?
>
> Do you mean. . . ?
>
> Let me ask you this again, so I'm sure I've got it right. . . .

Don't hesitate to repeat or rephrase questions. When you have doubts about the patient's accuracy, you can informally estimate precision in the history by going over the same material again, noting inconsistencies. Most beginning students are surprised and even dismayed at the variability of reports offered by patients at different times to different physicians, even by those patients who are considered "good historians." The patient's reconstruction of the illness is rarely as tidy as might be implied from reading edited case write-ups. Rather than having a logically organized and detailed view of their illness, patients often discover much of the history—the time course, the characteristics of symptoms, the relationships between events—in response to the interviewer's questions. They also refashion a new version of the story in reaction to how an interviewer implies that some data are interesting and relevant, while other data are unimportant. Thus histories change with time and with repeated questioning.

As the interview progresses, you may want to use more directive questions to investigate specific points. Closed or forced-choice questions lead to brief, specific answers:

> When did this discomfort begin?
>
> How many times did it occur this week?
>
> Does the blurring ever occur when you are having these headaches? Does the dizziness come before or after the onset of the headache? Do you ever get this dizziness without getting a headache?
>
> Has your husband ever hit you during one of these quarrels?
>
> Do you think about killing yourself?

Questions in this form allow clarifications of details but discourage elaboration.

Tactics for Clarification

For many patients, asking for a detailed report of the chronological course of the illness will help you gather additional important information, obtain a precise reconstruction of the sequence of events, and clarify important relationships between these events.

> Let's go back to the beginning. What was the first thing you noticed?
>
> Was there anything else bothering you then? What did you notice next? What were you doing at the time? And then what happened?

Relate the symptoms to actual events or places:

> Did you have any trouble at work this week?
>
> What happened at dinner yesterday?
>
> Let's focus on the most recent episode. Tell me exactly what was going on the last time you had this symptom.
>
> How many flights of stairs are there to your apartment? What is it like going up them?
>
> You said it hurt a lot. Can you compare the severity to other times you've had pain?

Or you may create a hypothetical situation:

> Suppose you had a big pizza right now. What would happen with your "indigestion"?
>
> How do you think it would feel for you to walk up that hill right now?

If the patient's responses are vague, you may offer a choice of answers or suggest answers. For instance, to identify the duration of symptoms, you might ask:

> You say the pain has been with you for a long time. Do you mean days or weeks or months? Does it come and go, or is it constant?

Guide your patients toward providing appropriate information. Politely let them know whether you need more data or if they are giving you more detail than is useful. Patients, after all, may have notions quite different from yours about what is relevant and how much information to provide. Often, past experiences with physicians lead patients to be rather brief, and you may need to encourage elaboration.

If the patient wanders or becomes repetitive or has difficulty focusing attention on an aspect of the history that seems important, you can redirect the interview:

> We should talk about this too, but right now let's go back to the chest pains. I need to hear about them in more detail. How long do they last?

Both garrulous and laconic patients may need more direction than provided by open-ended questions. The garrulous patient may need help focusing on important topics. The laconic patient (e.g., persons who have difficulty expressing themselves or who are reticent due to embarrassment or anxiety) may be uncomfortable when encouraged to initiate conversation or speak at length; a more structured, controlled interview, using directive questions to explore specific topics, often feels safer and easier to them and may eventually lead them toward freer expression. Patients who are forgetful or slightly confused also generally require highly structured interviews.

Precision

Strive for as reliable, reproducible, and objective data as possible, even with subjective complaints. Do not settle for vague terms—"rare," "frequent," "not uncommon," "mild," "severe"—when greater precision is required for symptom characterization. What is a "little worry," or a "little beer," or a "little blood"?

Do not assume that the patient's descriptive terms coincide with your own. Pains may be described as "sudden" when they develop and reach a maximal intensity over either a few seconds or a few days. "All the time" may mean constant, occurring for a few seconds every hour, or present on most days. "For the first time" may mean worse than ever before, yet not otherwise different from previous, milder episodes.

One patient's "terrible," "unbearable," "awful," or "severe" is another patient's "annoying," "troubling," or "strong." Often, patients' choices of words are as helpful in characterizing their personality style as in describing the severity of symptoms. A better guide to severity often is obtained by noting the degree to which a symptom interferes with the patient's usual activities. Thus ask a patient with knee pain how the problem affects work, sleep, and the ability to concentrate or enjoy daily activities; describe how far the patient could walk, and note when medication is used for symptom relief. Similarly, shortness of breath on exertion might be quantified in terms of (1) the distance walked; (2) whether the patient was walking on the level *vs.* on a specified incline *vs.* up a specified number of flights of stairs; (3) the time required to traverse the distance, or at least whether the patient was moving slowly *vs.* briskly; (4) whether the patient was walking with or without packages; (5) and the number and duration of required rest stops.

Surveying and Organizing

In the first few minutes of an interview, survey the patient's problems. By encouraging the patient to tell his or her own story, you not only help develop an alliance and gain a complete picture of the illness, you also obtain an overview of the issues that the patient wants to bring to your attention or feels are germane to understanding the presenting problems. You may discover the patient's agenda for the visit. A major hazard of interrupting the patient or discouraging elaboration in the early phases of the encounter is that you will proceed through the remainder of the interview without an awareness of important events and concerns that need to be explored.

After surveying the patient's problems, you may assert more direction over the interview by focusing and organizing the discussion. You may introduce your own agenda:

> I think we should carefully go over these new leg cramps, and then, if time allows, I'd like to hear more about your old shoulder problem. Does that seem reasonable?

> It seems that a lot of things have been bothering you recently and that you've been under a lot of stress since your father's death and this trouble with your husband. Let me understand more about how your personal life has been going this past year, and we'll return later to your joint aches and tiredness.

> I think we should use this first visit to go over your health problems and let me get to know you better. Then, I am going to review your records, and we can get together again in a few weeks. But is there anything you feel we need to get to today?

For each patient and setting, individualize your approach to the interview, striking an appropriate balance of either open-ended questioning and facilitation or directive questioning and exertion of control.

When time is limited, you should let the patient know about the constraints of the interview and should seek agreement on how to proceed.

> I know we had planned to do a complete checkup today, but it sounds like these new stomach pains deserve immediate attention and that we can't get around to everything in the hour we have. Let's make sure we check your blood pressure, though, and anything else you need to take care of today. How does that sound to you?

In setting priorities, urgent or important new problems (as defined by either doctor or patient) are generally addressed first, while attention may be deferred for chronic stable problems and other matters that are mutually recognized as less important. Obtaining or updating a full standard data base is often the last priority in taking a history. Some portions of a "complete" evaluation may be postponed to allow adequate time for more important topics. (Similarly, the physical examination should first address immediate health concerns. If time is limited, the clinician may defer attention to a "complete" checkup and preventive health measures.) But beware of passing over matters that concern the patient, even if you view them as trivial. Do not assume that bodily symptoms and recognized medical problems are of higher priority than psychosocial issues.

LISTENING

We listen through a theory, with a view to judgment and to action.

R. C. Cabot and R. L. Dicks
The Art of Ministering to the Sick (1936)

When you talk with the patient, you should listen, first, for what he wants to tell, secondly, for what he does not want to tell, thirdly for what he cannot tell.

L. J. Henderson
Physician and Patient as Social Systems (1935)

Listening and observing—as much as questioning—are important skills to master in becoming a better interviewer. Listening well does not mean just passively recording what patients say. You must attend carefully to how patients express themselves—why they say things in a particular manner and at a particular time in the conversation—and you must actively search for what their statements mean, as well as for what is not being said.

The patient's verbal and nonverbal expressions are rich with meaning but are not always easily recognized or deciphered. Audiotape and videotape recordings of interviews reveal that many details of the history and many important clues to the patient's concerns and feelings are regularly passed over. For instance, the patient who briefly mentions a nosebleed seems to have been asking indirectly if this minor symptom is connected with high blood pressure and strokes. A casual reference to "purple feet" turns out to be an allusion to profound fears about "gangrene like my mother had." Another patient hesitates for a moment, apparently overwhelmed by important thoughts or emotions, but the interviewer, rather than using attentive silence to encourage elaboration, changes the charged topic by asking a routine question.

The first few minutes of the interview are often particularly dense with associations and subtle implications. Listen carefully in order to hear the complexity of what is said and to become familiar with how patients express themselves. As a general rule, anything that a patient says is relevant, and your job, particularly in the early phases of the interview, is to appreciate the other person's logic. Often, the beginning interviewer searches only for hard facts about disease, ignoring statements that do not fit into a preconceived and overly circumscribed notion of what information is important.

Listen for how the patient puts together the story. What are his or her beliefs, attitudes, and feelings about this health problem? You need to understand the patient's view of the illness—notions about etiology, pathophysiology, prognosis, and proper management—so that you can provide appropriate personal care. Notice how the patient will mention various events with the implication that they explain why the illness began or got worse at a certain time. Attend to subtle expressions of concern and worry and encourage elaboration on these matters. What led the patient to come to the doctor now? What are the patient's expectations for the encounter; particularly what does he or she want you to do to help? Does this patient who complains of a headache want a computed tomographic scan for reassurance that he does not have a brain tumor? Or does he simply want pain medicine so that he can go about his normal business despite his headache? Or does he want a letter excusing him from work?

At the same time that you are cognizant of the patient's perspective on the illness, do not succumb to the trap of accepting this version at face value. For instance, a patient may believe that breast cancer is caused by trauma to the breast or may attribute a pneumonia to carelessly going out in the cold with wet hair, but you will find other background data more pertinent to understanding the etiology of the illness. While you attend carefully to the patient's viewpoint, you also need to make your own conclusions about the significance of historical facts. Eventually, the raw data you acquire from the patient will need to be reorganized according to a clinical perspective that determines which facts are relevant, how the facts relate to each other, what diagnoses are likely, and what action is required. You listen with your own theories about what the information means in terms of making a medical diagnosis. You also attend with theories for understanding the patient's personality, perceptions, and reactions to illness.

Listening to strong or unpleasant feelings, such as anger, envy, guilt, grief, and impatience, is sometimes difficult. Certain affects (emotions) may make you uncomfortable, and you may want to do something to make distressful feelings go away. But avoid premature reassurance or gratuitous advice based on a superficial appraisal of the patient. Listening is our first task and is often sufficient treatment. Listening is not inconsequential care. You are "doing something" very important by giving the patient the opportunity to share hard-to-bear feelings. Where else in the world can your patients go to talk so easily and privately about such feelings? Who else will listen so uncritically?

If a patient is angry or resentful toward you or your co-workers or makes insinuations about previous physicians or has recently changed doctors, inquire about it:

> Examiner: I get the feeling you are upset about being here today.
> Patient: No, I'm not upset . . . but I don't like having to wait around for hours.

> Examiner: Tell me more about what happened with your doctor.
> Patient: Well, I know I shouldn't say anything, but . . . .

Put yourself on the patient's side (or at least separate yourself slightly from guilt by association with the "bad" persons or institutions) and confirm your interest in the patient's feelings. The patient is then in a better position to tell you what he or she likes and dislikes about the process of obtaining medical care. You can learn about some of the hardships of being sick and getting medical help, about humiliations and inconveniences, about helpful acts of kindness and concern, and about this particular patient's expectations, perceptions, and reactions. Such information, in turn, can guide your actions and those of other clinical staff.

Listen for what is *not* discussed. Patients may exclude essential facts in the story, perhaps because of shame, a desire not to acknowledge upsetting problems, or a wish to suppress painful feelings. Where is the elderly person's family in this story of a lonely struggle with disability? Has the patient told you about a long illness without mentioning the diagnosis of cancer? Have a series of infuriating events been recounted without a hint that the patient might be angry?

Some patients "protest too much." They state their feelings so vigorously that one suspects that quite the opposite is true:

> I wouldn't let something like that bother me.

> I really don't care what they do.

Listen for anxiety. When patients come to the doctor, they are almost universally worried about their health. When you find yourself particularly tense in an interview, you may be responding to the patient's high level of anxiety. If you can acknowledge and explore your patients' concerns and can show that you respect their feelings and fears, the intensity of their distress will often be greatly diminished.

Even as you are pursuing a medical diagnosis, you simultaneously are learning about your patient's personality. In particular, listen for how the patient responds to or copes with the ubiquitous anxiety about illness: stoicism and denial, panic and helplessness, intellectualization, suspiciousness, and so on.

> I decided not to worry about it.

> I didn't know what to do.

> You've got to help me.
>
> Now don't try to tell me that I need to go to the hospital or take a bunch of tests.
>
> I figured it would go away. It really wasn't too bad, and I don't let things like that get in my way.

In assessing adaptation to the present illness, listen for how the patient seems either to minimize (or deny) or to amplify (or dramatize) the severity of symptoms and the need for help. Consider three patients with congestive heart failure. The first patient excitedly describes "a terrible gasping for air. I thought I was going to choke. My heart was jumping out of my chest. I was rushed to the emergency ward." The second patient calmly describes similar air hunger and palpitations, but reports that he dealt with it by sitting up for 20 minutes until he felt better, then lying down and going to sleep. On the morning after the episode, he makes an appointment for an office visit. The third patient comes in for a regularly scheduled checkup, but describes "a little trouble breathing and some fast heartbeats for a week or two" and adds, parenthetically, that he has spent many sleepless nights sitting upright in a chair: "I don't make a big deal out of things or go running to a doctor with every little problem." These three patients have nearly identical physical problems; critical listening will help you appreciate how their individual responses differ.

Reassurance and Advice

When patients express anxiety about the meaning of their symptoms, you may naturally want to alleviate their worry by reassuring them. However, you generally should not offer reassurance about symptoms that you do not yet fully understand and that require further investigation. A global or premature reassurance ("Everything is going to be fine" or "Don't worry") is usually neither truthful nor reassuring. Later portions of this text outline guidelines for effective specific reassurance based on a clear appreciation of the patient's concerns, as well as on a full medical evaluation.

A few honest, encouraging remarks, however, can be offered, even when the picture looks dismal:

> I think this will require some specific tests, but I am sure we are going to be able to get you some relief.
>
> I'm glad you're getting attention for this problem. I know we will be able to help you with it when we understand more about what is causing it.

Some unnecessary worry can also be alleviated. For instance, when a patient casually mentions spots before his eyes, your very detailed questioning may suggest to him that a serious problem is being investigated. If you conclude that the patient has a benign condition (such as "floaters"), you may be able to alleviate the anxiety promptly. Rather than going on to the next part of the history or waiting until the end of the workup, take a minute to explain your tentative impression and to reassure the patient. Try not to leave the patient dangling fearfully.

Avoid the temptation to give advice in early stages of the interview. When patients seek your counsel, but you are still trying to understand their problems and are not ready to give an informed opinion, or you feel that advice is inappropriate, you can *reflect* the question:

> Patient: Do you think I am being foolish?
> Interviewer: What do you think?

> Patient: What should I do?
> Interviewer: How do you feel about it?

Alternatively, you might say,

> I think we should talk more about this before trying to reach any conclusions.

> I'm going to do everything I can to help you with your decision, but ultimately you are going to have to make up your own mind rather than having me tell you what to do.

> I would like to discuss this with my supervisor before giving you any suggestions.

Self-Disclosure

In normal social conversation, we often respond to another person's story by telling about our own experiences. However, in clinical work, you should generally avoid reminiscing or otherwise giving personal information about yourself. You cannot predict how a patient will respond to such information and how the revelation will affect your relationship. A degree of anonymity about your personal life helps you maintain for the patient your desired stance of being impartial, objective, and nonjudgmental. Even more important, you want to focus attention on the patient, not yourself; self-disclosure puts patients in the position of having to respond to your experiences and feelings, rather than their own. Deflect personal inquiries by the patient.

> Patient: Have you ever had an abortion?
> Interviewer: Why do you ask?

> Patient: Did you ever go through a divorce?
> Interviewer: I think what is most important here is not my own experience, but what it is like for you.

Of course, patients are entitled to learn basic facts about you, such as your age and year in medical school. When they do inquire about such matters, answer them, but also ask them why they are interested. Finally, in very carefully selected instances, especially when you know the patient well, limited self-disclosure can be a valuable tool for strengthening a relationship.

AFFECT AND EMPATHY

That element of tragedy which lies in the very fact of frequency, has not yet wrought itself into the coarse emotions of mankind; and perhaps our frames could hardly bear much of it. If we had a keen vision and feeling of all ordinary human life, it would be like hearing the grass grow and the squirrel's heart beat, and we should die of that roar which lies on the other side of silence. As it is, the quickest of us walk about well wadded with stupidity.

George Eliot
Middlemarch

. . . he was all that others were, or that they could become. He not only had in himself the germs of every faculty and feeling, but he could follow them by anticipation, intuitively, into all their conceivable ramifications, through every change of fortune, or conflict of passion, or turn of thought . . . He had only to think of anything in order to become that thing, with all the circumstances belonging to it.

William Hazlitt (writing of Shakespeare)

The experience of being sick and of obtaining medical care is almost invariably colored by strong emotions. Encourage patients to express their *feelings* about the illness, as well as to tell the "facts":

How did all of this affect you?

What has it been like for you?

You said you were ashamed . . . [pause]

What do you mean by "depressed"?

Patients' emotional tone and other nonverbal behaviors may be a more reliable indicator of their feelings than their stated emotions. You may readily recognize anxiety from a patient's worried facial expression, sweaty palms, clipped speech, and restlessness. Similarly, a sad patient may exhibit a slumped, defeated posture, frequent sighing, slow speech, a furrowed brow, and eyes that are red and watery. Consider feeding back your observations to the patient in the form of a gentle confrontation:

You seem anxious.

I noticed that you looked a bit sad there when we were discussing your mother's illness.

Many patients will describe emotionally important events without verbally or nonverbally acknowledging the affective meaning. You may want to provide a simple interpretation of the patient's experience. Of course, you never totally understand your patients, but by listening carefully and responding in a respectful and unpretentious manner, you can offer statements that label their experience accurately and openly. You may simply name the feeling that a patient seems to be expressing:

I guess you were furious.

So you got quite upset.

Or you may convey your impression of feelings that were not directly expressed:

I could imagine that being difficult.

I wonder if you weren't very disappointed by the way your friends acted.

That must have really hurt, huh?

Try to respond promptly to clues about psychosocial distress: stay with the feelings. Do not postpone discussion to the time you plan to take the social history, lest you convey to the patient that such matters are unimportant to you.

Empathy begins with accurately perceiving your patient's experience. Listening and questioning are the key tools for achieving such an appreciation. Certainly, interviewers differ enormously in their innate ability to be empathic—their genuine interest in the patient, their facility at reading others' feelings, their ability to recreate within themselves another's experience and to resonate with it, and finally to convey such an appreciation effectively. Yet we can all strive for a basic understanding and respect for the patient's experience and learn ways to share our recognition. The interviewer's engagement in trying to appreciate the other person's experience communicates a fundamental interest and concern and becomes a source of comfort and support for patients and a validation of their feelings.

When patients do express important affects, your most basic tasks are to let patients know that you have registered their feelings and to show your interest. The simplest response is nonverbal: you reflect your sense that an important matter has been brought up by your facial expression or other gestures or through your tone of voice, perhaps while making facilitative comments. You may also communicate your understanding and interest by restating or summarizing what the patient seems to be describing:

So the news got you quite upset.

You've really been pleased with how things turned out.

Additional tasks in responding empathically include letting the patients know that you are affected by what is happening to them and conveying your respect and support. Empathic statements let patients know when you are touched by their experiences. Such statements can also indicate your acceptance of the patient's emotions, thus strengthening your rapport while encouraging further expression of affect:

It sounds rather frightening.

I'm sorry about how uncomfortable you've been.

You've had to face some terrible losses, and anyone in your position would be feeling this way.

You may even indicate your positive regard:

> You've been through quite an ordeal, and it's taken a lot of courage to do what you've done.

Novice clinicians often are concerned that inquiry about affect will seem intrusive. Patients, however, are generally grateful for your interest in their feelings. They are quite able to keep their expression of affect within comfortable bounds and to communicate clearly when they want to avoid further discussion. Therefore provide encouragement and a gentle pressure to express emotions, while allowing patients to avoid the topic or shift to neutral matters.

A much more common problem than being intrusive is neglecting to attend to affect. Patients often feel a natural pressure to discharge emotionally charged material, and they seek a safe setting, such as the doctor's office, in which they can communicate their feelings. The process of discharging is called abreaction, and is therapeutic in itself. Patients generally benefit from sensitive attention to feelings and from an opportunity to ventilate.

When patients express their emotions, your job is not to make uncomfortable feelings go away or to reassure the patient. In expressing such painful emotions as grief, shame, anger, loneliness, or sadness, patients are rarely creating or precipitating new problems over which you and they might lose control—opening a Pandora's box. They are recognizing existing problems and joining with you in a satisfying process of communicating their feelings and trying to cope better. So let patients cry. If you can be understanding and convey a sense of acceptance and appreciation for the patient, your attention will be comforting and supportive.

COMMON PITFALLS IN QUESTIONING

Various types of questions should be avoided. Some examples are given below.

Pitfalls To Avoid When Questioning Patients

Avoid "rapid-fire"

Avoid using multiple questions strung together:

> Do you ever see double, halos around lights, or flashes or spots before your eyes?
>
> Are you worried about cancer? Do you smoke?

The patient has no chance to give sufficient thought to each question and may end up answering none adequately or only replying to the last one.

Use unbiased questions

Avoid suggesting an answer ("leading the witness") or otherwise confirming preconceptions:

> You never have diarrhea, do you?
>
> Was it because you were walking too fast on a cold day?

You're having trouble with your knee, but otherwise your joints are fine, right?

Rather than: Does the pain radiate to your left arm?
Ask: Does the pain radiate anywhere?

Avoid jargon

Practitioners often use technical terms that are meaningless or confusing to patients.

Interviewer: Are you sexually active?
Patient: No, I'm only having relations with my wife.

Rather than: Have you ever had an MI?
Ask: Did you ever have a heart attack?

Rather than: Is there any family history of heart disease?
Ask: Does anyone in your family have heart trouble? . . . What kind?

Anticipate the patient's potential difficulty with medical terminology.

If I should use any unfamiliar terms or phrases, please stop me and let me know.

Clarify vague terms

Don't settle for imprecise descriptions. Clarify such terms as dizzy, tired, bloody, weak, blurry, constipated, or trouble sleeping.

Tell me more about what you see when your vision is blurred. Do you see more than one image? What if you close one eye or the other? Does the haziness come and go?

You said you have diarrhea. What were the stools actually like? Were they loose or watery? How often did you go to the bathroom? What are your bowel movements usually like? How often do you usually go?

Patients commonly adopt medical terms and previous diagnoses:

Then my hiatus hernia began acting up.

I get colitis whenever I get nervous.

Learn not to take such words for granted. Watch out for lay medical terms: a cold or flu, spells, allergy, heart attack, stroke, water pills. Commonly used words may have different meanings for you and the patient·

Interviewer: What kind of allergy did you have to codeine? What did it do to you?
Patient: It made me sick to my stomach.

Clarify lay terminology:

What are the heart pills called?

How did you learn you had an ulcer? . . . Did you have any x-rays of your stomach?

Beware of ascribing knowledge, behaviors, or feelings

Don't assume patients know basic anatomy and pathophysiology. Don't make assumptions about a patient's sexual experience or preferences. Don't take for granted that they want to work, get more education, be with their family, recover quickly, or learn more about their condition. Don't presume they are sad about a death or divorce or happy about a birth or promotion. When you need information on such matters, inquire! If you are not quite certain you understand your patient's feelings, rather than saying, "I know how that feels" or "That must have made you angry," you are safer saying:

> How did that feel?
>
> Was that hard on you?
>
> That sounds like it might have made you mad.

Don't assume that patients follow prescribed treatment. Assess compliance in a nonthreatening manner:

> How much of the medication were you able to take?
>
> How do you remember to take all those pills?
>
> Did you have any success cutting back on the cigarette smoking?

Similarly, assess health habits in a nonjudgmental manner:

> Rather than: How long have you had this drinking problem?
> Ask: Have you ever felt you had a problem with drinking?
>
> Rather than: Don't you know how bad smoking is?
> Ask: What is your understanding about the health consequences of smoking?
> Or: Does your smoking concern you?

Avoid social judgment

Questions can often convey demeaning attitudes:

> When did you finally get some good treatment?
>
> At your age, what do you expect?
>
> Don't you think you are a little young (old or heavy or thin) for that?

Don't equate poverty with laziness, lack of education with low intelligence, advanced age with dependency. Common targets for verbal and nonverbal disdain are welfare clients, alcoholics, drug addicts, criminals, homosexuals, unwed mothers, and the unemployed, as well as persons who are poorly acculturated, emotionally disturbed, ill-kempt, obese, aged, frail, or hopelessly ill. Other targets are people who are abused or abusive and those whose personality characteristics have earned them the clinical titles of "difficult," "hateful," or "problem" patients. Convey respect for the "least desirable."

Don't limit your attention to one problem

Finally, don't assume that the patient's initial complaint is his or her foremost concern. Once you have tracked down what seems to be the reason for the visit, check for other important but withheld problems. Patients may have multiple problems, and the most worrisome or embarrassing ones are often saved for last.

> Now you have told me about the headaches. Are there any other matters that concern you?
>
> Did we take care of everything?
>
> Anything else you want to mention?

DIFFICULT QUESTIONS AND CONFIDENTIALITY

The significance of some of your questions that are routine or are used to clarify the diagnosis may not be apparent to patients.

> Interviewer: Do you take birth control pills?
> Patient: Why do you ask?

> Interviewer: Because oral contraceptives can affect your health and may have something to do with the headaches you are having.
> Patient: Really? In what way does the pill affect you?

When you ask unusual questions or sense that the patient is uncomfortable or balking at your inquiry, explain the logic of your query. Share your intentions in the interview:

> It's important for me to know how you are using alcohol because it may influence many parts of your body and also may affect some of the tests we take.

> The reason I am being nosy about just what kind of work you do is that certain jobs can lead to specific problems with your health.

Doctors learn to ask about charged topics that would not be mentioned in ordinary conversation and that might even seem out of place among intimate friends and family.

> Many people don't talk about these things outside of the doctor's office, but it's no surprise that it's on your mind.

Among the topics you will encounter and may find troubling are sexuality, bowel and bladder function, alcohol and drug abuse, criminal behavior, spouse and child abuse, illegitimacy, adultery, terminal illness, and death.

How is it that physicians can obtain personal information without causing great resistance, shame, or discomfort on the part of the patient? One important factor is the recognized role of the physician—the mandate to seek and use information only for the patient's benefit. Patients generally appreciate that you are not exploring embarrassing topics for your own prurient interests. You will become more comfortable with asking difficult questions (and, in turn, communicate your ease to patients) when you have gained experience in using such personal information in clinical work. But also consider explaining why you are asking.

The physician's privileged role is strengthened by the rule of privacy in the clinical encounter. You may want to speak directly to your patient's concerns about confidentiality:

> This information can be of importance in your treatment. Of course, everything you say is in confidence.

> We need to discuss this matter but I will not write it down in your record.

Another even less tangible factor that permits the doctor to explore intimate matters is the trust that patients develop from a sense that the physician is sincerely concerned, but also neutral, nonjudgmental, and respectful. In the course of an interview, the physician may repeatedly demonstrate positive regard and a sensitivity to the patient's vulnerabilities, or may provoke distrust, shame, and guilt. When you have established a trustful relationship, patients often accept and even expect what might seem like intrusiveness, just as they readily permit the intimate contact of the physical examination.

INTERVIEWING OLDER PATIENTS

Patients older than 75 years of age frequently seek medical help alone or are brought to the doctor by caregivers—family members, friends, or paid help. Interviewing older patients can be different and sometimes difficult unless attention is paid to their special communication needs. Older patients may speak more slowly, have voice tremor and roughness, hearing loss, diminished naming and comprehension skills, and vision impairments that prevent them from picking up on nonverbal clues in doctor-patient conversations. They also typically have multiple chronic conditions that require attention.

In your encounter, respond attentively and respectfully to the patient rather than just addressing yourself to the escorts.

- Question and advise the patient in a quiet room with chairs arranged to allow for direct, close-up communication (see Fig. 2–1).
- Speak louder.
- If needed, repeat questions to assure comprehension.
- If needed, engage the patient's permission for the family to share in the transmitted advice and directions, which should be given both verbally and in writing.
- Engage the patient even while separately addressing caregiver concerns.

Most important, throughout the interview the patient should be encouraged to actively participate and should not be ignored because of his or her age or because of caregiver concerns. During questioning, when older patients may wander and reminisce, do not hurry. Listening to reminiscences is important for patient self-esteem and in establishing a relationship and learning their concerns. These reflective stories sometimes reveal the patient's personal concerns (e.g., of being alone).

> Patient: I was a navy pilot after high school.
> Doctor: Tell me, what was that experience like?
> Patient: Well, . . .[The reminiscence takes some 10 minutes]

USING INTERPRETERS IN INTERVIEWS

An estimated 14 million people in the United States lack basic English language skills, many of whom seek medical aid at clinics and hospitals where you will be working. Interpreters may be needed to get an accurate history, develop a therapeutic doctor-patient relationship, and provide health education. You may try to "take the history" yourself by using whatever language skills you have, or you may use interpreters—family or friends who accompany the patient, hospital personnel, or, preferably, trained hospital interpreters. Regardless of who you use, negotiation with the interpreter is important.

The roles interpreters assume vary. An interpreter may participate in a traditional question-answer mode, a neutral translating role; conversely, an interpreter (one with a health care job or connections in the patient's community) may advocate and negotiate for the patient or reassure or alarm the patient by controlling information you have transmitted. Given the various roles the interpreter may want to exercise, it is most important to negotiate what you want and expect.

- Tell the interpreter what you hope to accomplish.
- Decide, with the interpreter, on translating techniques (simultaneous, consequential, or summary).
- Encourage interpreters to ask questions when uncertain and to comment when they notice misunderstanding. Such negotiations can ensure effective history-taking and patient care.
- Ask the interpreter, "How is it going?" to get comments and "interpretations" of the patient's reactions.
- Allow and encourage questions.

SUGGESTED READINGS

Battle M: Guidelines for providers in cross cultural settings, Boston, 1995, Massachusetts General Hospital (privately printed).

Greene NG, Majerovitz SD, Adelman RD, Rizzo C: The effects of a third person on the physician-older patient medical interview, *J Am Geriatr Soc* 42:413, 1994.

Huntly RA, Helfer KS, editors: *Communication in late life,* Boston, 1995, Butterworth-Heinemann.

Pacific Medical Center: Cross cultural health care project: a report, Seattle, 1994.

Ryan EB, Meridith SD, MacLean MJ, Orange JB: Changing the way we talk with elders: promoting health using communication enhancement model, *Int J Aging Hum Dev* 41:89, 1995.

Silliman RA: Caring for the frail older patient: the doctor-patient-caregiver relationship, *J Gen Intern Med* 4:237, 1989.

Waitzkin H, Britt T, Williams C: Narratives of aging and social problems in medical encounters with older persons, *J Health Soc Behav* 35:322, 1996.

Woloshin S, Bickell NA, Schwartz LM, et al: Language barriers in medicine, *JAMA* 273:724, 1995.

CHAPTER 4

ELICITING INFORMATION FOR DIAGNOSIS AND MANAGEMENT II: THE CONTENT OF THE MEDICAL INTERVIEW

The most important difference between a good and indifferent clinician lies in the amount of attention paid to the story of a patient.

SIR FARQUHAR BUZZARD (1933)

This section of the text identifies the specific information you need to acquire to make a diagnosis and to plan management.

THE PRESENT ILLNESS

After you have introduced yourself and the process of the interview and have settled comfortably in the office, inquire about the present illness (or present problems). Your introductory remarks may lead the patient to describe the reason for the visit, requests, and details of the present illness, or you may need to ask directly.

> Could you tell me what brings you in today?

Reason for the Visit

For your written or oral presentation of the case, you should specify the patient's reason for the visit, a brief phrase that identifies the focus of the present illness and serves as part of the headline for your presentation. The reason for the visit can often be stated in the patient's own words:

> Patient: My urine has been burning since yesterday.
>
> [Reason for visit]: Burning on urination for 1 day.
>
> Examiner: Do you come with any particular questions about your health?
>
> Patient: The chest pains have been worse this week, and I think my blood pressure must be up.
>
> [Reason for visit]: Worsened chest pains for 1 week.

The term *chief complaint* is similar to the *reason for the visit*. The former term is frequently used in write-ups of inpatients but often makes little sense in ambulatory care. In the first place, a patient may have several both-ersome symptoms. You may not want to force the patient to select one problem as most important. Second, not all patients come to the doctor with complaints (e.g., headaches, weakness). For example, some will be feeling well but will be concerned about their health and bring requests ("I want my cholesterol checked"). Patients might come for a routine or follow-up visit ("The doctor said to come back in a year"). Others have administrative reasons ("I need a blood test to get married" or "I need these disability forms to be filled out").

Requests

Requests refer to what the patient hopes to accomplish in the visit.

> Examiner: How did you hope I could help you today?
> [or]: How did you want me to help you with this problem?
>
> Patient [whose reason for visit is "chest pains for the past month"]: I want a good checkup, especially of my heart.
>
> I want to know if I have heart disease, like my brother.
>
> I want an EKG.
>
> I want some medicine for this chest pain so that I can work [or sleep or exercise or go to a wedding next Saturday].
>
> I want to know what this chest pain is about, and if I should worry about it.
>
> I need to have my heart checked so that these disability forms can be completed.
>
> I want a referral to a heart specialist.
>
> Doc, I can't do jury duty with this pain. Would you write me a note?

The requests (along with triggers and attributions discussed later in this section), though not regularly recorded in a traditional medical history, offer important information about the personal meaning of being ill and obtaining help. Moreover, you will need to understand the request to arrive with the patient at a mutually satisfactory care plan and to provide an appropriate and effective explanation about the diagnosis and treatment.

Requests may be complex and often are not easily elicited. Consider a young woman patient who complains of being tired. She might, for example, be seeking some of the following:

A Patient's Requests _____

Explanation and reassurance
Is this the first sign of cancer, like on the TV program last week?
Do I have "mono" like my girlfriend?
Am I working too hard?
Can this be due to the birth control pills?

Testing
Please check my blood for thyroid problems.
Don't you think I should get a chest x-ray?

Medications
Should I be taking vitamins or iron?
Maybe I ought to take some antibiotics.

Psychosocial assistance
The kids are wearing me down. I just wanted to talk.
I need help controlling my anger.
I need help finding a day-care center.
I can't sleep because of the noise outside; do you think I should find a new apartment?
I can't sleep since my boyfriend left; am I going crazy?

Administrative matters
If you sign this form, I can get a few days off from work.
Please fill out these disability papers.
I'm too tired to walk up here to your office. Can you get me a taxi voucher?

No request from the patient
I came because my husband insisted. He wants to know if I'm really sick.

Probing is often required to elicit requests:

> Patient: I want a checkup.
> Interviewer: What did you want checked?
> Patient: I want to know if I have any signs of multiple sclerosis.

At the very beginning of the interview, requests may not be freely expressed. They are sometimes shared more readily further on in the visit when the patient feels more trusting of the doctor. Questioning about requests may be reserved for this later time or repeated then.

Triggers

For the tired young woman described above, consider how your appreciation of her reason for presenting would differ if she had had the problem for a few days, a few weeks, or a year. A useful and often overlooked question for understanding the patient's perspective is "Why now?" Particularly when you are investigating a minor or long-standing illness, inquire about the trigger for the visit:

> What led you to get help now?
> How did you happen to consult with us today?
> When did you decide to come in and get checked?
> What got you to come in?

Such questions can reveal the patient's requests and attributions and often begin to unravel a complex series of biomedical and psychosocial events that led the patient to present with a problem.

In the hospital, a patient's reasons for being under care usually seem obvious. You may feel that your outpatient's reasons are also obvious, but surveys indicate that only a fraction of the patients who experience an episode of illness consult a physician. For every patient who presents with a cold or chest pain or swollen legs—minor problems as well as more serious ones—there are three or four who handle the problem without formally seeking medical help. Except perhaps for patients whose physical distress has truly become intolerable, the complaint itself is rarely a sufficient explanation for why this patient came in today rather than last week, next week, or never.

> I read about cancer in the paper and decided I better get this checked.
>
> My wife got fed up with my getting up at night and insisted I come in.

Typically, patients develop physical symptoms but do not bring them to the attention of a physician unless other factors intervene. Intervening factors are often psychosocial: the course of symptoms does not follow the patient's expectations ("My buddy says that this cold should be gone in four days"), the patient otherwise becomes concerned about the meaning of the symptoms ("My brother felt like this when he got 'mono'"), or a visit is provoked by the combination of the symptoms with psychological or social matters (such as grief, family conflict, anxiety states, isolation, frank psychiatric disorders, lifelong patterns of help-seeking behavior, or hoping to feel well for an upcoming social event or vacation). Many patients with psychosocial difficulties cannot readily articulate the role of these factors in their decision to seek help; the alert physician must make a psychosocial diagnosis along with a biomedical one. Understanding "triggers" helps you appreciate the patient's situation and what kind of help this patient wants and needs.

Characterizing the Symptom

You investigate the present illness (or present problems) by asking the patient to elaborate on the reason for the visit:

> Tell me more about what it's been like.
>
> Tell me the story of this illness.
>
> Can you describe what it feels like?

"Dimensions" To Characterize Symptoms

Location
Where is the symptom located?
  Can you show me by putting your finger on the spot?
Has it changed location?

Does it radiate or move?

Quality or character
What does it feel like?
> Sharp or dull? Crampy? Tingling? Throbbing?

What does it look like?

Chronology (frequency, onset, duration, course)
When were you last feeling well?
> When did it begin?
> When did you first notice anything wrong?

Have you ever had anything like this before?

How long does it last?
> What's the longest it lasts? The shortest?

Is it constant?
> Does it come and go?
> Suddenly or gradually?

How do you feel between attacks?

How often do you get it?
> What's the most often you've had it?
> The least often? The average?

How has it changed since it started?
> Is it getting more or less frequent?
> More or less severe?

Severity or amount
How bad is it?
> Does it interfere with your activities at home?
> At work?
> Does it disrupt your sleep?

How much? (e.g., number of loose stools, cups of sputum)

Aggravating (or precipitating) and alleviating factors
What were you doing when it first began?

What brings it on? Under what circumstances do you get this problem?

What do you do when it happens?

Is there anything that you do that makes it worse? Better?

Is it related to:
> Eating (before, during, or after meals; size of meals; type of food; swallowing)
> Body position (lying down on your back, stomach, or side; sitting up; standing) or changing position (standing up, lying down, turning over in bed)
> Movement of separate parts of the body (e.g., arm, leg, neck) or to physical activity (walking, climbing stairs, exercise, strenuous work)
> Pressure on one part of your body
> Coughing or deep breathing
> Mood (anger, excitement, sadness, other emotions)
> Any other activities at work or home?

How soon after you eat (change position and so forth) do you feel better? Worse?

Have you treated yourself (e.g., with heat, cold, immobilization, diet, rest, activity, prescription medication or over-the-counter preparations)? Has the treatment helped?

Have you gotten help from other practitioners (doctors, chiropractors, pharmacists, spiritualists, friends)?

Associated symptoms

What other problems are associated with this one? [Your questions may include the complete *review of systems* for any system related to the problem.]

Disability and adaptation

How has it affected you?
Has it affected your physical function (e.g., work, rest, sexual activity)?
Your mood or thinking?
Your social relationships?
How does it affect the people around you (e.g., family, friends, co-workers)?
How have you managed?
Whom do you turn to for help?
   For emotional support?

Attributions

What ideas have you had about this problem?
   What have you thought was wrong?
   What do you think caused this problem?
   What has it meant to you?
   What have others made of it?
What brings it on?
   Why do you think it started when it did?
   What have others made of it?
   Do you know anyone with a similar problem? What is it like for them?
How do you think it should be diagnosed? Treated?
Do you have any thoughts on what it might lead to?
   Does it seem serious?
What concerns you the most about it?
[If your patient initially denies having attributions, you should ask again later in the interview. You can encourage a response by saying, "Most everyone has some ideas about what might be causing this sort of thing."]

An old mnemonic for the major dimensions of a symptom is "O P Q R S T": onset, provocation/palliation, quality, radiation, site, and temporal profile.

As you develop facility in pathophysiological and clinical reasoning and in the process of differential diagnosis, you will become increasingly aware of additional information that is essential to characterize a complaint, including not only the biophysical "dimensions" of a symptom but also the relevant risk factors and the "pertinent positives and negatives" from the review of systems.

An Example of the Present Illness

Later, when giving an oral or written presentation of the present illness, you will want to organize the data into a coherent story that, insofar as possible, argues in favor of a particular disease or syndrome, while allowing the reader to consider major diagnostic possibilities:

- Reason for visit:

Mrs. Platt is a 23-year-old female office worker who complains of 3 months of "spells" in which she sees flashing lights, sometimes followed by a mild headache.

- Present illness:

The patient has enjoyed generally good health until about three months ago, when she first experienced "spells" which started with a vague sense of nausea and with lights flashing before her eyes, followed occasionally by a headache. The spells begin in the morning when she awakens, often on weekends, and occur every week or two. The lights are described as dazzling zigzag lines seen in both eyes, but occurring either in the right or left visual field. No vomiting, weakness or paresthesias are noted. The initial symptoms resolve gradually over ten minutes, and roughly half the time are followed by a mild unilateral throbbing headache. The headache occurs over the entire half of the head and becomes increasingly severe over the next half hour. She never needs to stop what she is doing or lie down, but she tries to avoid bright light and loud noises. Two aspirin give moderate relief, and she usually feels better in two to four hours.

She initially thought she had developed an eye strain from using a copying machine. She became concerned and made this appointment when she read a brochure on glaucoma.

She notes no relationship of her spells to diet, alcohol, menses, or stress, and she does not use oral contraceptives.

There is no family history of migraine.

THE STANDARD DATA BASE

The standard data base consists of the following: the past medical history, social history, family history, and review of systems.

In this section of the interview, you gather the background information that is collected on each new patient, regardless of the reason for the visit. The past medical history (or past history) is a life record of health, disease, medical treatment, and health-related practices. The social history is a broad profile of the individual's personal and social background. The family history is a description of the family's patterns of illness. Finally, the review of systems is a detailed inventory of symptoms.

Some of the standard data base will already have been collected in the earlier phases of the interview in conjunction with your investigation of the patient's immediate problems. Indeed, in an ideal history of the present illness, you elicit all the past history, family and social history, and review of systems pertinent to understanding the reason for the visit. In actual practice, your inquiry into the standard data base may uncover additional facts that you will later realize to be essential for characterizing the presenting complaint, and you will incorporate this information in your write-up of the present illness.

The standard data base is collected by asking a series of routine questions and by pursuing new problems that emerge. Systematic data collection ensures you and the patient that important medical facts are not overlooked and gives you a more complete picture of the patient's medical history. For patients in ambulatory care, you may not have time to get all this information on your first visit, so you may gather only the most essential data and arrange to finish up at future visits.

In learning basic clinical skills, you want to develop habits of thoroughness and systematic inquiry. You should obtain as "complete" a standard data base as is feasible. Eventually, as you develop a more flexible style that can be adapted to the clinical setting, you will vary the content of your history appropriately.

Past Medical History

The basic questions for a very detailed past medical history are arranged in a hierarchical fashion below; relatively specialized inquiries are indented under broader or fundamental questions, and the queries that are essential to a complete interview are in **bold**. Tailor your investigative strategy to the patient and the clinical setting, pursuing the more detailed issues when you obtain positive responses to general questions or when circumstances demand greater thoroughness and precision. For instance, when you are considering the diagnosis of acquired immune deficiency syndrome, you would ask about transfusions and intravenous drug abuse, even though the patient denied any operations, serious injuries or illnesses, or the use of recreational drugs.

Questions For Obtaining a Complete Past Medical History

Hospitalizations
Have you ever been hospitalized?
  What for? When? Where?

Operations and injuries
Have you ever had any surgery or operations?
  What for? When? Where?
Have you ever been involved in a serious accident?
  Did you break any bones?
  Have a serious head injury?
Have you ever required a transfusion?

Pregnancies
Have you ever been pregnant?
  How many times?
  Any miscarriages or abortions?
Any problems or complications with the pregnancies?
  Toxemia?
  Did you take any hormones during the pregnancy?
How were the births?

Illnesses

Have you had any other serious illnesses?

　　When? Tell me more about it.

Let me ask you some specific questions. Have you ever had:

　　Anemia or bleeding problems?

　　Needed a transfusion?

　　Heart problems or heart failure?

　　Murmurs or rheumatic fever?

　　Heart attacks or angina?

　　High blood pressure?

　　Pneumonia or tuberculosis?

　　Asthma, emphysema?

　　Stomach problems or ulcers?

　　Liver or gallbladder problems?

　　Hepatitis or jaundice?

　　Bladder or kidney infections or stones?

　　Venereal disease?

　　　　Gonorrhea, syphilis, or herpes?

　　Arthritis, rheumatism, or gout?

　　Infections or inflammatory disease of the uterus or fallopian tubes?

　　Thyroid problems? Diabetes?

　　Cancer?

　　Seizures?

　　Nervous or emotional problems?

　　　　A nervous breakdown?

　　　　Attempted suicide?

Medications

Do you use any medicines or drugs?

　　What are their names?

　　What are they for?

　　How long have you been taking them?

　　Do you know their size or strength?

　　[For medicines taken regularly:]

　　　　When do you take them?

　　　　　　How often do you miss a dose?

　　[For medicines taken as needed:]

　　　　How often do you take them?

　　　　　　How many in a week (or day or month)?

　　Have the medications helped?

　　　　How?

　　Have you had side effects?

Do you take anything for sleep or your bowels?

Pain medicine?

Vitamins or minerals?

Birth control pills?

Medicines that do not require a prescription?

Are you using any alternative or complementary therapies—treatments not traditionally prescribed by physicians—such as special vitamins or minerals, herbal remedies, diets, and so on?

Allergies and adverse reactions
Do you have any allergies?
  What kind of allergic reaction did you have?
Have you had any allergic or adverse reactions to medicines?
  Penicillin or sulfa?
  Injections used in x-ray studies?

Habits
Do you smoke?
  Cigarettes? Pipe? Cigars?
    How much? For how long?
    Do you inhale?
    Did you ever try to cut down or quit?
      How? What happened?
    Did you ever smoke?
      How much? For how long?
Do you drink alcohol?
  [The CAGE Test (see Asking About Alcohol in Chapter 10):]
    Have you ever felt the need to **C**ut down on drinking?
    Have you ever felt **A**nnoyed by criticisms of drinking?
    Have you ever had **G**uilty feelings about drinking?
    Have you ever taken a morning **E**ye opener?
  Did you ever drink regularly?
  What do you drink?
    When do you drink?
    How much do you drink?
What about recreational drugs?
  For instance, marijuana ("pot")?
  Cocaine ("coke") or heroin?
  Others?
    Are you using them now?
      How often?
  Did you ever use them regularly?
  Have you ever injected drugs?

Exposures
Are you exposed to any health hazards in your work or personal life?
  Physical, emotional, and sexual abuse are increasingly recognized as common problems in our society. Have you or other members of your family been harmed or threatened?
  Has a partner physically hurt you or frightened you?
    Forced you to have sexual relations?
    To engage in sexual practices you disliked?
    Have arguments led to pushing, shoving, slapping, hitting, or kicking?
    Have any partners hurt you physically?
    Has a partner used any kind of weapon, such as a gun, knife, or club, to hurt you?
Are your work conditions safe?
Are there risks of accidents, injury, or exposure?
  Are preventive measures used?

In your job or leisure-time activities, do you work with or around any hazardous materials—substances that might make you sick?

How about in your past jobs or hobbies?

    Chemicals, dusts, or fumes?

    Radiation?

    Lead?

    Solvents?

    Asbestos?

Do your job or hobbies involve:

    Prolonged sun exposure?

    Loud noises?

    Physical stress?

    Emotional stress?

        What about tension on the job?

  Do you know what to do to protect yourself from hazardous exposures?

      What do you actually do?

[Further inquiry is based on an appreciation of the patient's presenting problems and on the risks associated with particular occupations]

Travel

Have you traveled outside the United States in the past few years?

    Where?

        Outside this state?

Diet

Are you on a special diet?

Have you tried to lose weight? How?

  Do you do anything to control your weight?

Do you try to avoid cholesterol or saturated fats?

    How often do you eat red meat?

    How about poultry and fish?

    What about dairy products, such as eggs, butter, and whole milk?

    Fried foods?

    Have you had your cholesterol checked?

Do you limit your intake of salt?

  Do you usually salt your food?

[When further inquiry is appropriate:]

    What do you usually eat

      For breakfast?

      For lunch?

      For dinner?

      For snacks?

    Where do you eat these meals?

      Who does the cooking? The shopping?

    Do you drink caffeine-containing coffee or tea?

      Caffeinated tonic or soda?

      How much?

    What about sources of fiber in your diet?

[For women who are perimenopausal or menopausal:]

    Do you take calcium supplements?

Health maintenance

[This section is also called *health risk profile, health promotion,* or *preventive health care* and is not included in many traditional history formats. Some clinicians include habits and diet under this section]

Periodic health examination

Do you have a regular doctor?
   How often do you get routine medical checkups?
When was your last dental exam?
Do you get your eyes checked?
   Have you been examined for glaucoma?
Have you had your cholesterol measured?
[For women]:
   Do you check your breasts for lumps?
   Have you gotten breast x-rays (mammograms)?
   Have you been getting regular "Pap" smears?
[For older adults]:
   Have you had your stools checked for signs of bleeding?
[Other screening procedures to consider include testicular self-examination, audiometry, fasting glucose, hematocrit, electrocardiogram, skin test for tuberculosis, syphilis serology, HIV testing, cultures for gonorrhea and *Chlamydia,* and sigmoidoscopy or colonoscopy.]

Immunizations

Did you get immunizations as a child?
   Measles, mumps, rubella?
   Polio?
   Tetanus and diptheria?
      Have you had a tetanus booster in the past 10 years?
[For women in childbearing ages]:
   Have you been checked to make sure you have had German measles (rubella)?
[For the elderly and other persons considered at high risk for respiratory infections]:
   Have you had an annual flu shot?
   The pneumonia vaccine?
[For persons at high-risk]:
   Hepatitis B vaccine?

Injury prevention

Do you use seat belts?
Do you have smoke detectors at home?
[For parents of young children]:
   Are you familiar with ways to prevent children from poisoning themselves?
      Do you know how to reach the poison control center?
   Have you checked your hot water temperature?
[For the elderly and their helpers]:
   Has your home been checked for hazards?

Exercise

Do you do anything for exercise?
   How do you keep physically fit?

Contraception/sexually transmitted disease
Are you having sexual relations? With men, women, or both?
[For heterosexually active women in childbearing years and their male partners]:
    Are you using any method of birth control?
        [If yes]:Are you satisfied with this method?
        [If no]:Are you concerned about pregnancy?
Are you concerned about sexually transmitted diseases, such as AIDS?
    What precautions do you take?
    Do you use condoms to prevent diseases?

Social History

> *The competent physician, before he attempts to give medicine to his pa-*
> *tients, makes himself acquainted not only with the disease which he*
> *wishes to cure, but also with the habits and constitution of the sick man.*
>
> *Cicero*
> *De Oratore II*

At various times in the initial clinical review, you have the chance to get acquainted with a stranger who is seeking your medical help. Be as inquisitive about this unfamiliar person as you are about bodily complaints. Know your patients. When patients mention important people in their lives or refer to their work or other major activities, inquire further. Give reign to your curiosity. In getting to know the person with whom you are talking, you foster a mutually satisfying relationship and you acquire data that are important for diagnosis and management.

Many other questions are relevant to special groups at risk. For instance, in examining older adults, screening for common impairments in functional status may aid the physician in preventing serious problems. Among the topics that deserve attention are nutrition and weight, visual impairment, hearing loss, memory problems, incontinence, depression, and activities of daily living (see Chapter 16).

The more we know about our patients, the better we can care for them. A basic social history is essential for providing care that joins patients' personal needs with the technical treatment of their disease. Consider a 45-year-old man who falls from a roof, injuring his back and arm. He has enjoyed excellent health all his life, recently passing an "executive physical" with flying colors. In the emergency ward, he is noted to have a vertebral compression fracture that will necessitate bed rest, as well as a fractured arm that is treated with a cast. We need know little more to make a diagnosis or to plan immediate treatment. However, if we want to understand the meaning of illness to this patient and if we want to work with him toward his rehabilitation, we know practically nothing. How does he ordinarily use his arm at home and at work? Will he lose his job if he cannot function normally for a few months? Is he happy to get away from work or frantic to be back?

Does he have insurance, savings, pressing bills, a family to support? What will prolonged bed rest be like? Does he ordinarily spend his free time reading and watching television or playing tennis and working in the garden? Has he ever been bedridden before? How can he be transported to physical therapy appointments? Other questions would come to mind for a patient of a different age, sex, occupation, illness, and so on.

The social history (also sometimes called the patient profile, psychosocial history, or personal history) is the section of the medical record in which you present a brief biography of the patient. Following the often nebulous admonition to care for the "whole person," you sketch out an answer to the question, "Who is this person?", by addressing three topics:

1. The patient's current life (living situation, personal relationships, work, and leisure)
2. Past life (important events in the patient's background or upbringing, such as geographical, ethnic, and class "roots," as well as information about growing up, education, work, relationships, and difficulties with major developmental tasks)
3. The personal and social significance of illness and other stresses (e.g., the impact of major losses).

Additionally, your social history should systematically investigate the psychosocial issues that may help explain the patient's illness or that bear on its management. For patients with "problems of living" or other emotional or social disturbances, this portion of the history may form the core of the present illness.

Basic Content

At a minimum, the social history should describe where the patient was born and raised, his or her highest level of educational attainment, current occupation, marital status and number of children, major stresses, and a statement about general satisfaction with life. If the registration data of the office or hospital record does not otherwise indicate how the patient is paying for medical services, this information should be sought. Commonly useful specific questions for a basic social history are the following:

Questions For Obtaining a Social History _____

Introduction
I'd like to know a little more about you—your background, your work, your family.

Upbringing
Where were you born?
Where did you grow up?
  Where else have you lived?
Where were your parents from?
How did your parents support themselves?
When did you leave home?

School
What about school?
How far did you go?

Military
Have you ever been in the military?

Work and finances
Have you worked outside the home?
What kind of work have you done?
Are you working now?
   What kind of work is it?
   Do you like it [inquiring about the setting, the co-workers and boss, and the physical environment]?
[For housewives, as well as many people who are retired or are not working or who have nontraditional styles of work, a good question is:]
How do you spend your day?
[Alternatively:]
How do you support yourself?
   What other jobs have you had?

Residence
Where are you living?
What is your living situation like?
   Who is with you?
How long have you been there?
How are things at home [seeking information about the physical setting and social situation]?
Are you satisfied with your housing?

Family and relationships
Who are the important people in your life?
[Alternatively:] Tell me about your family.
   How are they?
   What are they like?
   What is your relationship like?
Are you married?
   How is your spouse?
   Are you satisfied with your marriage?
   Have you been married previously?
Do you have children?
   How are they?
   Do you see them?
Do you have other family?
   How are they?
   Do you see them?
How has illness affected your closest relationships?

Leisure
What do you do for fun? What do you do in your free time?
Do you have hobbies?
Do you participate in sports?

Do you do anything for exercise?
How do you spend your vacations?

Religion

What is your religious upbringing?
Are you a regular churchgoer? (or) Do you go to temple regularly?
Do you participate in religious activities?
Are your religious beliefs important to you?
  How?

Satisfaction and stress

How are you feeling about the way your life is going?
  Your personal and family life?
  Your work or career?
Do you have hopes or plans for changing it?
What goals do you have for the immediate future?
  For the more distant future?
Have there been recent changes in your life?
  New stresses?
Have you had any major setbacks or disappointments in the past few years?
  Any losses?

Medical costs

Do you have insurance for your medical bills?
  How will you handle the expense?
  How will you handle the loss of income [from a new disability]?

Many of the questions of a standard social history may seem dry and factual, but you should try to understand what these events mean to the patient. Especially when a striking happening is noted—a death or chronic illness of a sibling or parent, a new occupation or a move to another part of the country, the beginning or end of a major relationship—you will want to know not only that it occurred but also how the patient reacted.

What did it mean to leave school at age 16?

How did you cope with the divorce?

What has it been like being retired?

An occasional patient will ask, "What does all this personal stuff have to do with my heart problems?" A response might be:

I think I can be more helpful when you and I share more of an understanding of what has been going on in your life.

This is part of getting to know you better so I can be a good doctor for you.

It's hard to appreciate how your body is reacting without also knowing something about what you've been going through.

With other patients, this question can provide an opportunity to discuss the relevance of psychosocial issues:

I cannot be sure at this point how important some of these matters are [an honest disclaimer], but the pressures at work do seem significant in your life. I wonder if they may have had something to do with your getting sick. Understanding them might also be important in your getting better [a statement of relevance]. What do you think?

A guide to pursuing a more detailed social history is provided in the section titled Psychosocial Assessment in Chapter 10.

In What Part of the Interview Does One Obtain the Social History?

Some clinicians prefer to begin the interview by obtaining a basic social history. They feel more comfortable exploring the patient's medical history after learning some biographical data. Most clinicians, however, find that patients are eager to begin the encounter by telling the story of their illness and that the social history emerges comfortably later in the interview, especially as greater trust develops. Consider trying out both approaches for yourself.

Many important features of the social history are best obtained in the course of acquiring a description of the present illness and past medical history. While discussing medical problems, the patient is likely to mention the key people and places that provide a context for illness, as well as his or her personal reaction to events. You then have a fine opportunity to explore important aspects of the social history and to demonstrate your interest in the patient's social setting and feelings. The interviewer simply needs to encourage elaboration at the appropriate time:

> So you live in East Boston. Did you grow up there? Where does the rest of your family live?
>
> You're pretty fed up with your work. What other kind of work have you done? How did you like it?
>
> So this is your first child. How has being a parent affected you? Your wife?
>
> This has been a long, taxing illness. How have you managed? What has been most difficult for you? For your family?
>
> How has it affected your relationships to the people closest to you? Your work? Financially?

Likewise, the patient's reporting of psychosocial topics brings out further biomedical data that deserve elaboration:

> So your mother has been sick with complications of diabetes . . . Does anyone else in the family have diabetes? Are there other illnesses that run in your family?
>
> That sounds like pretty strenuous work. How has this problem with leg cramps been during the day when you are working?
>
> So you have had two kids . . . Are you interested in having more children? Do you and your wife do anything for birth control?
>
> We've been talking about your difficulty in getting by with your family on welfare. I'm wondering how you have managed to follow the cholesterol-lowering diet when you are having trouble making ends meet.

For experienced clinicians, the interview may weave back and forth between biomedical history and psychosocial topics, one subject flowing naturally into the next. Eventually, all areas of the history are covered, but not in any strict order. Beginning clinicians, however, generally need to proceed through the bulk of the interview in the standard order in which it later will be recorded, thus assuring themselves that all important topics are covered. Beware, however, of passing over significant social problems that patients bring up, lest you appear to be uninterested or unconcerned. Try to follow the patient's lead, putting aside your agenda. At a minimum, acknowledge important matters and indicate that you want to hear more about them later:

> This divorce sounds like quite a lot of stress for you. Let's try to finish up talking about your breathing problem, but then I would like to hear a lot more about what's been happening with your ex-husband.

Family History

The family history is a record of the major medical conditions of the patient's close relatives, focusing primarily on genetically transmitted disease. In obtaining this portion of the standard data base, you should inquire about the health of parents, siblings, and children. You will generally also ask about grandparents, except when your patient is elderly. Pay particular attention to treatable or preventable illnesses with a known inheritable component, to early deaths, and to clusters of diseases. Occasionally, you will want to sketch out a family tree of all known relatives (e.g., when a genetically determined pattern of illness is suspected).

The family history may be valuable in suggesting or supporting a new diagnosis (e.g., when a patient's condition is similar or related to that of a parent). Information about disease in the family might also lead you to screen the patient and relatives for inheritable disorders and to treat the patient as "high risk" for familial problems (e.g., breast cancer). You may suggest prenatal screening of a fetus.

The family history also provides a critical piece of social and psychological information. The illnesses of one's family are of foremost concern to most people as they think about their own health. Patients are likely to fear that they will develop the very disorders that their parents, grandparents, and siblings have experienced. New physical symptoms are commonly attributed to familial diseases, and patients will often harbor concerns about the prevention or early detection of such conditions (e.g., "I want to be checked for diabetes. My aunt has it" or "I wonder if this depression is going to be like my mother's."). A patient may tolerate a serious condition because of the family history ("I'm a nervous girl—it runs on my mother's side of the family" or "We've all gotten arthritis when we got old"). Conversely, patients with a family history of one ailment (e.g., heart disease) may somewhat unrealistically conclude that they do not have to worry about other common ailments (e.g., cancer).

Finally, the health history of family members (or of other persons who live or work with the patient) may be helpful in diagnosing contagious illnesses or conditions caused by hazardous exposures.

While eliciting the family history, the interviewer often finds excellent opportunities to explore relationships within the family or to investigate other aspects of the social history. Listen, for instance, to the emotional tone when your patient reports a death. Please note, however, that the family history section in the medical record is only intended to describe longevity and disorders among persons who are genetically related to the patient. While some physicians use this section to record psychosocial background about the family and the medical condition of the spouse, the convention in this text is to include such data in the social history.

Questions for Obtaining a Detailed Family History

Are your parents living?
  How is their health?
    Any problems?
    How is it being treated?
  How old were they when they died?
    What was their illness like?
  What other kinds of health problems did they have?
Do you have brothers or sisters?
  How old are they?
  How is their health?
Your children?
  How old are they?
  How is their health?
Are there any health problems that run in your family?
Has anyone in your family had:
  A problem like you have?
  Anemia or bleeding problems? [In African-Americans, inquire about sickle cell anemia]
  Heart troubles, angina, or heart attacks?
  High blood pressure?
  Tuberculosis, asthma, or emphysema?
  Kidney troubles or kidney stones?
  Arthritis or rheumatism?
  Thyroid problems or diabetes?
  Cancer?
  A drinking problem?
  Nervousness or emotional problems?
  Weight problems?
    How old were they when the problem developed?
Do you have any other concerns relating to your family's health?

Review of Systems

In this portion of the standard data base, you inquire about common symptoms referable to each organ system. The purpose of this inventory is to screen for disease processes that have not as yet been discovered in the history. A systematic and thorough review, organized to scan for common complaints referable to each system of the body, will jog the patient's memory about symptoms and diseases that have not already been mentioned and will remind the interviewer about topics that may have been overlooked. Inquire in detail particularly about areas relevant to the patient's main health problems.

The review of systems is traditionally conceived of as a series of highly directive interrogations. Initially, you should learn to perform a terse, rapid, yet rather complete and methodical inventory. We encourage you to learn to use a standard list of specific questions. Until you have memorized these questions, you may want to come to the interview with a checklist that can later be entered in the patient's record. In the early stage of your clinical training, you will need such a detailed screening tool to assure that you have inquired about key topics. Also, your familiarity with a comprehensive review of systems helps you appreciate the ways in which various disease processes present—as symptoms and clusters of symptoms.

As you become more familiar with patient assessment, you will learn to gauge your questioning to the patient and the clinical setting, including your time constraints. For instance, only a brief cardiopulmonary symptom review would seem appropriate for an athletic young woman who needs a checkup for entering graduate school. You might inquire about symptoms of parasitism if she had just returned from a year in South America. On the other hand, an exhaustive symptom check might be appropriate for a cancer patient or an elderly diabetic. Similarly, the language of these questions needs to be adapted to the individual patient.

Questioning proceeds from the general to the specific:

How are your eyes?

Any trouble with your vision? With pain or discomfort around your eyes?

Do you ever see double?

You pursue the more specific concerns whenever the patient gives a "positive" response to a general question or when the clinical setting demands a detailed search for symptoms.

Table 4-1 gives a list of questions you can use in your review of systems. First, the more general and routine screening questions are noted, under which are indented more specific inquiries. Even more specialized questions need to be learned for certain circumstances.

Text continued on p. 62

Table 4-1	Questions for Obtaining a Detailed Review of Symptoms

Symptom	Questions
Constitutional	
General health	How is your general health?
Energy	Do you seem to have enough energy?
Sleep	Difficulty sleeping?
	Trouble falling asleep?
	Trouble staying asleep?
	Feeling tired when you get up in the morning?
Appetite	How is your appetite?
Weight	How is your weight?
	What would you like it to be?
	Is it changing?
	How much? Since when?
	What is the most you have weighed?
	Least?
	Have you followed any diet?
Fevers, chills, sweats	Have you had fevers or chills?
	Shaking chills?
	Does your whole body tremble and your teeth rattle?
	Sweats?
Skin	Any problems with your skin?
Pruritus	Itching?
Sores	Ulcers or sores that don't heal?
Pigmentary changes	Moles that have changed shape or color?
Bruising	Easy bruising or bleeding?
Hair, nails	Problems with your hair or nails? Change in your body hair?
Head	
Trauma	Have you injured your head?
	Been knocked unconscious?
Headaches	Any problem with headaches?
Dizziness	Dizziness?
	Do you feel faint or lightheaded?
	Does the room seem to spin or do you feel like your head is spinning?
Syncope	Do you ever pass out or feel like you are about to pass out?
	Do you actually lose consciousness?
	For how long?
	Do you fall? Hurt yourself?
Eyes	How are your eyes?
Visual problems	Are you satisfied with your vision?
	Do you wear glasses? Did you ever?
	Why?
	How do you use your glasses?
	When were they last checked?
	Do you have any problems such as:

Table 4-1—cont'd

Eyes—cont'd	
Blindness	Loss of vision?
Blurring	Blurring or double vision?
Inflammation	Redness or irritation?
	Discharge? Excess tearing?
Spots, flashes	Spots or flashes?
	Halos around lights?
Ears	How are your ears?
Deafness	Are you satisfied with your hearing?
	Can you hear well?
Otalgia	Do you have pain in your ears?
	Discharge? Itching?
Tinnitus	Do you have any buzzing or ringing in your ears?
Nose	Have you had any troubles with your nose?
Rhinitis	Runny nose?
	Do you have hay fever?
Epistaxis	Nosebleeds?
Sinusitis	Sinus problems?
Mouth and throat	How about your mouth or throat?
Dental problems	Any problems with your teeth?
	Toothaches, cavities?
	Trouble chewing food?
Dentures	Are you satisfied with your dentures?
Sores	Any problems with sores in your mouth?
	Sore tongue?
Hoarseness	Hoarseness or changes in your voice?
Dysphagia	Difficulty swallowing?
Neck	Any problems with your neck?
Pain	Stiff neck or pain in the neck?
Lymph nodes	
Swelling	Any problems with enlarged glands or nodules?
Breasts	Any problems with your breasts?
Mass	Do you check your breasts for lumps?
	How often? Did you notice anything?
	Would you like to learn to check yourself?
Tenderness	Have you noticed any tenderness in your breasts?
Discharge	Any discharge?
Respiratory	Any chest problems?
	How is your breathing?
Exercise tolerance	How far can you walk on level ground without stopping?
	Do you have to stop to rest and catch your breath?
	Walking on level ground?
	Climbing a flight of stairs?
	Can you climb two flights of stairs quickly?

Continued

Table 4-1—cont'd

Respiratory—cont'd

Orthopnea	Do you have trouble lying flat in bed? What happens? How many pillows do you sleep with under your head?
Paroxysmal nocturnal dyspnea (PND)	Do you ever get short of breath when you are lying in bed at night? What do you do when you wake up with breathlessness?
Wheezing	Do you ever wheeze?
Cough	Do you have a cough?
Sputum	Do you bring up sputum? How much? What color? When? How often? For how long?
Hemoptysis	Do you ever cough up blood?
Pleurisy	Does it ever hurt to breathe?

Cardiovascular

	Have you had any heart problems?
Palpitations	Do you feel your heart beating fast or irregularly?
Pain	Do you get pain or pressure over your chest? Tightness?
Dyspnea, orthopnea, PND	[See Respiratory]

Gastrointestinal tract

	How about your stomach and bowels?
Pain	Stomach pains or cramps? Bloating?
Indigestion	Upset stomach, indigestion? Belching? Food intolerance?
Heartburn	Heartburn? Regurgitation of acid into your throat?
Nausea, vomiting	Nausea or vomiting? What does the vomitus look like? Coffee grounds? Blood?
Diarrhea, constipation, change in bowels	Diarrhea or constipation? How often do you move your bowels? Are they hard or soft? What consistency? What color? Have your bowel movements changed?
Melena	Black or tarry bowel movement?
Rectal problems or bleeding	Hemorrhoids or rectal problems? Itching? Pain? Gas? Bleeding?
Jaundice	Ever had jaundice or turned yellow?

Urinary tract

	Any trouble with your urine?
Dysuria	Pain or burning when you urinate?
Polyuria, nocturia	Are you urinating more than usual? Do you have to get up at night to urinate? How often?
Pyuria, hematuria	Blood or pus in your urine? Gravel?

Table 4-1—cont'd

Urinary tract—cont'd

Urgency, Incontinence	Trouble starting or stopping urination?
	Losing your urine?
	When you cough or sneeze?
	Feeling you have to go in a hurry?
	Change in the size or force of the stream?
	Dribbling or difficulty emptying your bladder?

Female genitalia

	Problems with your vagina or uterus?
Vaginitis, sores	Have you had any vaginal discharge or itching?
Venereal disease	Have you had any sores or infections around your vagina?
Menarche	How old were you when your periods began?
Menses	Are your periods regular?
	How long between periods?
	How long do the periods last?
	How many pads or tampons do you use?
Dysmenorrhea	Do you get cramps or bloating with your periods?
Metrorrhagia	Do you ever bleed between periods?
Premenstrual	Do you regularly get any troubling physical or emotional
syndrome	symptoms in the week or so before your period begins?
Menopause, hot	When did you stop having periods?
flashes	Have you had hot flashes?
Sexual dysfunction	Are you having sexual relations?
	Do you relate sexually to men, women, or both?
	Are you satisfied with your sexual life?
	Any loss of interest in sex?
	Are you able to reach a climax or orgasm?
	Have you had pain on sexual relations?
	Do you have any questions or concerns related to sex that
	you would like to discuss today?

Male genitalia

	Any problems with your penis?
Sores, discharge,	Have you had any sores on your penis?
	Discharge or drip?
Scrotal pain	Pain or swelling in your testes?
Hernia	Hernia?
Sexual dysfunction	Are you having sexual relations?
	Do you relate sexually to men, women, or both?
	Are you satisfied with your sexual life?
	Any loss of interest in sex?
	Difficulty getting or maintaining a good erection?
	Difficulty controlling ejaculation?
	Do you have any questions or concerns related to sex that
	you would like to discuss today?

Continued

Table 4-1—cont'd	
Joints and extremities	How are your joints? Your legs?
Cramps	Have you had cramps or pains in your legs?
	When you walk?
	At rest?
Varicosities, phlebitis	Have you had problems with the veins in your legs?
	Tender or swollen?
Edema	Do your ankles swell?
Arthralgias, arthritis	Do your joints ache?
	Do they get red or tender?
	Do they swell or get stiff?
Low back pain	Low back pain?
Endocrine	
Heat or cold	Do you find that you prefer room temperatures cooler or
intolerance	hotter than others?
Polydipsia	Have you had excess thirst?
Central nervous system	
Cranial nerves	Any trouble with your sense of smell or taste?
	[See Head, Eyes, Ears, Nose, Throat, reported earlier.]
Paralysis	Weakness or paralysis?
	Trouble moving your arms or legs?
	Twisting or pulling of your face?
	Trouble getting in or out of a chair or bed?

Interviewing Technique in the Review of Systems

The bulk of the review of systems is conducted as a brisk interrogation in which the patient is asked simply to answer "Yes" or "No" about having experienced specific difficulties or symptoms: "Have you ever had. . . ?" or "Are you having any trouble with. . . ?" Most of the answers should be "No"; you inquire further about each "Yes." Try to avoid repeating questions that have been asked previously.

Your questioning technique allows you some control over the amount of detail provided by patients and over the quality of the doctor-patient relationship in this portion of the interview. If you quickly follow each patient response with another question or a comment, such as "O.K.," you discourage elaboration and maintain a dominant role. If you pause and listen after the patient replies, you foster clarification and amplification, as well as a collaborative relationship.

When you begin learning to take this part of the history, you will probably want to obtain the review of systems after the family history, just before beginning the physical examination. You can introduce this section of the interview by saying:

Table 4-1—cont'd

Central nervous system—cont'd

Paresthesia	Numbness or areas with unusual sensations?
	"Pins and needles" sensation?
	Burning in your feet?
	Altered sense of hot or cold?
Clumsiness	Clumsiness or dropping things?
	Bumping into things?
Balance	Loss of balance?
Gait	Trouble walking?
Involuntary	Shaking or trembling?
movements	Twitching or jerking?
Seizures	Fits or seizures?
Attention, memory	Loss of memory or periods of confusion?
	Trouble concentrating?
	Getting lost?
Language, speech	Slurred speech or trouble talking?
	Trouble reading?
Thought disorder	Upsetting or unusual thoughts going on in your mind?
Nervousness	Nervousness or trouble relaxing?
Depression	Crying or sadness?
	Depression?
	Thoughts about suicide?
Boredom	Bored or losing interest in life?

Finally, you might ask:
Do you have any other concerns about your body?
Did you want to mention anything else?

> Now I'm going to ask you a series of routine questions about your body.

As you become more proficient in your clinical skills and have memorized the review of systems, you may want to integrate most of this section of the history with your physical examination. Inquire about common symptoms referable to a system around the same time as you are examining that body part. However, make clear to the patient that you regularly ask such questions during the physical examination. By posing your questions before examining the relevant body part, you avoid giving the impression that your inquiry is a response to abnormalities that have just been discovered, thus sparing your patient unnecessary worry.

Today's review of systems, especially for uncomplicated outpatients, can be administered largely with relatively open-ended prompts (e.g., "How are your eyes?"). The patient is first advised that he or she will be given a "body quiz," and then is asked to respond if he or she has any symptoms related to the part of the body that is mentioned:

Tell me about your eyes. How about your ears? Stomach? Bowels?

Among sophisticated and unsophisticated patients alike, familiarity with the body is common, so your reference to a body part will stimulate the patient's associations about most impairments and previous diseases. Clinical experience helps you decide when to engage in more specific inquiry.

Ideally, the patient will give a quick negative answer to the majority of your questions, while a few portions of your inventory will reveal important new medical facts. Not infrequently, however, a patient will give positive responses that have an uncertain significance: a mild discomfort on urination that has occurred four times over 2 years; a troublesome itch that lasted for 5 days about a month ago, but now has resolved; two nosebleeds in the past few months. Asking about duration and severity may help you label some symptoms as trivial or significant, but only clinical training and experience will tell you which complaints to take seriously. However, if you believe you are gathering too many minor complaints, consider only asking more general questions (e.g., "Any chest problems?"), while also directing the patient to report only on recent or current problems (e.g., "Have you had any *recent* difficulties?" or "Are you having trouble now with. . . ?") or on those causing significant disability ("Have you had *serious* problems with. . . ?").

Occasional patients will respond affirmatively to many of the symptoms you mention or will be reminded of a variety of related concerns, causing this section of the history to drag on and on, bewildering the interviewer with details. Such a phenomenon is called a "positive review of systems" and may be suggestive of the phenomenon of somatization (see the later section, The Doctor and the Somatizing Patient in Chapter 13). For such patients, the review of systems may best be conducted by avoiding leading questions and by using only very general screening questions about immediate concerns:

What other problems are particularly troubling you now?

What is bothering you the most these days?

In today's busy clinical practice, however, a detailed review of systems is sometimes obtained through a written patient questionnaire. Patients are asked to complete it before the clinical encounter. Then, the doctor reviews it with the patient.

CHAPTER 5

MORE INTERVIEWING TECHNIQUES

How does one become a good doctor? As I understand it a good doctor is one who is shrewd in diagnosis and wise in treatment; but, more than that, he is a person who never spares himself in the interest of his patients; and in addition he is a man who studies the patient not only as a case but also as an individual....The good doctor, whether general practitioner or specialist, is also a man who studies the patient's personality as well as his disease.

HUGH CAIRNS

TRANSITIONS

Guide your patient through the interview process. If a man comes in with a backache and you begin asking about hypertension, diabetes, and cancer (as part of acquiring the standard data base), he may be confused and worried. Explain the transitions between sections of the interview.

Now, let's go on to some routine questions about your general health.

Similarly, when you choose to organize the flow of the interview, help the patient understand what you are doing:

You have told me some about your headaches and stomach pains, and also said that you are having lots of troubles with your parents. Let's now talk some more about what is going on with you and your parents, and then later we can come back to the other problems.

At the end of the history or physical examination, make a smooth ending, explaining what will happen next:

Good. Now I think I have the information that I need before giving you your physical exam. Is there anything else you would like to tell me before we begin the next step?

Those are all my questions for now. Let's go on to the physical examination. I would like you to get completely undressed now, including your shoes, socks, and underwear, and to put on this gown. I'll step out and then come back in a few minutes to examine you.

PATIENT EDUCATION

Educate your patients. The word, "doctor," originally meant "teacher." The entire interview is an opportunity to inform your patient about the diagnosis, treatment, and prognosis—to provide "patient education." For example, when a patient has rheumatic complaints, you might say:

I'm going to be asking you some questions about your general health because many common diseases may significantly affect your joints and muscles.

65

Do you know what we mean by arthritis?

Some medications can affect your joints, so it's important for me to know if you're currently taking any.

Listen for topics about which the patient has uncertainties and concerns or would otherwise benefit from further knowledge. Find out what the patient understands:

What do you know about bursitis?

WHEN PATIENTS QUESTION DOCTORS

So much instruction about the interview has to do with questioning and listening to patients. Often forgotten is how the dialogue has to do with explaining. Explanations not only address the topics on the doctor's agenda, such as medical advice, but also answer the stated and unstated questions that patients bring. The most familiar questions asked by patients are about illness. Most patients ask their doctors questions to clarify their diagnosis, treatment options, and preventive measures (see Quick Tips: Common Questions Patients Ask Doctors). Encourage patient assertiveness by inviting such questions:

Do you have any questions you would like to ask me about your diagnosis and treatment?

Are there other questions you think I should have asked you?

Many questions express requests:

Don't you think I need an antibiotic?

What about an x-ray?

Would you fill out this Medicaid form?

Patients (or families) may also have questions that embody complaints about their care or concerns about possible mistakes in their treatment:

Why wasn't the cancer found sooner?

Why didn't you call back?

They may state their distress bluntly:

You killed him! He wanted to come in but you said to wait.

The test stopped my heart. The doctor didn't even apologize!

When patients are aggrieved—feeling victimized by medical actions or inactions—they often only want the doctor to apologize, explain carefully what happened and, if appropriate, admit error. Such conversations are difficult for the clinician when the patient or family is hostile. The presence of a third party, such as another colleague, may help with particularly sensitive discussions. Regardless, the events of care and treatment should be carefully

---

QUICK TIPS

Common Questions Patients Ask Doctors

- What do I have, doc?
- What shall I take?
- What's to stop this from happening again?
- Will it continue?
- Why did this happen to me?

---

reconstructed, the understanding and concerns of the patient and family reviewed, their feelings or complaints acknowledged, and regret expressed. Apology can help to reestablish a good relationship.

ENCOURAGEMENT AND SUPPORT

An impartial attitude—an ability to suspend judgment about people—will allow you to develop a therapeutic alliance and to respond to the needs of patients with many different backgrounds, values, beliefs, and behaviors, some of which you may not approve or like. A neutral stance in your relationship with patients may also help you avoid such pitfalls as providing premature advice and reassurance, making social judgments, or inaccurately ascribing knowledge, behaviors, or feelings. However, you should also find opportunities to demonstrate your interest and regard and to provide encouragement and support. For instance, when a patient shares news that is unambiguously pleasing, offer a positive response:

> Patient: And I'm looking forward to my first grandchild in June.
> Interviewer: Isn't that nice.

> Patient: I've finally lost the 10 pounds I've been trying to get off.
> Interviewer: That's great! What's your secret?

Strengthen your rapport, when possible, by praising the patient:

> It was a good idea to come in today.

> That's great. You've really given me a clear picture of the problem.

> You've put a tremendous effort into helping your sick mother, and she's really lucky to have you.

You can be supportive about how patients are coping with difficulties without necessarily validating their assessment or approach:

> I can see that you are working hard on this problem and doing your best to help your children.

> You've been struggling under terrible circumstances. You've tried everything you can think of.

At times, you may want to directly state your desire to be supportive:

> I see what a tough time you're having, and I want to help you with these problems.

SUMMARIZING

Having completed the initial history, there is always the likelihood that some of the patient's major concerns have not been touched upon or that you have not correctly understood some of the patient's story. A brief summary is useful at the end of the interview to "reopen the door." Give the patient the opportunity to modify your summary.

> Okay, to summarize, it seems you have been in good health but have been bothered recently by leg cramps when you walk long distances. You have some close relatives with poor circulation, so I will be certain to check you for any sign of that problem. Is there anything you feel I may have missed? No? Then let's begin the physical exam.

SETTING PRIORITIES

A thorough clinical evaluation touches on a great many subjects. You may be wondering how such a lengthy list of topics and themes can be accommodated in a reasonable amount of time.

The answer is, in part, that experienced clinicians can manage multiple tasks quickly, efficiently, and even concurrently, while students need more time. Learners should also remember, however, that all the suggested information need not be collected in one visit. Particularly in ambulatory care, the scope of topics is wide and the mandate is comprehensive, but many items can be covered at different times as the patient returns for additional visits. The diagnostic and treatment plan can include not only tests or medications, but also further information-gathering and communication. Typically, a clinician will make sure that urgent matters, as defined by the doctor and the patient (e.g., acute pain and other new, severe, or worrisome symptoms), are cared for immediately, and then focus on less pressing matters (e.g., management of subacute and chronic problems), if feasible. Time might be set aside in the future to complete these tasks, to carry out additional tasks related to chronic care (e.g., monitoring compliance, reviewing patient education about self-care), or to address long-term issues of health maintenance and disease prevention (e.g., doing the routine Papanicolaou smear and rectal examination or encouraging smoking cessation). Similar priorities are set for hospitalized patients, for whom clinicians usually focus almost entirely on more immediate concerns.

THE FIRST FEW MINUTES—A RECAPITULATION

The first few minutes of the interview set the stage for successfully taking a good history. Reviewing videotapes of interviews conducted by medical students and house officers, we find that major deficiencies and inefficiencies in the conduct and outcome of patient encounters can often be traced to this initial period.

For most encounters, the first few minutes of the interview should allow patients to describe the broad outlines of why they came and what they hope to accomplish. Patients often describe their attributions with slight or no prompting. With a little encouragement, they reveal triggers and requests. The role of the interviewer is to facilitate the patient's presentation, usually by asking a few open-ended questions and providing encouragement, and to listen carefully. Beware of starting your interview with close-ended questions or by otherwise focusing the patient's story on specific symptoms or other aspects of the history. A major temptation for beginning interviewers (and a normal consequence of being anxious) is to rapidly identify a chief complaint and to direct attention to a quickly formulated diagnostic hypothesis or to a familiar line of questioning. The patient's attempt to convey his or her version of the full history is interrupted or diverted. As a consequence of such premature focusing, the patient is discouraged from elaborating on his or her own perspective about the problem, and the interviewer tends to overlook or not be given statements or clues about additional problems, major psychosocial factors related to the presenting complaint, and the patient's view of the illness. Therefore, early in the interview, avoid the temptation to close in on what you perceive as the patient's major problem. Keep your mind open for other hypotheses. Listen attentively for a broad picture of the patient's condition: use the initial moments as a time for surveying and then for planning how to explore this broad picture.

CHARACTERIZING THE SYMPTOM—A RECAPITULATION FOCUSING ON PAIN

As a reminder of the process of characterizing a symptom and a basic primer on pain assessment (a neglected topic in clinical training) we offer the following review of how to investigate a complaint of pain. For each pain (remember that patients may have more than one pain), include the following:

Pain Assessment

Location (well localized or diffuse) and **radiation** (dermatomal or peripheral nerve root distribution)

Quality (e.g., aching, burning, shooting, colicky, crampy)

Chronology

  Time of onset

  Temporal pattern—especially intermittent versus continuous; frequency and duration of intermittent pain; and course

Intensity—can be quantified by patients using a numerical scale of 1 to 10 (where 1 = barely noticeable and 10 = worst imagineable or worst experienced); consider also using a visual analog scale. Note how the pain changes over time.

Aggravating and alleviating factors, including relationship to position, motion, local pressure, activity, eating, anxiety, and so forth. Pain that is related to movement or pressure is called "incident pain." Include responses to all treatments (and alternative therapies), both previous and current.

Associated symptoms, particularly paresthesias (e.g., numbness, tingling, hyperesthesia, allodynia [pain from light touch], and weakness or muscle wasting). For chest pain, ask about cardiopulmonary symptoms. For abdominal pain, ask about gastrointestinal and genitorurinary symptoms.

Disability and adaptation—describe functional impairment, especially the effect of pain on sleep, mobility, and other aspects of daily life. Describe the effect of the pain on mood and enjoyment and other aspects of psychological function.

Patient and family perspective—attributions (patient and family's understanding of the pain, its meaning, cause, appropriate diagnostic and therapeutic management, prognosis); requests (what the patient and family want done, particularly distinguishing between requests for relief versus those for a clear diagnosis); views of the illness and its management; personal and cultural attitudes about pain and its treatment, including, if relevant, attitudes about opioid tolerance and dependence, concerns about drug diversion, and consideration of the cost of treatment.

THE PATIENT'S PERSPECTIVE

A final reminder about the importance of the patient's perspective: students often forget to ask about requests and attributions. In outpatient medicine, you regularly need this information to place the present illness in proper context and to make an assessment and negotiate a plan. By the end of your interview, make sure you understand the patient's reasons for coming now, what he or she is thinking about the diagnosis and course of the illness, and what he or she expects and desires of you. If your patients bring up important problems as you are ushering them out the door—"Oh, by the way. . . ." or "There's just one more thing I meant to tell you"—look back at how you conducted the interview and why the patient's concerns were not expressed earlier.

COMMUNICATION OF INFORMATION BEFORE, DURING, AND AFTER THE PHYSICAL EXAMINATION

> *In the last analysis, we see only what we are ready to see, what we have been taught to see. We eliminate and ignore everything that is not a part of our prejudices.*
>
> *Jean Martin Charcot*

Before examining a patient or performing any procedure, explain your intentions and ensure the patient's acceptance. Beware that your notion of an appropriate examination may be different from the patient's. Some patients do not expect to undress, let alone undergo rectal or pelvic examinations. Others expect measurement of their weight and blood pressure on every visit or may feel that you have neglected to check them properly if you do not listen to the heart and lungs and palpate the abdomen, even though you believe that the visit requires only talking or attention to a limited portion of the physical examination.

Give the patient clear directions about undressing:

Please take off everything but your stockings and underpants. You'll need to remove your overclothes and bra.

Would you take off all your clothes above your waist?

Please strip to your shorts only.

Respect privacy. In general, cover at all times those parts of the patient's body that are not normally exposed, unless you are examining that part. In the hospital, curtains around a patient's bed should be arranged with attention to privacy. For an office visit, a gowned or partially undressed patient should not be visible to other persons. Doors to an examining area should not be opened casually. Before entering the examination room, knock on the door and wait until the patient acknowledges that it is permissible to enter the room. Similarly, if a patient is undressing behind a curtain in your office, ask if he or she is ready before you pull back the partition.

During the physical examination, especially when you linger over any of the diagnostic maneuvers, the patient may become particularly worried about what you have found. Don't conduct the examination in silence. Make a habit of offering brief explanations of what you are doing while you do it. You will be reducing mystification, enhancing the patient's medical knowledge, and communicating respect by involving the patient in the care process. When the examination is normal, let the patient know. Everyone appreciates this good news, both during the examination and at the end of the consultation.

Now I'm going to look back into your eyes to check the blood vessels . . . Everything looks fine.

I'm going to listen carefully to your heart now . . . Fine. I can hear some parts better if you now lie on your left side . . . Sounds perfect.

Potentially embarrassing or painful portions of the examination (e.g., the rectal and pelvic) can be made much more comfortable if you maintain a calm, respectful manner and explain as you go along. Your tone and choice of words help shape the patient's experience:

Now I'm going to touch you around the outside of your vagina . . . That looks normal . . . You may get a twinge when I press firmly here . . . That ovary is fine . . . Now, I'm going to check you around your rectum, and you may feel like you want to move your bowels for a moment . . . This may feel a little strange . . . you may feel some pressure here. . . .

Finish the examination with a transition statement that explains what is going to happen next. Excuse yourself in order to discuss the patient with your preceptor.

O.K., we are all done with the physical exam now. I'm going to step out for about 15 minutes to talk with Dr. Goodson. We'll be back to talk to you some more, and he'll want to listen to your heart. Why don't you make yourself comfortable in this chair. Do you need anything before I go? A magazine? The bathroom is across the ball.

A NOTE ON CHAPERONS

A chaperon will be required for all pelvic examinations performed while you are in training. The chaperon will preferably (but not necessarily) be a woman, especially when the examiner is a man.

Chaperons are needed for three reasons. First, students need technical assistance, especially while learning the examination. A physician or nurse-practitioner should be present for supervision during this difficult portion of the physical examination. Second, many women find that having another person in the room makes them feel less vulnerable and reduces possible sexual overtones. (However, it should also be noted that some women find the presence of this additional person intrusive.) Third, should patients view the examiner as acting inappropriately during the procedure, a chaperon provides some medicolegal protection. Women practitioners generally do not use chaperons for the pelvic examination (though, technically, both male and female examiners could be accused of assault or improper behavior).

Similar issues pertain to the examination of the male genitalia, particularly for minors and for some adults with emotional or intellectual difficulties, but physicians, including female physicians, generally do not use chaperons for this portion of the physical examination.

CHAPTER 6

CONSULTING WITH YOUR PRECEPTOR

You and your instructor will now identify the patient's major problems and make an assessment and tentative plan for each of them. This process is further described in Chapter 8, Recording.

The format of your consultation with the preceptor should be clarified before you see the patient. When and where will you meet? If questions arise earlier in the examination, where can the preceptor be found? Will the instructor review the history? Where? Should the patient remain in an examining gown so that the instructor can readily check on the physical examination?

INTRODUCTION TO ORAL CASE PRESENTATION

Your consultation with your preceptor generally begins with your oral presentation of the patient's history and physical examination. Your goal is to provide a terse, lucid account of the essential features of the case, organized and delivered in such a way as to be readily followed in a single hearing by the listener.

Before you begin your presentation, take a few minutes to organize your thoughts and identify salient features of your clinical encounter. Consider the following six guidelines for your presentation:

1. Follow a familiar format, such as the expanded form used in written case presentations:
    a. Patient profile and reason for visit. In one or two sentences, you describe the patient and why he or she sought help. The patient profile generally includes the patient's age and sex, and, if relevant, marital status, race, occupation, and any major medical issues, particularly those that are important to understanding the presenting problem. Your opening statement serves as a headline, identifying the central topic or topics of the presentation. It generally should indicate the duration of the problem.

This 58-year-old married, unemployed waiter with a history of hypertension presents with a 6-week history of urinary frequency and urgency.

This 79-year-old retired postal worker and widower with diabetes, peripheral vascular disease, and peripheral neuropathy presents with a fever and a draining wound on the sole of his right foot for 2 days.

b. Present illness. This section of the history is the major focus of an oral presentation. Include the essential information for diagnosing and managing the patient's medical and psychosocial problems. If more than one major problem is evident, begin with the most important one and later describe less pressing concerns.

In describing a problem, you generally should include all the standard data base that is immediately relevant. For instance, in describing a patient who you believe has just had a heart attack, you would include under the present illness the following: previous hospitalizations or surgery for cardiac problems; history of hypertension, congestive heart failure, angina, or other heart conditions; risk factors, such as smoking, sedentary life-style, or hypercholesterolemia; family history of coronary artery disease; and any symptoms (e.g., nausea, vomiting, diaphoresis, palpitations, and lightheadedness) whose presence or absence is helpful in establishing this diagnosis.

c. Standard data base (past medical history, social history, family history, and review of systems). Except for the relevant portions of the standard data base that are included in the description of the present illness, this section of the history is generally presented in a few sentences:

The remainder of the history is unremarkable except for a significant occupational exposure to asbestos and the recent discovery of a lung cancer in his older brother.

d. Physical examination. Again, you should follow a familiar format, beginning with general appearance and vital signs, then proceeding in an orderly fashion from head to toe, and concluding with a neurological examination. Mention only those physical findings that, by virtue of being either present or absent, help establish a diagnosis or particularly deserve the listener's attention. Otherwise, simply indicate that an organ system was normal or unremarkable. For example:

He is a well-appearing middle-aged man in no apparent distress. The vital signs were unremarkable. The head, eyes, ears, nose, throat, and nodes were normal, as were the heart and lungs. However, the abdomen revealed a 13-cm suprapubic mass that was firm, smooth, nontender, and dull to percussion. The abdomen was otherwise soft, flat, nontender, and without masses, organomegaly, or demonstrable ascites. . . .

e. Assessment *and* plan. While you may not be expected at earlier stages of training to offer a differential diagnosis or to suggest a detailed diagnostic and therapeutic plan, you should at least try to identify major problems and to make general suggestions about what further steps might be appropriate. Bring to your preceptor's attention your own concerns and identify any parts of the history and physical examination about which you are uncertain.

2. You are advised not to simply give a verbatim report from the patient or to recite the entire history and physical examination. You need to select the essential information from the interview and physical examination and organize it into a coherent story that can be quickly grasped by your preceptor. Your opening statements should give a broad picture of the patient and the illness, and you should follow with a logically organized presentation of the details required for understanding the case.

   While your presentation ideally should provide all the major relevant information required to understand and manage the patient's problems, do not feel that you have to address every question. Your preceptors can ask for elaboration on matters that interest them.

3. In organizing the presentation of the present illness, three approaches are commonly employed. All three may be used in various parts of the same presentation.

   First, in "symptom-characterization," one focuses on a key symptom and provides an orderly description of its "dimensions." For instance, in a patient with recent onset of exertional angina, careful description of the pain is the central feature of the present illness.

   Second, in a "chronological report," the events that constitute the present illness are set forth as they evolved over time. Such an approach might be used for a patient with a long history of angina who now develops a change in the pattern of chest pains.

   Third, usually in conjunction with one of the previous two methods, "hypothesis-testing" or "problem-solving" serves as the logic for presenting data. Here, one of the diagnoses under consideration becomes the focus of attention, and the presenter leads the preceptor through a consideration of various facts that are useful for confirming or disconfirming such an hypothesis. Thus, for a patient with a presumed pneumonia, the presenter would describe the symptoms of cough, sputum production, and fever, but then might turn to a consideration of the presence or absence of various risk factors for this particular diagnosis (e.g., a history of smoking, chronic lung disease [including a personal or family history of cystic fibrosis and emphysema], conditions associated with aspiration or a compromised immune system, exposure to tuberculosis or other pathogens [including travel to areas where certain infections are endemic], history of immunization for influenza or pneumococcus, and so forth). If a diagnosis other than pneumonia were being considered seriously, the presenter might next focus on the data that would tend to confirm or deny this alternative hypothesis (e.g., if pulmonary embolus is a possibility, has the patient had dyspnea, pleurisy, hemoptysis, previous pulmonary emboli or blood clots, symptoms or signs of thrombophlebitis, or such risk factors as prolonged immobility, birth control pills, or other medical conditions associated with a tendency to form clots?).

Hypothesis-testing or problem-solving is a fundamental consideration whenever clinical data are presented, and the inclusion of any data in an oral presentation should be justifiable in terms of its usefulness in determining the patient's problems. Problem-solving logic is also used to decide which details to describe in the physical examination. Thus, in presenting a patient who you feel might have had a pulmonary embolus, you would take care to note the presence or absence of any features of the physical examination that are typically associated with that diagnosis or that would tend to suggest a competing hypothesis.

While the use of symptom-characterization or a chronological report for organizing a presentation is easily grasped by students, the problem-solving approach is much more difficult to understand and apply. The choice of an appropriate hypothesis may require considerable clinical background. Similarly, the presenter needs a substantial familiarity with medicine to know which information is relevant to evaluating an hypothesis, namely what data will help confirm or disconfirm a tentative diagnosis. Therefore, until you develop greater clinical expertise or have the opportunity to read in some detail about a particular case, your oral presentations are likely to omit key data or to include information that is not very useful for problem-solving. Consequently, your preceptor may ask you questions that either seem irrelevant (because you do not understand their role in figuring out the case) or that you wish you had included (now that you realize their importance), while perhaps finding little interest in portions of your presentation (that are not germane to the major diagnostic issues).

4. Speak crisply and clearly. Try to engage your audience.

5. Practice and review your presentations. Seek feedback.

6. Except for the most complex cases, you should be able to give an oral presentation in 5 minutes or less.

See Chapter 18, Oral Case Presentation, for further guidelines and recapitulation of basic material presented here.

GETTING GOOD SUPERVISION

You will learn more if you take an active role in determining what kind of supervision you get.

For all your clinical work, let your preceptors know that you are eager for feedback. While your oral and written presentations will be the basis for much supervision, your interviewing and physical diagnostic skills should also be observed directly. Ask your preceptors to view your interviews and physical examinations, and get help especially with those skills about which you are uncertain. The preceptor might sit in on your patient encounter, review videotapes, or have you demonstrate portions of the history and physical examination on a patient or volunteer. (The preceptor should also occasionally demonstrate his or her skills by interviewing and examining the patient with you.)

Ask the preceptor to clarify expectations about your performance. For instance, what should your oral and written presentations be like? How long? What format? What kind of reading should you do, and how should it be reflected in your written case presentations? Seek prompt feedback and ask to redo problematic presentations.

Until you know more about clinical medicine, you will have difficulty deciding what information is relevant to understanding the present illness as well as how to formulate an assessment and plan. You will need guidance from your preceptor. Before preparing your write-up, make sure your preceptor helps you identify the patient's major problems and the foremost considerations in the differential diagnosis. Ask about how to organize your write-up. For patients who have a number of problems, ask the preceptor which issues you should focus upon in your reading. Seek suggestions for your further study, such as appropriate textbooks or journal articles. Seek out references on "evidence-based medicine" that can support intelligent decision-making among the patient, instructor, and yourself.

Try to maintain an active role in your patient's care, assuming as much responsibility as your capabilities allow. Your supervisor must carefully oversee your clinical work, but you benefit from opportunities to practice new skills and to take on increasing responsibility. If you realize from your supervision that you omitted a key portion of the history or physical, ask if you can go back to complete your examination, rather than passively watching your preceptor obtain the missing data. Try to formulate your own assessment and plan, rather than having one prescribed solely by the preceptor. After you and your preceptor have agreed on a diagnosis and plan, ask to be the first to discuss them with the patient. Be the one to call or write the patient about laboratory test results. Try to arrange to see the patient on follow-up visits or to telephone later to inquire about how the patient is doing.

Learn from patients. Always read about your patient's problems. Well-chosen books and articles help you integrate your daily patient care experiences with basic and clinical science knowledge.

Finally, discuss your cases with other students and physicians. Volunteer to present cases for teaching rounds. Use every opportunity to practice your oral presentations and to learn from others.

CHAPTER 7

THE EXPOSITION PHASE: INFORMING AND COUNSELING THE PATIENT

It is our duty to remember at all times and anew that medicine is not only a science, but also the art of letting our own individuality interact with the individuality of the patient.

ALBERT SCHWEITZER

You now need to explain to the patient what you have concluded and to discuss further diagnosis and treatment.

A major task in the exposition phase is informing the patient. It is difficult to provide a good explanation—one that effectively communicates new information and addresses the patient's questions and concerns.

EDUCATIONAL STRATEGIES

Studies of patients' recall of their doctors' explanations suggest that only a very small portion of delivered information is retained. Be respectful of the potentially enormous discrepancy of medical knowledge between you and even the brightest, most well-informed patients. The explanations given to patients in a few minutes involve concepts you have learned over long periods of intensive study.

Use educational strategies to help your patients learn essential information:

Strategies To Help Your Patient Learn Essential Information

Set aside enough time. Don't put off the exposition until the last few minutes of the interview. Good explanations take time.

Keep the message simple. Physicians' explanations are often overloaded with elaborate discussions of pathophysiology, differential diagnosis, and alternative approaches to management. Such "mini-lectures" reflect major preoccupations for doctors and medical students, but may have little interest or use for most patients.

Use lay terminology. Choose language that is simple, straightforward, and concrete. If you introduce technical terms, explain their meaning. Translate complex concepts so that they are readily understood by the patient.

Focus on key points. The scope of discussion should be based on realistic expectations of what your patient can adequately comprehend, depending on his or her intellectual background, the complexity of the material, the limited time, and the common difficulty of learning new material in the somewhat anxiety-ridden setting of the physician's office. To cover a few essentials well is a reasonable and honorable goal for most interviews; use follow-up visits to share more information.

When you do present a large amount of information, lead off with key points, since your initial message is often best retained. You generally will want to begin with a simple summary of your conclusions, putting forth your main messages in a clear, brief, well-organized fashion. Later, if you introduce crucial matters, beware that they are not lost amidst the complicated dialogue; stress the importance of any matters that you particularly want the patient to remember.

Categorize information. When communicating a complex message, you can help the patient organize new knowledge and remember it by explaining what kind of information you are providing. In general, these categories are the diagnosis, diagnostic studies, treatment, and prognosis:

> I want to begin by discussing what we think is wrong and what studies you need, and then I can tell you how to take care of this problem. . . .
>
> First, I want to tell you what the main problem seems to be. . . .
>
> Now, I would like to discuss some studies that may help us figure out what is wrong. . . .
>
> Now you know what is causing the problem, so let's discuss what we can do about it. This is the treatment I propose. . . .
>
> This is what we expect will happen with the treatment. . . .
>
> Now I want to review what else you need to do to take care of this problem. . . .
>
> O.K., that's the main problem. Let's go over this other matter. . . .

Similarly, try to wrap up your discussion of one topic before going on to another, so that your patient sequentially focuses full attention on one matter at a time.

Repeat and stress key points.

Engage and motivate patients and seek feedback. The task of providing good explanations cannot be carried out well by simply deciding what patients should listen to or by guessing what they want to hear. You need your patient's help to decide what to talk about. Moreover, patients learn better and take more responsibility for their care when they are actively engaged in the process of learning about and planning for diagnosis and treatment.

In providing information, listen for patients' responses to what you say. Encourage their comments and questions. Check whether your major points are understood.

> What do you know about this illness?
>
> Now let me see if we both see things the same way. What is your understanding about the cause of this problem? Why have we decided on these studies?

Have patients describe key responsibilities and rehearse plans:

> Let's go over the plan. How are you going to monitor your blood sugar now?
>
> How are you going to take the medicine?

The patient's response will guide you to further discussion, either to clarify essential points or to expand the range of topics to be considered.

Feedback is important not only for explaining, but also for arriving at a satisfactory diagnostic and treatment plan. Try to avoid dictating plans. Make suggestions, not commands. Acknowledge the importance of the patient's participation. Support the patient's sense of responsibility and communicate your appreciation of his or her role.

> What kind of problems do you anticipate with this plan?
>
> What else do you need to know in order to manage things until our next visit?
>
> You've been doing a fabulous job in looking after your health. How can I help you now?
>
> You've got a lot to do now. I know it's not easy.

Consider having the patient propose a plan:

> How would you suggest we proceed now?
>
> How do you want to handle this?

Be encouraging. Patients learn better when they are given praise. Recognize their strengths and acknowledge their efforts. Communicate positive regard. Be enthusiastic and hopeful.

> You've got it just right. That's great!
>
> You've really mastered a tough task here.
>
> I admire you for sticking to it, and I think that's a sign that you'll really be able to take care of this problem.
>
> You're making fine progress. Congratulations!

Provide written instructions. For even the simplest regimens, written instructions will usually be valuable, both at the current visit and in future encounters. Offer pamphlets that have been developed to inform lay persons about illness and its management.

Ask your patients whether they can *read and understand these instructions.* Significant numbers of patients—roughly a quarter of the United States population—cannot read or are unable to comfortably comprehend patient education materials, even those written in relatively simple language. For those patients who are literate in other languages, written materials ideally are available for them in their native language. For many other patients who speak and understand a language but cannot read it, consider nonwritten means of communicating health-related information: previously developed or individually prepared audiovisual materials, including picture books, slide presentations, and audio or video cassettes. Knowing a patient's reading ability is important when using written materials to promote patient education and adherence, but also when using health questionnaires, consent forms, advance care directives, and insurance forms.

Make an effective conclusion. As the interview comes to an end, choose a few key points to repeat and emphasize. Repetition is a valuable educational strategy through-out the interview, but is particularly worthwhile in closing, since your parting messages are often particularly well retained by the patient. You may restate the diagnosis and reiterate your major advice.

> Your blood pressure is a bit low now. Remember to stop the pink pills, called Prinivil or Zestril. Keep taking the white ones each morning, the "water pills" called hydrochlorothiazide.

> O.K., the plan is for you to try to notice when you get these chest pains during the next 2 weeks. You'll keep this notebook about what has happened, and show it to me when you come back.

The conclusion is also a time for a brief message that motivates the patient, as described in the next section. Well-chosen words can inspire patients, helping them attend to complex regimens and suggestions for behavioral change. You also motivate the patient and reinforce your therapeutic relationship by ending with praise and encouragement.

BASIC CONSIDERATIONS IN EXPLANATIONS

Two broad questions are useful in thinking about the task of providing a good explanation and determining the scope of your discussion. First, what does the patient want to know? Ask the patient. Already, you should have noted explicit or implicit questions. Based on your knowledge of the patient, especially your elicitation of requests and attributions, what should be said? Are there discrepancies between the plan you are proposing and what the patient wanted? Remember that occasional patients want little explanation, others require a great deal.

Second, what does the patient need to know to care properly for herself or himself? The answer is often that patients need only rather brief explanations of the diagnosis, further studies, and choice of treatment, but require very clear, concrete, specific, and detailed information on how to follow a plan. For instance, you may need to provide careful instructions on how to elevate the legs, when to take a pill in relation to meals, what to do when a prescription runs out, where to get a test.

Follow-up visits and telephone calls will give you the opportunity to learn about misunderstandings. A fasting blood test is taken after the patient has had a morning cup of coffee. A patient makes a second visit to the emergency ward, not having been warned that a rash might still spread for a few days after treatment is begun. A "noncompliant" patient stops an important medication because he feels better or worse or encounters side effects. The patient who never filled your prescription for the relief of a headache later says that he "really just wanted to know if it was a brain tumor." If you do not discover such misunderstandings, you probably are not carefully monitoring outcomes.

TASKS FOR THE EXPOSITION PHASE AND CLOSING OF THE INTERVIEW

We now examine the major tasks for the final phase of the interview. Please note that the tasks overlap and do not have to be carried out in a particular order, but they are presented schematically in a sequence in which they are commonly accomplished. Also, as an introduction to the exposition phase, we present detailed suggestions and multiple examples, but do not mean to imply that all tasks should be carried out in every interview.

Explaining the Diagnosis and the Proposed Plan _____

Explain your diagnosis

The cough, temperature, and your feeling terrible are signs of what we call "bronchitis."

These headaches are caused by the medication you took for your heart condition.

On examining you, we found a heart murmur. Have you ever been told that before? Do you know what it means?

Explain the significance of the various symptoms and signs

The swelling of your legs comes from the accumulation of fluid there. This is another result of your liver problem.

We do not think your arthritis is causing this new leg pain. We think it's from a muscle strain.

Explain the results of tests and other investigations

The chest x-ray was entirely normal.

The blood test shows that your red blood cell level is low again. You are anemic.

Explain how you arrived at the diagnosis

By looking at your urine under a microscope, we see that you have an infection in your bladder. The infection can cause the bleeding you've noticed recently.

The tenderness is right over a tendon in your shoulder. This condition is called "tendinitis."

Explain the proposed plan

Explain elements of the plan—tests, x-rays, referrals, medications, diet, limitations on activity (especially going to work), and so forth—and alternatives. Explain the purpose of each element in the plan.

A blood test will help us check the fat in your blood.

These drops will treat the infection in your ear canal.

I know you were thinking about a chest x-ray, but we don't really think you need one to treat this bronchitis properly. We do want to prescribe cough medicine so that you can be more comfortable and sleep at night. How does that sound?

There is a small chance that this illness could be an early sign of a more serious condition, and I think you should have a few more tests to make sure that it is only a "cold."

> This swelling in your legs can be treated in a variety of ways. First, the more time you spend with your feet elevated and the less time you spend standing up, the better it will get. Second, you can wear heavy support stockings—the kind the nurses often wear in the hospital—though most people don't like to wear them in this hot weather. Third, you may get some relief by eating less salt and otherwise reducing the amount of the mineral sodium in your diet. Finally, we can give you medicines that tend to reduce the excess fluid in your body.

If any unusual or unfamiliar procedures are planned, explain them in detail. Patients particularly want to know if they are likely to experience any discomfort.

> The ultrasound will show us whether you have any stones in your gallbladder and help us understand why you're having these problems. The test is done by holding a special microphone against your stomach, aiming at your gallbladder. It doesn't hurt. You just have to lie still. You won't be able to eat on the morning of the examination.

In explaining the purpose and likely outcome of diagnostic and therapeutic interventions, you should indicate any permanent results of a medical or surgical procedure (e.g., a scar or an ostomy), any risks that are reasonably foreseeable, and, particularly for major decisions, the availability of any reasonable alternatives. Highly remote risks need not be disclosed, but there are no clear rules about what risks and what alternatives ought to be presented to which patients. In general, patients should be straightforwardly informed about major risks and benefits, using language that is understandable to them and that helps them to evaluate therapeutic decisions. For further discussion, let the patient guide you into deciding what level of detail is appropriate.

Educate the patient

Help the patient become an active participant in the care process. You will find opportunities for education throughout the interview, but especially in closing:

> Has bronchitis been explained to you?

> What is your understanding of emphysema?

> Since your mother has pneumonia, let me tell you what we mean by pneumonia and how it is managed.

> We recommend that some people get a shot each year to prevent the flu. Did you ever get a flu shot? Would you like one this fall?

Provide Reassurance Where Appropriate

Now that you have performed a thorough history and physical examination, you can provide credible reassurance. Insofar as you have elicited requests and attributions and have understood the patient's experience of the illness, you will be able to address the patient's specific concerns directly.

> You don't have pneumonia.

> I know you are concerned about diabetes, and I am glad to say we find no sign of it.

> There's no reason to think you have cancer, but we suggest you get some routine tests again this year.

If you find yourself trying to relieve anxiety with global reassurance (e.g., "You have nothing to worry about" or "Everything is going to turn out O.K.") or that you are guessing at the patient's concerns, go back to basic questions about the patient's perspective.

Give encouragement. Everyone likes to hear that he or she is well.

> Your general health seems excellent. Compliments to you!

> Otherwise, you seem in great shape.

> You're taking good care of yourself and you're enjoying your life. That's great!

Seek Questions and Concerns

Keep your initial explanation brief. Let patients' questions lead you to areas that require clarification or elaboration. Make it clear that you are interested in the patient's thoughts and feelings.

> Do you understand how you can take care of this matter?

> Does what we've said make sense to you?

> Are you feeling better?

> Do you have any questions?

> What else would you like to know?

> Have we accomplished what you wanted for this visit?

Be honest. If you are stumped by the patient's questions, say so directly.

> I don't know, but I can find out.

> Let's ask Dr. Ehrlich what she thinks about that.

If you make a significant mistake, don't hide it. Disclose the mistake and apologize for it.

Shared Decisions: Negotiate a Mutually Satisfactory Plan

Patients and their physicians inevitably have somewhat different viewpoints on the nature of a clinical problem and on the goals and methods of care. Conflict is inherent in such a situation. When significantly divergent perspectives are not reconciled, both participants in the clinical process tend to be dissatisfied, and the patient may be noncompliant.

Negotiation is a style of conflict management that reflects an application of egalitarian values to the doctor-patient relationship. The clinical process is viewed as a partnership, a collaboration between two persons who have differing expertise but who enjoy mutual respect, share a desire for consensus, and seek a common goal of health improvement.

What do you want to do?

What do you think about this plan?
   What parts do you find acceptable?
   What parts seem unacceptable?

Do you have any alternative ideas?

Earlier in the interview, you should have identified the patient's requests, and your proposed plan should have taken these into consideration. At this stage, you may need to further characterize the patient's goals and preferred methods of achieving those goals. If the proposed plan or range of plans does not suit the patient, you need to negotiate. Similarly, in seeking questions and concerns regarding the diagnosis and proposals for management (and later, regarding the details of the plan), you are refining your appreciation of the patient's views, and you may either arrive at a management scheme that better suits the patient or you may identify points of conflict that require further negotiation.

Negotiation is facilitated by an atmosphere that encourages patients to express their perspective and to acquire the information necessary to make informed decisions.

While we wait for the *H. pylori* blood test to come back, we can deal with your stomach distress in three ways. One, you can continue with the antacids, and as long as you feel better and are getting over your discomfort, we won't need to think about further tests. I know you are concerned about an ulcer, but regular antacids should be adequate treatment for that condition. Two, you may want to try a drug such as omeprazole, which will cut down on acid secretion in your stomach and may work better than what you have already tried. Three, we can go right ahead now with endoscopy—look down your throat into your stomach to see if an ulcer is present. What do you think about these options?

You have enlargement of the prostate. It is preventing your bladder from emptying well—that's why you've had to get up at night so often to urinate. There is no sign of any more serious problem. You could get relief of your symptoms by having a prostate operation now. Alternatively, you could just put up with your problem and wait to see if it gets worse or bothers you enough that you want to reconsider having an operation. What are your thoughts?

Remember that patients are ultimately responsible for their own care. Approach the negotiation process with flexibility, including a recognition that one's own wishes may not be fully met. Once these preconditions are established, the first step in successful negotiation is to clarify the nature of the conflict. What are the divergent goals and methods? Next, how can conflict be resolved, minimized, or merely recognized and accepted? (See the section Conflict: Its Negotiation and Management in Chapter 14.)

Provide Specific Information About the Plan (see Quick Tips: About the Plan)

Be Explicit

If you want your patient to change his or her diet, give specific information. Avoid vague advice, such as "cut down on fats." Provide instructional booklets or refer the patient to a dietitian who can give detailed instructions.

Similarly, if you want to prescribe exercise, be precise:

> You should now take a 1-mile walk each day. Try to walk briskly so that you are done in about 20 minutes. Record how long it takes you.

> For your first few days at home after the heart attack, you should stay in your apartment. You can walk around as much as you want. For now, you shouldn't do any housework or other hard work or heavy lifting. For just a few more weeks, you shouldn't engage in sexual relations. After this weekend, however, I'd like you to go downstairs twice a day and to take a leisurely walk around the block, weather permitting. For now, go slow on your walk, and stop to rest if you are not feeling well. If you develop any discomfort, such as chest pain or shortness of breath, call me. . . . Okay, now let me hear how you understand this plan.

Explain Prescribed Medication

Regardless of whether patients ask for detailed information about a new prescription, you should indicate its name, purpose, schedule (e.g., number of pills and when they should be administered), and how long the medication should be taken, as well as any common side effects. A description of the appearance of medications can also be helpful.

QUICK TIPS

About the Plan

- Be explicit and precise.
- Describe proposed diagnostic procedures.
- Explain prescribed medications—name, purpose, schedule, and how long the medication should be taken. Describe the medication's appearance.
- Explain the expected outcomes; stress the importance of following the plan.
- Ask the patient to repeat your explanations and instructions to ensure his or her understanding. You may ask the patient to bring in medications for review occasionally.
- Help the patient remember what you have said—write it down or help the patient write it. Provide instructional brochures. Provide medication charts, calendars, or trays.

> I am giving you a prescription for tablets of hydrochlorothiazide, which is a water pill, or diuretic. It will lower your blood pressure. You should take one pill every morning. You may find that you urinate a little more than usual for the first week or two after you begin the tablets, but that will stop soon. Otherwise, you are unlikely to notice anything different except that when your blood pressure is taken, we expect it will be lower.

You may need to take this medicine for the rest of your life to keep your blood pressure controlled. It is important that you take this regularly. If you are ever thinking of changing or stopping the medicine, please discuss the matter with me beforehand.

Now, let's make sure you and I have this straight. How will you take the pills?

Some people get a little sick to their stomach with Motrin. Take it on a full stomach—after a meal—and you can usually avoid this problem.

Your urine will turn orange while you're taking Pyridium.

With any new medication, patients commonly are concerned about such issues as drug dependence, toxicity, cost, whether it can be taken with previously prescribed medications, and whether it can be taken with food or alcohol. What should the patient do if side effects develop? For any chronic medication, explain why it needs to be taken regularly and the consequences of stopping treatment.

This medicine is meant to keep the fluid out of your lungs. If you stop taking it, the fluid may reaccumulate and you will get short of breath again and may get seriously ill. I think you should continue taking the pills even if you are feeling fine.

Beware of vague or readily misunderstood instructions. "Take with meals" can be understood as meaning to administer before, during, or after meals. Moreover, patients may eat at various times of day or may skip meals. "Four times a *day*" may be understood to mean that medication is not given at *night.* "Every four hours" may be interpreted to mean four, five, or six times in a day.

Tailor your prescription to the patient. If a pill should be taken four times a day, figure out with the patient what times for administering the medication would be convenient or most easily remembered. Link times for taking a drug with regular events in the patient's life: arising in the morning, brushing teeth, eating meals, watching the evening news, going to bed, and so forth.

Explain the Expected Outcome of the Treatment Plan

You should be feeling better soon. The bronchitis usually goes away in 4 or 5 days. Even so, keep taking the erythromycin for a full week.

What is the value of treatment, the consequences of noncompliance? Consider stressing the importance of following the plan.

High blood pressure may not make you feel bad, but it can cause damage to your heart and circulation if you do not treat it properly. You may not feel differently with the treatment, but we expect you to be more healthy and to live longer. You can reduce your risk of having a heart attack or stroke.

Ask the Patient to Repeat Your Explanations and Instructions

Now, let's go over it again. How are you going to treat this cough?

May I quiz you about what you know about this illness?

What is your understanding now about the cause and treatment of your condition?

Whenever a long-term treatment plan is initiated (e.g., a low-salt diet, a drug regimen for hypertension, a program for diabetic urine testing), ask the patient on subsequent visits to go over what he or she recalls about the illness and to report what was actually done:

What are you taking for your blood pressure now?

How did it go?

What kind of problems did you have with this new diet?

You will find it useful to have your patients occasionally bring in their medications for review. You might ask a new patient to bring in all of his or her medications, as well as empty pill containers that are still around the house.

Help the Patient Remember

Patients are usually too anxious to remember much of what is said in the office. Write down directions and points that need to be reinforced, or help your patients write these down for themselves. Enlist others—the office nurse, technical assistant, nurse-practitioner, or physician assistant—in the educational endeavor. Provide instructional brochures. Involve the family.

Medication charts, calendars, and trays can help patients keep track of their pill-taking. To facilitate identification of medications, you might tape an actual pill to a medication list. Make sure pill containers are labeled with clear and up-to-date instructions.

Seek Further Questions and Concerns

Do you think this treatment is reasonable?

Do you foresee any difficulty in starting on this treatment?

Do you think you will have any trouble remembering to take the pills? [Following the diet? Getting to the hospital for the tests? Paying for the medicine? Giving up this old habit? Changing your use of free time? Finding the time for this regimen?] Do you have other concerns?

Before we wrap up, do you have any questions or concerns?

Such an invitation might be considered training in patient assertiveness. Another invitation is for the patient to comment on the interview process itself:

Are there any other questions you think I should have asked you?
Anything else I should explain more?

Listen for and explore the personal meaning behind the patient's questions and responses.

Patient: Well, that's my life.
Doctor: What do you mean?

Patient: Heart conditions are serious.
Patient: Does it have any side effects?
Doctor: Anything in particular worrying you?
Patient: Well, I heard these drugs could make you impotent.

Motivational Interviewing: Counseling on Behavioral Change

Sometimes, your plain advice is sufficient to get patients to change their behavior. However, many of the tasks that physicians prescribe require considerable motivation and behavioral change: remembering to take medications,
following an unpleasant, complicated, or time-consuming regimen, altering
a diet, modifying a long-standing habit, and keeping regular appointments.
The clinician's well-meaning advice, perhaps accompanied by a lecture on
the seriousness of the matter or an appeal to the physician's authority and
wisdom, is often ineffective.

Getting patients to change behaviors that contribute to ill health is often difficult, yet enormously important. Many habits—smoking, overeating,
excessive drinking, and using drugs—lead to disease and disability, and nonadherence to various treatment recommendations can lead to complications
or poor outcomes. Miller and Rollnick and Prochaska et al. analyzed the
process of decision-making in altering behavior and the tactics that influence
change in medical practice and have delineated the following stages:

- Precontemplation
- Contemplation
- Preparation
- Action
- Maintenance

Termination or relapse can occur at any stage. An appreciation of the patient's stage in behavioral change can help guide the clinician to effective interventions and also help to avoid interventions that are only appropriate at
other stages. The following section lists some ways to help your patients
change behavior.

Suggestions for Behavioral Change

**Develop an alliance with the patient around the issue of changing be-
havior.** Does the patient want to change? Is current behavior seen as a problem? If
not, why not? Are you trying to dictate what to do, while the patient acquiesces, or is
the patient clearly in charge of his or her life, joining with you in trying to understand
behavior and in finding ways to change it?

What do you want to work on? Your smoking? Your weight?

What are your thoughts about approaching this matter?

Reinforce behavioral change as the patient's personal responsibility. If
the patient wants to change, does he or she want help from you? How can you be of
assistance? Convey your personal interest in helping. Solicit patients' ideas about how
they can be helped, as well as about what difficulties will be encountered. Beware of
alienating patients by foisting unwanted advice upon them.

Stress the importance and the seriousness of the problem and the benefits of behavioral change. Educate patients about the health consequences of their behaviors and about the process of changing. You can be firm and clear about what you know, yet not be authoritarian about what the patient should do.

Explore the forces that encourage or discourage change. What factors in this patient's biological and psychosocial makeup seem to predispose to unhealthy behavior? What factors seem to promote well-being, and how can they be strengthened? What are the barriers to change, and what resources are available for overcoming them? For example, your history on a smoker might include the following:

When did you begin smoking?

Why do you smoke? How do you feel about smoking? Why do you want to continue to smoke?

What is your understanding of the risks of smoking? Are you concerned?

Have you had any symptoms or illnesses related to the smoking?

What benefits do you see in stopping? What problems?

Have you ever tried to stop? What happened?

What difficulties do you foresee in cutting down or stopping? In maintaining progress or staying quit?

What would help you change now? How can you increase your determination?

What treatment options are you aware of? Would you like to know more about them? What do you think about these treatment approaches? Do any of them appeal to you?

What kinds of strategies could you use when problems arise after you cut down or quit?

What kind of support do you have for changing? For maintaining changes?

How could I help you?

Fashion educational and motivational efforts to suit each patient. In exploring the factors that encourage or discourage change, pay particular attention to health concerns that hold salience for this person. Use these clues to motivate the patient and tailor an approach to his or her particular situation. You can target your attention to the patient's specific fears (e.g., not having enough breath to play baseball or affecting a child's health and habits) or you may link smoking to current health problems (e.g., recurrent bronchitis). For this patient, would it make more sense to cut back on smoking or to try quitting entirely?

Similarly, identify and reinforce strengths (e.g., "You've put a lot of energy into taking good care of your body, especially by jogging, and that's great!"). Anticipate problems and help overcome them by teaching skills or suggesting specific strategies (e.g., what to do or think about when the patient feels a strong desire to restart smoking).

Invoke social supports and address social factors that mitigate against change. Involve your patient's loved ones for social support. Work with your patient to come up with alternatives to replace their harmful habits. You may present various treatment options, such as nicotine replacement therapy and a variety of health care and community services that support behavioral change (e.g., referral to group therapy, a hypnotist, or a worksite-based program for smoking cessation). Reading material may also be useful.

Use positive suggestions.

When your airways start to recover from the smoking and you start clearing out your lungs, your breathing will get better and better and you will feel healthier and stronger.

You will be able to look back on this and feel great about what you have accomplished. I think you'll really feel proud.

Be encouraging and supportive. Let patients know you appreciate and accept their feelings about modifying or continuing behaviors and their difficulty in changing. Avoid being judgmental, pejorative, or punitive. Respect all attempts at change, and praise all desirable efforts, even those the patient perceives as a failure. Recognize the most minor progress, focusing on success so that the visit is a positive experience for the patient. When progress is slow, reset goals to more attainable levels, lest the patient become discouraged. Develop alternative strategies and renegotiate a plan. Express optimism about future progress. Convey your continued interest and support—your eagerness to work on the problem with the patient.

Set realistic goals and commitments. By the end of the visit, you and the patient should set realistic, specific goals and seek agreement on pursuing them until the next appointment.

You don't seem ready to give up your smoking habit now, but I wonder if you couldn't cut back from two-and-a-half to two packs a day?

Consider the following steps for concluding your discussion about behavioral change:

1. Seek a clear commitment.

So you are ready to quit, and you have a good plan for staying quit. When's the day?

2. Have the patient directly state his or her intentions. Consider having the patient make a written "contract," stating his or her intentions.
3. Engage the patient in the process of monitoring progress (e.g., recording cigarette use or sending you a postcard when specific goals are met).
4. Plan prospectively for difficulties and rehearse strategies for overcoming them.

How will you handle it when you go to the lodge and they're all smoking?

5. Recognize and accept the possibility of relapse or failure. Beware of making the patient ashamed to return. Anticipate how the patient may feel about failure.

Let's see how you've done in the next month. If this doesn't work well, we'll figure out what went wrong and we'll know how to do better next time.

6. Be encouraging.

That's great. You've got a good plan and you're ready to help yourself.

7. Restate the importance of change, using a message tailored to the patient.

You don't want to end up with emphysema like your father.

8. Ensure follow-up. Ask for suggestions on how you can be helpful. For some patients, frequent visits are helpful for maintaining interest and resolve. Consider a telephone call or a postcard before the next visit as a method of assessing progress and encouraging continued attention to behavioral change. Continue surveillance not only to monitor progress but also to maintain it (e.g., after the smoker quits).

An approach similar to the one just given for smoking cessation might be used in establishing a complicated chronic drug-administration schedule or promoting other behavioral change. What does the patient think and feel about this health problem and its treatment? What might motivate this particular patient to follow a difficult regimen? What kinds of obstacles can be anticipated, and how can they be addressed? What strengths and supports can be enlisted? How can the regimen be made simple, convenient, and otherwise easy to follow? What skills can the patient be taught, and what other resources might facilitate change? How else can the physician be encouraging and helpful? What steps will the patient pledge to take? How will the regimen be monitored? What kind of follow-up contact is useful?

Counsel on Health Promotion and Disease Prevention

"Health maintenance" or a similar term belongs on every patient's list of problems. Identify the health concerns that your patients bring to the visit. Investigate their individual risks and educate them on measures to promote health and to prevent disease and disability. Identify and explore adverse health behaviors and help patients change. Similarly, be encouraging about healthful behaviors.

Make Provisions for Follow-up Care
Explain Plans for Follow-up

If you don't get better, or if you start coughing up thick, green or yellow sputum, or if you should get a fever over 101° will you let us know?

We will want to check your heart again in 2 weeks. Can you come back then?

Tell the Patient When to Come Back and Why

We would like to check your lungs again in about 6 months. You can get your flu shot then. How does this arrangement sound? Come back sooner if you are having any difficulties, of course. If you give this slip to the secretary, Mary Lou, on your way out, she will give you an appointment.

Some problems do not require follow-up, but most patients will be offered "routine visits" for preventive care.

Arrange for Transmitting Information on Clinical Studies

Let the patient know how test results, normal and abnormal, will be communicated.

> We will write you about the results of your tests.
>
> I will let you know right away if anything abnormal turns up. If you don't hear from us within a few days, it means that your tests were all okay.
>
> Ms. Chaput, the nurse, will call you about your results.
>
> If you want to get the results before our next visit, please call my secretary, Rita, a few days after the test so that she can get the report and we can get back to you.
>
> I should have the biopsy report 4 days after the procedure. Let's sit down and talk about it then.

In general, unless patients are going to be seen soon after a test is taken, they deserve to be notified about the studies or to know a convenient method for obtaining the results. Serious "bad news" should usually be given in person, as should the results of major procedures, especially when a very serious or life-threatening condition is suspected. For instance, a visit to review the biopsy of a breast tumor might be scheduled a few days after the procedure, assuming that the pathologist's report will be ready by then. If the tumor is benign, you can always call the patient immediately with the good news and cancel the appointment, but if the report indicates malignancy, you will not be in the awkward position of giving distressing information over the telephone.

A formal letter or a phone call about test results underscores the value you attach to patients having information about their medical conditions and helps engage them in self-care. A form letter—"Your mammogram on 4/6/98 was normal"—suffices when "routine" screening studies are normal.

Be Available for Later Questions and Problems

Let your patients know that they should feel free to contact you or your preceptor if they have any questions in the future. Give them your preceptor's professional card with your name added and encourage them to call if problems develop before the next visit.

Use the Acute Illness Visit to Discuss Ongoing Care

Take the opportunity to talk about the use of health services and about the importance of health promotion. Explain how phone calls and appointments are managed, both for emergencies and routine matters.

> I'm glad you came in today. This is how you can reach us in the future.
>
> If you develop such a bronchitis again, you can reach us anytime at. . . .
>
> I think you can treat this on your own the next time. Here are a few things that I'd suggest you would call me about, if they should happen.
>
> I suggest you return for a checkup in 2 years. We can repeat your "Pap" smear then.

Say Goodbye

As the interview comes to a close, warn the patient:

> Well, we're going to have to finish now. Is there anything else we need to discuss?

Remember to allocate enough time so that you can end your interview effectively. Rather than introducing new topics or opening up further dialogue, conclude with a message that wraps up and reinforces what you have previously discussed. During the last few minutes, you will probably want to summarize one or two major points and repeat a few essential instructions. Your final words can also serve to motivate the patient. You send off the patient with an inspiring message, often with an appeal to previously identified concerns about current medical problems or future health. Additionally, consider solidifying your relationship with patients through closing comments that provide encouragement, praise, personal appreciation, and assurance of your continued involvement.

Finally, say goodbye, perhaps accompanied by physical touch, such as a handshake.

> It was nice to meet you. We'll talk again when you come back in a couple of weeks.

> I'm pleased to meet you. I might not see you again, so I want to wish you well.

Termination

While practicing physicians may maintain long-term relationships with patients and enjoy an illusion that the association will last forever, students and house officers frequently must break off their contact with patients as a rotation ends or a phase of training is completed. The process of ending a relationship is called termination.

Not saying goodbye can leave patients confused and feeling neglected or unappreciated. In many social situations where two persons part, they soften any upset about the separation by acting as if they will see or talk to each other sometime: "I'll probably be back in Boston in the next few months, so I'll look you up then" or "Let's do lunch sometime." Unfortunately, such socially acceptable practices fail to acknowledge the importance of relationships and the difficulty of separation.

Practice saying goodbye to your patients, including ones to whom you do not feel particularly attached, and give them all the opportunity to say goodbye to you. Unless you are very sure that you will be able to maintain the relationship despite your incredibly busy, demanding training, it is better to part without implying or stating that you will continue the contact, which can set up the patient for serious disappointment or misunderstanding.

In saying goodbye, you will often learn, probably to your surprise, how significant you have been to patients and what they value about the relationship. Even if you did not feel appreciated, many patients develop deep attachments to the medical and nursing staff who care for them. Some patients, of course, will not miss you and may have much more important rela-tionships with other clinicians or may be used to changing doctors fre-quently. You will also encounter persons who clearly cared about you but have difficulty acknowledging such an attachment, and they will be helped by your recognition that the relationship was meaningful.

SUGGESTED READINGS

Choices and changes: clinician influence and patient action workbook, New Haven, Conn, 1996, Bayer Institute for Health Care Communication.

Miller WR, Rollnick S: *Motivational interviewing: preparing people to change addictive be-havior,* New York, 1991, Guilford Press.

Prochaska JO, Norcross JC, DiClemente CC: *Changing to good,* New York, 1994, William Morrow.

Rollnick S, Heather N, Bell A: Negotiating behavioral change in medical settings: the development of brief motivational interviewing, *J Ment Health* 1:25, 1992.

CHAPTER 8

RECORDING

Patients tell stories; doctors write histories.

ANONYMOUS

The best memory is a record made at the time.

SIR WILLIAM GULL
APHORISMS

Careful observation and systematic recording are fundamental to the scientific method in clinical work. The medical record must be legible and should be constructed in a standard format that is familiar to readers, allowing them readily to find the data they need.

Three distinct kinds of information are included in the medical record:

1. **Data base.** This term describes all the clinical facts that are gathered for understanding the patient's condition. The data base includes the reports of the patient and other informants (history, "symptoms"), as well as the observations made by clinicians through physical examination ("signs") or laboratory methods. In the "problem-oriented" medical record that is used by many clinicians, reports from patients or other persons are termed "subjective" data, whereas the findings of physical examination and laboratory tests are called "objective."

2. **Assessments.** These are opinions about the significance of the data base, including interpretations of the history, physical examination, and laboratory tests; impressions about the diagnosis and prognosis; hypotheses about etiology and pathophysiology; discussions of consultations and reference material; and thoughts about further diagnostic efforts or treatment.

3. **Plans.** This category refers to actions that are actually being undertaken as a result of the clinical evaluation. Plans include diagnostic procedures, treatments, and education of the patient. Once a diagnostic or therapeutic step is undertaken, it becomes a fact in the data base, and hence a possible influence on later assessments and plans.

FORMAT FOR THE WRITE-UP

The written case presentation is a specialized literary form. The format may vary from one institution to another, while each clinician develops an individual style, but the following should serve as a useful model. See also the case example in Appendix A.

Identifying Data

The patient's name and identification number should be written on the top of each page of the write-up. The date of the interview should also be noted on the first page.

The patient's full name, date of birth, address, and telephone number, as well as the name, address, and telephone number of the nearest relative or person to be notified in case of problems, should be readily available in the record. Since these are often recorded by a registration clerk, you usually do not need to repeat them in your note.

If the patient was referred by a physician or other health care worker or a social agency, note the name, address, and telephone number of the referral source at the top of the first page. Consider noting the referral as part of the reason for visit.

A title that identifies the writer (e.g., "Third-Year Student Evaluation," "Senior Resident's Note," or "Rheumatology Consult") is often placed at the head of the write-up when the medical record contains notes from many persons.

Patient Profile and Reason for Visit

In this headline sentence, you describe the patient in terms of age, sex, race, marital status, occupation, and any other particularly important descriptive data, including major medical conditions that are important background for appreciating the present illness. You then state, often in the patient's own words, the reason for the visit.

> This 25-year-old, Asian, single, female graduate student complains of "blood in the urine" for 2 days.
>
> This 51-year-old, white, male truck driver with insulin-dependent diabetes, whose father died last month, presents for a checkup.
> ▲

For hospitalized patients, you generally report the reason for the admission (the chief complaint on presentation to the hospital), even if you are seeing the patient later in the hospital stay. For instance:

> This 88-year-old, remarkably healthy, widowed union organizer who underwent a right mastectomy for breast cancer 8 years ago, was admitted 10 days ago for right hip pain and inability to walk after she slipped in the bathtub.
> ▲

Source and Reliability

This section is usually unnecessary and may be omitted. Your reader will assume that your source of information was the patient and that the patient was a reasonably reliable historian. However, if a significant part of the history was obtained from another source (e.g., family member, friend, translator, medical records) or the reliability of the history is questionable (e.g., the records are incomplete or the patient is confused, demented, psychotic, retarded, hostile, uncooperative, unrealistic, hard of hearing, or otherwise unable to understand or communicate well), make a note to that effect.

> Spanish-speaking patient interviewed with her sister who speaks English well and seemed to be a careful translator.

> Patient a poor historian due to failing memory; source is mostly her husband and the hospital record.

▲

If a few points in the history were obtained from sources other than the patient, you can integrate this information into the next section, the present illness, without including a section on sources:

> The patient reports feeling weak for about 5 days, though her husband notes that she was already failing 2 to 3 months ago.

▲

Present Illness

Here you thoroughly but succinctly describe each presenting complaint or reason for the visit, including the dimensions of symptoms, the patient's perspective, and all other information relevant to assessment and management of the problem.

Like a journalist preparing a newspaper article, you want to offer an impartial report, based on the patient's own words, yet you must select and arrange the raw data to create a story that makes clinical sense to you and your readers. You cannot simply list facts. You translate the patient's words into the language of a case report, and you reconstruct the patient's account. A good written history of the present illness is based on an understanding of the patient's illness and is organized to reflect a process of reasoning about the significance of the various symptoms. Your description—the way you order the data and relate facts to each other—should suggest and justify a particular diagnosis or a set of diagnoses, giving the information that helps the reader appreciate that other diagnoses are unlikely. Some guidelines for organizing the story have been discussed in Chapter 6.

You should generally draft a problem list before writing up the present illness. Guidelines for deciding on what is a problem and on when to lump problems together or to separate them are provided later in this chapter under Assessment and Plan and in Chapter 17, The Medical Record. If there are two or more problems that belong in the write-up of the present illness, rank them by importance or arrange them in a logical order, and then present them separately, using a problem title and number at the head of each subsection (e.g., #1 Dysuria, #2 Shoulder pain).

You also generally need to plan out an assessment (see Assessment and Plan) before making a final draft of the write-up of the present illness, as the organization and content of the section are best handled with a clear sense of the diagnosis or differential diagnosis.

The Standard Data Base

Past Medical History

See the format used in the case example in Appendix A. The patient's medical history is arranged under a set of standard headings and subheadings described previously:

- Hospitalizations (date, reason, hospital)
- Operations and injuries (date, name of procedure or injury, where treated)
- Pregnancies (including abortions)
- Illnesses (name, when diagnosed, and sometimes a brief description of the problem)
- Medications (name, dose, route, timing for all prescribed or over-the-counter medications. Refer to a pharmacology textbook for the standard format and Latin abbreviations.)
- Allergies (allergen and nature of allergic response), especially drug allergies
- Habits
    Tobacco
    Alcohol
    Other recreational drugs
- Exposures
- Travel
- Diet
- Health maintenance
    Periodic health examination
    Immunizations
    Injury prevention
    Exercise
    Contraception/sexually transmitted diseases

In this section of the history, a brief note, usually not a full sentence, is used to outline the data in tabular form, for instance:

    Operations—1968, cholecystectomy, Boston City Hospital
    Tobacco—none

Social History

The social history is the only portion of the standard data base that is presented in prose format. Use full sentences to give the patient's biography, following the categories of information described in Chapter 3.

Family History

Use either a tabular format or a pedigree diagram (Fig. 8-1).

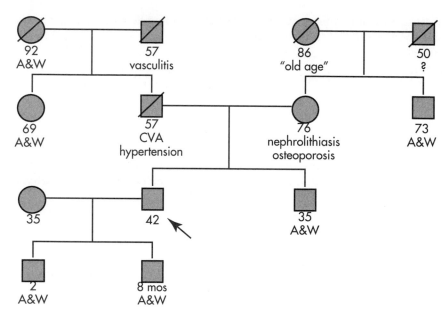

Fig. 8-1 Pedigree diagram. In pedigree diagrams, males are represented by squares and females by circles. A diagonal line through a symbol indicates that the person has died. Siblings are arranged from left to right in order of birth with the firstborn (eldest) sibling on the far left. A number within or below a circle or square represents the person's current age or age at death. The patient is designated with an arrow. *A&W,* Alive and well.

Tabular Format:

Maternal grandmother died age 86 of "old age"
Maternal grandfather died about age 50, unknown cause
Paternal grandmother well at age 92
Paternal grandfather died age 57, vasculitis
Mother well at age 76—nephrolithiasis, osteoporosis, PAT
Father died age 57, cerebral bleed from vascular malformation; hypertensive
One brother alive and well, age 35
Two sons, age 8 months, 2 years, alive and well

Review of Systems

In recording this section of the history, separate the positive and negative findings, as in the case example shown in the Appendix. Give a brief description of any positive findings. Your readers will generally skim the review of systems (ROS), so use underlining, colored ink, or an asterisk in the margin to identify any significant abnormalities. More advanced students will often mention only positive findings, noting that "the remainder of the ROS was negative in detail," but for your own learning purposes, your initial written reviews of systems should report both positive and negative findings in detail.

Data acquired in the course of obtaining the review of systems may be recorded in other portions of the standard data base or in the section on present illness. For example, if the patient is reminded in this portion of the history of a previous surgery, a note would be placed in the part of the past medical history (PMH) that is devoted to operations. Similarly, complaints may be unearthed that are relevant to the reason for the visit and should be recorded under the present illness. Occasionally, the review of systems will divulge a complaint that deserves to be treated as a new problem in the present illness. The actual review of systems section of the record is used only to describe problems that are minor, insignificant, or of questionable importance. When symptoms have already been recorded in previous portions of the history, simply state, for instance, "See PMH" or "See Problem #2."

Physical Examination

Begin with vital signs and general appearance, then skin, then proceed essentially from head to toe, ending with the musculoskeletal and neurological examination. See the case example in Appendix A.

Laboratory Work

Results of laboratory evaluations are included if they are already available when you are making an assessment and plan. The usual order is:

1. Hematology, beginning with the complete blood count, often written in a grid:

$$\frac{\text{Hematocrit}}{\text{Platelets}} < \text{WBC Differential}$$

For example:

$$\frac{41.6}{180,000} < 14,600 \quad 72P \quad 6B \quad 18L \quad 3M \quad 1E$$

2. Urinalysis (appearance, specific gravity, dipstick for pH, protein, sugar, ketones, blood, and other tests; microscopic analysis of sediment)
3. Serum chemistries, beginning with the electrolytes, which also may be written in a grid, including the blood sugar:

$$\frac{\text{Na}\ |\ \text{Cl}}{\text{K}\ |\ \text{HCO}_3} < \begin{array}{l}\text{BUN}\\ \text{Glucose}\\ \text{Cr}\end{array}$$

For example:

$$\frac{140\ |\ 97}{3.9\ |\ 25} < \begin{array}{l}26\\ 137\\ 1.2\end{array}$$

4. Chest x-ray and other x-rays
5. Electrocardiogram
6. Bacteriology—Gram stains and other stains and cultures
7. Special studies (e.g., examination of cerebrospinal fluid)

Hospital Course

When you evaluate patients who have been in the hospital for a day or more, you may record data from the hospitalization (including test results, opinions of consultants, and the response to treatment) either at the end of the present illness or in this separate section. If you use this separate section, the present illness should include only that information that would have been available at the time of admission.

Assessment

Having obtained the history and performed a physical (and perhaps laboratory) examination, you are now ready to make an assessment (or impression, or differential diagnosis).

The assessment consists of two basic steps. First, create a list of all the problems you have identified in the history, physical examination, and laboratory tests. Problems may include any physical or psychosocial complaints or symptoms, any findings from the physical or laboratory examination, as well as diagnoses, syndromes, or other matters that deserve some diagnostic evaluation or management. For example, one patient's list might include the following:

1. Health maintenance
2. Sore throat, fever
3. Hypertension, controlled on medication
4. Marital discord
5. Smoking
6. Family history of colonic carcinoma
7. Allergy to penicillin (hives)

In the simplest cases, your title for the problem may essentially convey your assessment:

Upper respiratory tract infection
Cystitis
Paronychia, left third finger

▲

If a definitive diagnosis cannot be made, your problem title may be a symptom, perhaps accompanied by an impression, based on your current knowledge:

Muscular weakness and fatigue, etiology undetermined
Itchy throat, possible allergic symptoms
Chest pain

▲

Health maintenance is usually the first or last problem. Otherwise, problems should be ordered in terms of seriousness and priority. Related problems should be grouped together. Further guidance on identifying and naming problems and on using the problem-oriented medical record system is contained in The Medical Record in Chapter 16.

The second step in making an assessment is to give your opinion about the significance of each problem and indicate which further diagnostic and therapeutic efforts should be considered. As noted above, for simpler cases, the title of the problem may convey your assessment, and as you become a more experienced clinician you will not bother explaining your diagnosis or management for very straightforward or routine matters. However, for pedagogical purposes at this stage in your training, and whenever somewhat complex or unusual problems are addressed, your assessment should explain how you arrived at a particular diagnosis or differential diagnosis, and let your reader know what you intend to do about the problem.

A good way to begin your assessment is to summarize the data base that you feel is relevant to understanding the problem. You should include key symptoms, risk factors, signs, and laboratory tests.

In summary, this 61-year-old woman with lupus and recurrent urinary tract infections, including pyelonephritis, now presents with dysuria, suprapubic discomfort, fever, an otherwise benign physical exam, and a urinalysis with pyuria, hematuria, and bacteriuria.

▲

In your assessment, you may discuss the etiology, pathophysiology, severity, prognosis, differential diagnosis, diagnostic considerations, and treatment options for the problem. You may speculate on the relation of this problem to others. Cite references, including either journal articles or textbooks. In general, your assessment should identify the most likely diagnosis and review the data that support this diagnosis. Alternatively, identify and discuss the several leading diagnoses. Also, mention conditions that you have considered and deemed less likely but that are important to recognize and manage (e.g., diagnoses that may be uncommon but ought to be "ruled out" because they are serious or benefit from prompt treatment). You may also describe what further data are needed and how such information will help pin down a diagnosis.

The clinical picture is diagnostic of cystitis.

Upper urinary tract infections may present similarly, but further tests to clarify whether the upper tracts are involved will not affect our immediate treatment. She has no history or symptoms particularly suggestive of nephrolithiasis, and an IVP performed 6 years ago showed no evidence of structural abnormalities in the urinary tract.

Until the results of today's culture are available, treatment consists of an antibiotic that covers common urinary tract pathogens, particularly *E. coli.* She is allergic to sulfa, so we will choose ampicillin. With her history of recurrent infections, we will give her a 2-week course and recheck her urine in about 3 weeks. If she develops subsequent infections, we will try to distinguish between recurrence of the same pathogen and acquisition of a new one.

▲

Plan

While the assessment calls for opinions, the plan describes your actual management of each identified problem. There are three categories of plans:

Diagnostic (Dx): Further observations, questioning, examinations; obtaining medical records; laboratory tests (blood, urine, cardiogram, sputum, and so forth); x-rays; referral to a specialist.

Treatment (Rx): Medication; advice on activity and diet; letter to school or work; surgery; referral to a community agency.

Patient Education (Pt Ed): Instructions to the patient on self-care, occupational hazards, changing life-style; education on diagnosis, prognosis, and management; advice on when to make return visits or contact you.

▲

Beware of confusing Dx in this section (which stands for *diagnostic plans*) with the diagnosis. Diagnostic plans are actions taken to further evaluate a problem, whereas the diagnosis is part of the assessment and represents an opinion about the significance of findings.

In the medical record, the following format is used to identify each problem and record the assessment and plan:

#1 Cough, fever
Assessment: Influenza. In view of the patient's mild disability, as well as the absence of high fever, purulent sputum, or worrisome findings on pulmonary exam, a serious chest infection is unlikely. A chest x-ray is unnecessary, and the patient agrees that symptomatic therapy is indicated.
Plan: Diagnostic—none
   Treatment—Glyceryl guaiacolate with codeine 5 ml po q4h prn 120 ml, refill x1
   Patient education—Discuss course of illness, use of medication, and need for flu shot and reexamination. Call if fever, cough, or dyspnea worsens or if symptoms not resolving within a week

#2 Glaucoma
Assessment: Asymptomatic, open-angle glaucoma without evidence of significant visual damage
Plan: Diagnostic—Refer to Glaucoma Clinic for further evaluation
   Treatment—per Dr. Hutchinson in Glaucoma Clinic
   Patient education—Discuss meaning of glaucoma and importance of follow-up while asymptomatic

▲

For all medications, carefully record the name (generic and, if used, brand name), dose, route, timing, quantity prescribed, and number of refills allowed. Refer to a pharmacology textbook to learn the standard format and common abbreviations for prescribing medications.

Remember to indicate clearly the advice on when to return next:

Return to the clinic in 3 months to see Ms. O'Leary, the nurse-practitioner.
Follow-up by phone, 2 weeks.
Call in 5 days if not better; otherwise, return as needed.

▲

Your Name

Give your name and, if appropriate, identifying data (e.g., Harvey Cushing, HMS II).

FOLLOW-UP NOTES

Progress notes include descriptions of new problems and the course of previously noted problems, an update on selected portions of the physical examination, results of laboratory tests, a description of plans that have been carried out, and a revised assessment and plan. Each problem can be updated with a "SOAP" (Subjective, Objective, Assessment, Plan) format note, as described in the following example. New problems can also be introduced with this format.

Subjective: All the relevant data from the patient's report or other sources of history
Objective: All relevant findings from the physical examination and laboratory tests
Assessment: Your impression or differential diagnosis
Plan: Dx—Diagnostic plans (not the diagnosis!)
　　　Rx—Therapeutic plans
　　　Pt Ed—Patient education

For example:

#1 Cough, fever
　S: Resolved in 3 days with cough medicine
　O: Lungs clear; no sputum
　A: Influenza, resolved
　P: Dx—None
　　　Rx—None
　　　Pt Ed—Suggest flu shot next November; return to clinic prn recurrent cough
　　　　　and sputum

#2 Health maintenance
　S: Does breast self-exam erratically
　O: Breasts—no masses, discharge
　A: Needs annual breast x-ray
　P: Dx—Xeromammogram
　　　Rx—None
　　　Pt Ed—Encourage monthly self-exam
　　　　　—Review self-exam with nurse
　　　　　—Advise on value of x-rays, especially with her family history
　　　　　—Follow-up during November visit

▲

A list of current medications and other treatments is useful in a progress note. This information is generally placed in a separate section, sometimes at the top of the page. Such a tabulation can also be part of the subjective notes (especially for outpatient visits, since the list represents the patient's report) or part of the objective notes (especially for inpatients, since the list is obtained from the doctor's orders or the nurses' medication sheets).

An alternative approach for organizing follow-up notes on patients with complicated disease courses is to describe the subjective data under separate problem titles, but to give only a single objective section or physical examination section, followed by separate, problem-oriented assessments and plans. This is similar to the standard format for an initial evaluation or hospital admission note. For example:

29 April 1998
Routine follow-up visit

#1 Hypertension
   S: Continues faithfully to take his medications, hydrochlorothiazide 50 mg q AM, but has been eating lots of salty foods

#2, 3 Obesity, hypercholesterolemia
   S: Seeing nutritionist regularly and has lost 6 lbs in 4 weeks
   Tolerating diet well

#4 Asthma
   S: One episode in 2 months, related to visiting friends who have two cats; uses inhaler twice a week; satisfied with current regimen
   O: 168/98 R arm large cuff 172/96 L arm P72 R16
   Cor—S_4, no significant murmur
   Lungs—clear, but forced expiration produces mild wheezing

Assessment

#1 Hypertension, not adequately controlled
   P: Dx—None
   Rx—Discontinue hydrochlorothiazide
      —Begin enalapril 5 mg one tab daily #30; refill × 5
   Pt Ed—Discuss toxicity of new medication, especially postural hypertension
      —Follow-up 10 days

#2, 3 Obesity, hypercholesterolemia, making good progress
   P: Dx—12-14 hour fasting lipids
   Rx—None
   Pt Ed—Encourage and congratulate. Discuss maintenance of diet and anticipate problems during upcoming vacation

#4 Asthma, stable, well-controlled
   P: Rx—Continue albuterol inhaler
   Pt Ed—Follow-up prn worsening symptoms

▲

The use of the SOAP format helps remind you in your oral and written case presentations to always distinguish between four logically distinct clinical realms: (1) the history (called subjective), while obviously obtained and organized by you, is presented as the patient's report and should not contain your observations or impressions; (2) the objective data (your observations and the results of laboratory examinations) are "facts" that should be separated from the patient's reports or your interpretations; (3) the assessment is your opinion of the clinical meaning of the collected data; and (4) the plan is what is actually done, a description of action based on the assessment.

CHAPTER 9

READINGS

The interview between doctor and patient has been the subject of many studies, some of which may interest you. Approaches to describing or understanding the clinical encounter include the following: the investigation of nonverbal communication or metacommunication (including proxemics and the characterization of "body language"); linguistic studies and the microanalysis of language and behavior; sociological schemes describing illness behavior, roles, power, and information-transfer; anthropological explorations of ethnic and cultural factors in the presentation of symptoms and of the social meaning of illness; psychological and social psychological attempts to understand helping relationships, empathy, attributions, requests, and expectations; and clinical psychiatric assessment of specific diagnoses, personality types, defenses, "problem patients," and emotional reactions to illness and care-seeking. All of these frameworks can help inform your practice, cultivate your instincts, and add perspective to your work.

As introductory clinical texts and articles, we recommend the following:

1. Enelow AJ, Forde DL, Brummel-Smith K: *Interviewing and Patient Care,* ed 4 New York, 1996, Oxford University Press.

   This text offers an excellent framework for understanding the process of obtaining information and for learning basic interviewing skills. Techniques for successful questioning are detailed, and problem areas are identified. For students seeking more introduction to the clinical interview (after reading or rereading this book), Enelow and Swisher's book is our first choice.

2. Rogers CR: *On Becoming a Person: A Therapist's View of Psychotherapy,* Boston, 1961, Houghton Mifflin.

   See the section "How Can I Be of Help," especially the chapter, "The Characteristics of a Helping Relationship," for an introduction to "humanistic" or "client-centered" therapy. Rogers identifies "unconditional positive regard" as the key quality in a helping relationship.

3. Smith R: *The Patient's Story: Integrating Patient-Doctor Interviewing,* Boston, 1995, Little, Brown.

   A text contrasting a patient-centered versus a doctor-centered process with illustrative interview dialogue.

4. *The Medical Interview,* Lipkin M, Putnam SM, Lazare A, editors: New York, 1995, Springer-Verlag.

   A comprehensive multiauthored text with detailed bibliography.

5. Platt FW: *Conversation Repair: Case Studies in Doctor-Patient Communication,* Boston, 1995, Little, Brown.

6. Cassell EJ: *Talking With Patients,* vol 1, *The Theory of Doctor-Patient Communication,* vol 2, *Clinical Technique,* Cambridge, Mass, 1985, MIT Press.

   A detailed, lively account of how language operates in clinical settings and of how an appreciation of linguistic processes can improve clinical care. This book is nicely written and is full of helpful clinical observations and suggestions.

7. Kaufert JM, Putsch RW: Communication through interpreters in health care: ethical dilemmas arising from differences in class, culture, language, and power, *J Clin Ethics* 8:71-87, 1997.

8. Woloshin S, Bickell NA, Schwartz LM, et al: Language barriers in medicine in the United States, *JAMA* 273:724-728, 1995.

9. Feldhaus KM, Koziol-McLain J, Amsbury HL, et al: Accuracy of three brief screening questions for detecting partner violence in the emergency department, *JAMA* 277:1357-1361, 1997.

10. Alpert EJ: Violence in intimate relationships and the practicing internist: new disease or new agenda? *Ann Intern Med* 123:737-746, 1995.

11. Annas GJ: A national bill of patients' rights, *N Engl J Med* 338:695-699, 1998.

12. Balint M: *The Doctor, His Patient, and the Illness,* rev ed, New York, 1972, International Universities Press.

    An outstanding advanced text on psychosocial aspects of outpatient general medicine. Balint, a psychoanalyst, studied family practice in Great Britain by holding weekly seminars with general practitioners. The material is very practical and readable, and very intelligent.

13. Peabody F: The care of the patient, *JAMA* 88:877-882, 1927. Reprinted partially in Stoeckle JD, editor: *Encounters Between Patients and Doctors: An Anthology,* Cambridge, Mass, 1987, MIT Press.

    A classic paper on the ideal doctor-patient relationship.

14. Szasz TS, Hollender MH: A contribution to the philosophy of medicine: the basic models of the doctor-patient relationship, *Arch Intern Med* 97:585-592, 1956. Reprinted in Stoeckle JD, editor:

Encounters Between Patients and Doctors: An Anthology, Cambridge, Mass, 1987, MIT Press.

An introduction to three models of the doctor-patient relationship—activity-passivity, guidance-cooperation, and mutual participation—and how the relationship is influenced by the condition of the patient.

15. Francis V, Korsch BM, Morris MJ: Gaps in doctor-patient communication: patients' response to medical advice, *N Engl J Med* 280:535-540, 1969. Reprinted in Stoeckle JD, editor: *Encounters Between Patients and Doctors: An Anthology,* Cambridge, Mass, 1987, MIT Press.

An influential early study of doctor-patient communication that underscored the impact on patient satisfaction of the doctor's explanation about illness and treatment.

16. Lazare A: Shame and humiliation in the medical encounter, *Arch Intern Med* 147:1653-1658, 1987.

Patients frequently experience shame and humiliation, and these feelings may have great impact on the doctor-patient relationship. Physicians, too, experience these affects. Therapeutic implications are discussed.

17. Berger J, Mohr J: *A Fortunate Man: The Story of a Country Doctor,* New York, 1967, Pantheon Books.

A moving portrait of a British general practitioner and a stimulating inquiry into the nature of medical work.

18. Stoeckle JD, Barsky A: Attributions: uses of social science knowledge in the doctoring of primary care. In Eisenberg L, Kleinman A, editors: *The Relevance of Social Science for Medicine,* Amsterdam, 1980, D Riedel.

19. Lazare A, Eisenthal S, Frank A, et al: Studies on a negotiated approach to patienthood. In Gallagher EB, editor: *The Doctor-Patient Relationship in the Changing Health Scene,* DHEW pub no (NIH) 78-183, Washington, DC, 1978, US Department of Health, Education and Welfare. Reprinted in Stoeckle JD, editor: *Encounters Between Patients and Doctors: An Anthology,* Cambridge, Mass, 1987, MIT Press.

The last two references serve as background papers for the clinical approach described in this text. They are available from the Primary Care Program Educational Office, Ambulatory Care Center 6, Massachusetts General Hospital, Fruit Street, Boston, MA 02114.

ADVANCED
TOPICS

CHAPTER 10

MORE TACTICS FOR ELICITING INFORMATION

The process is not physical, it's mental, and if your mind says you're weak, you'll be tired physically. Your mind is where you control everything. What you think is what you are.

ALEX GRAMMAS, MANAGER
MILWAUKEE BRAVES

ATTRIBUTIONS: WHAT PATIENTS THINK IS CAUSING THEIR ILLNESS

The physician must appreciate what illness means to the patient. This meaning is often embedded in what the patient thinks has caused the illness—the illness attributions. Essential interviewing tasks include listening for, eliciting, and attending to attributions.

What Does "Attribution" Mean?

Before discussing how to elicit attributions, some definitions deserve attention. The term "attribution" is used to denote either a *process*—the cognitive act of explaining a cause ("I think my arthritis came from too much stress at work")—or the *cause* itself—the "self-diagnosis," "self-labeling," or simply "naming" by the patient ("Doc, this pain is in my heart"). Arthur Kleinman, a psychiatrist-medical anthropologist, refers to patients' attributions or explanations as "explanatory models" (see Suggested Readings at the end of the chapter).

Where Do Attributions Come From?

When individuals experience bodily distress, they automatically search for a cause, an explanation. Ascribing cause to uncertain bodily sensations—"My stomach aches; I think I ate too fast and too much"—helps make sense of the experience and provides a sense of control; uncertainty is reduced. The attribution may also suggest action to take, for example, self-treatment ("I'll try some Maalox") or seeking of lay or medical advice ("What do you think, Doc?").

Patients' notions of the cause of their conditions derive mainly from three overlapping sources: (1) lay knowledge about illness, culled from the newspaper, magazines, television, radio, and the patient's lay networks, especially from how family and friends interpret a problem; (2) cultural beliefs about health and illness, learned while growing up in a particular group (e.g., Anglo-Saxon, Asian, Hispanic, or African) and perhaps diverging from the prevailing scientific view; and (3) personal meanings that patients have developed from their own experience with illness (e.g., when illness may be defined as a threat or challenge, or viewed as a personal fault). Personal meanings often derive from incidents of illness among family and friends (e.g., a man whose father recently died of cancer of the lung may interpret minor chest symptoms as signs of a serious illness).

The attributions that individuals entertain about their distress may contain any of several causes, for example:

1. Events before the onset ("I got sick after losing my job")
2. Behaviors of the individual or other persons ("He's been so aggravating that now I'm sick"; "I keep thinking cancer, knowing how much I smoke")
3. The physical environment ("If it hadn't been so cold, I wouldn't have caught this")
4. Medical disease and its perceived biological basis ("My brother had heart trouble, you know; I wonder if that's what I'm getting"; or "It's old age")

Some individuals are quite sophisticated in their attributions, making specific self-diagnoses. ("I think I have an ulcer"; "I think I have angina"). Perhaps surprisingly, individuals may have more than one, even several, explanations of their distress, and may simultaneously express contradicting theories.

Often inseparable from patients' views of the cause of their bodily distress—the etiology, pathophysiology, and diagnosis—are notions about appropriate diagnostic and therapeutic management and prognosis. For example, a patient may present with a request ("I want a chest x-ray") or a concern ("I hope this isn't something real serious") that reflects an attribution ("This cough could be a sign of tuberculosis").

Moreover, while attributions are ideas or explanations, not affects, they convey mood or personality. For example, anxious or depressed patients may tend to assign grave meanings to minor events. Self-blame in the attribution process often conveys underlying guilt or shame. "Defensive styles" for coping with anxiety can be described as habitual patterns of attribution: denial is a process of minimizing or ignoring seriousness (as when a doctor treats his own heart pain as indigestion); projection assigns causality to outside forces; and so forth.

"Medical student disease," as described in an essay by the sociologist David Mechanic, provides a useful model of the attribution process, particularly the development of attributions that diverge from the prevailing medical model. This "disease" is a very common psychosomatic illness that occurs when a medical student interprets normal bodily sensations or minor illness as a sign of a serious condition, often a disease recently encountered in school. Three factors seem important in producing worrisome attributions about an innocuous matter. First, the student, like most patients, lacks the medical knowledge necessary to evaluate the symptom correctly (i.e., as an experienced clinician). Second, external cues direct attention to the symptom and the possibility of a fearful underlying problem. Students often suspect a disease that was recently encountered in medical school or that affected a family member. (An analogous situation for patients is when the media draws attention to a medical condition. For instance, when Happy Rockefeller and Betty Ford were found to have breast cancer, many women interpreted their breast lumps as malignant and rushed to the doctor. Recent publicity about Lyme disease has similarly triggered many consultations. [See the following section on "triggers."]) Third, stress plays a role; the "disease" commonly occurs before major school examinations or is associated with general anxiety. This third factor often helps explain why a worrisome attribution was selected rather than a trivial one, and why the symptom was taken seriously at this time. Thus, incomplete knowledge, external cues or triggers, and stress should be considered in interpreting patients' attributions, especially when the latter seem unusually serious.

The Importance of Attending to Attributions

In the following medical tasks, a recognition of attributions may be useful.

Communication of Information

A good explanation of a patient's diagnosis, treatment, and prognosis should refer to what the patient already thinks is wrong. The practitioner should acknowledge concordance as well as differences between the patient's attributions and the clinician's diagnosis. Agree with the patient, if appropriate, but also explain what the illness is not (as viewed by the patient), while explaining what the doctor thinks it is:

> Like you, I think this is just a cold.

> I know you are concerned about a tumor, but I believe this is a tension headache.

Recognizing and working out the difference between the patient's attributions and the clinical diagnosis promotes patient satisfaction and compliance and also helps you negotiate an appropriate therapy.

> I know you have thought that depression is only psychological, but it also has a biochemical basis for which medication can help.

> I appreciate that you attribute your fatigue to your recent heart attack, but I think your new medicines are causing this.

Effective Reassurance

In managing symptomatic states (pain, dyspepsia, headache, vertigo) and emotional reactions to disease (depression, anxiety), attributions are regularly important. The attribution is the source of worry and anxiety that often brings patients to the doctor and is the focus of their requests for diagnosis and treatment. Many patients desire reassurance instead of or in addition to treatment that relieves symptoms.

Effective reassurance requires learning what the patient thinks is causing the problem. Too often, clinicians offer global or general reassurance ("Everything seems fine" or "You have nothing to worry about") or advice, which often is not reassuring ("Don't let this get you upset" or "You shouldn't let these matters get to you. Leave everything to me"). Effective reassurance is specific: directed to the patient's particular concerns ("This is not a sign of the cancer worsening; this is a sign of the cancer spreading, but it is not as serious as you imagined. We have a rather simple and highly effective treatment for this problem").

When you encounter patients who seem to have been adequately treated and reassured, yet who continue to suffer and seek further care, consider the possibility that they are harboring worries that have not been fully addressed. Elicit their attributions and requests.

Personal Support

Patients are sometimes hesitant to reveal their attributions and attendant worries, although such notions may be the impetus for consulting the physician. Reluctance may stem from the fear that lay beliefs will be ridiculed by the sophisticated medical practitioner. Nonjudgmental listening and responding to attributions and concerns, therefore, help define a therapeutic relationship that is open and supportive.

Ongoing Care and Compliance

Diagnostic and therapeutic actions become the substrate for further attributions. Patients commonly have notions about the significance of their physician's behavior ("He didn't seem to pay much attention to my foot pains, so it's probably nothing"), test results ("He said the urine was fine, so I can't have diabetes or cancer"), and treatments ("This is the same medicine my uncle got after his third heart attack, so I must have a serious heart condition"). Such views may play a significant role in patient satisfaction, compliance, and well-being.

Of particular importance is the patient's view of medications ("These pills make me sick"). Clarification of the patient's view of the action and side effects of drugs may be critical in ensuring optimal compliance.

How to Elicit Attributions

In the course of a routine interview about a problem, many patients will state their attributions directly or will make comments that imply their notions. Often, listening well is sufficient to identify attributions:

Yes, this pain has been with me all morning. I woke up with it, right here and here, and it hurts when you touch. You know it's just been 2 years since Bill died with lung clots.

I've been having these headaches and feeling tired. I guess I've been working a lot the last couple of weeks and not getting much sleep.

Common hints about attributions, as well as opportunities to inquire about them, come from statements about:

1. Triggers:

Patient: . . . so my mother said I better get checked.
Doctor: What was she concerned about?

2. Requests:

Patient: . . . so I figured I'd better get a blood test.
Doctor: What did you hope we could check with the test?

3. Concerns:

Patient: . . . so I got kind of worried.
Doctor: What concerned you?

Attributions may otherwise be elicited by direct questions:

What do you think may be causing your pain?

What do you think might be doing this?

Any idea what is happening to your body (stomach, bladder, other area)?

What do you think you've got?

Answers are not always forthcoming. Patients may be reluctant to disclose their thoughts and may protest that the doctor should answer such questions: "Gee, Doc, that's what I came to see *you* for." Responses that bypass this resistance are:

Everyone has some idea.

What do other people in your family think is the matter with you?

I understand that you don't know, but what do you think is the matter?

Yes, I'll examine you and tell you what I find but I'd like to know what you've been thinking.

Summary: The Uses of Attributions

Attributions reveal the patient's perspective on illness, providing an entrée into the often fascinating world of the patient. Attributions help explain the illness behavior ("triggers" or why the patient came to the doctor). They reflect emotional reactions to bodily complaints (e.g., worry) and strategies for coping with illness (e.g., denial). By appreciating attributions, the doctor learns about the basis of the patient's behavior; by responding to them, the doctor facilitates, personalizes, and enhances care of the patient.

WHY NOW?—TRIGGERS IN THE DECISION TO SEEK MEDICAL CARE

Doctor: Chest pain?
Patient: Yeah, Doc. You see my brother had a heart attack last week.

Bodily distress by itself seldom brings the patient to the doctor. Most of the enormous quantity of physical disturbances experienced in everyday life (and reported in surveys) is ignored, self-diagnosed, and either tolerated, self-treated, or dealt with through the advice of family, friends, or relatives. More-over, many patients experience symptoms that they (and physicians) con-sider serious and deserving of medical attention, yet they do not visit a doctor or they delay such a consultation. Conversely, many patients present with minor complaints that have been well tolerated for days, weeks, or months, and the reasons for now bringing these symptoms to a physician's attention are not obvious. The extra, final push to contact a physician often comes not from the nature of the symptom itself, but from events, called trig-gers, most of which, surprisingly, are social and psychological rather than biomedical.

Triggers are the events that answer the questions, "Why now?" or "Why did this person come in when others might not?" Especially when patients come with problems that have been present for a week or longer, an appre-ciation of the trigger often makes the underlying purpose of the visit intelli-gible. The trigger usually is closely connected with the patient's attributions and requests, and thus the physician's exploration of how the patient de-cided to come to the doctor often provides an important perspective on that person's experience of illncss, coping, personality, care-seeking patterns, and social, economic, and psychological barriers to using medical services. An exploration of triggers may also help the physician assess the degree of dis-ability or distress associated with a symptom as, for instance, when a well-tolerated disability suddenly is brought to attention because a visiting rela-tive insisted on having the doctor check it.

Common Triggers

Based on studies in our medical clinic by Irving Zola, we list six common trig-gers: (1) interpersonal crises, (2) social interference of symptoms, (3) sanc-tions of another person, (4) perceived threat of the symptoms, (5) altered barriers to care, and (6) the nature and quality of symptoms. Some examples of each type are illustrated in the following examples.

Interpersonal Crises

A woman who had been overweight for years came to the doctor for a diet. The in-terview revealed that the decision to get help was made after a highly valued friend remarked at a party that the patient had gotten "so heavy no one could sit next to you." The devaluation by an esteemed friend made her seek medical aid to lose weight and to share her sense of shame. In treatment, the "hurt" in the interpersonal relation was acknowledged, and the patient enrolled in a diet workshop.

A middle-aged postman presented with an irritating rash on his leg which he had experienced for 2 months. On the morning before he called for an appointment, he had a heated argument with his wife and was reprimanded at work. He said he "just got fed up" with the rash and decided to get it checked.

▲

Commonly, patients are more likely to seek attention for a medical problem when they are feeling anxious, sad, overwhelmed, lonely, confused, and so on. Personal crises and other problems of living may heighten people's sensitivity to bodily complaints and their tendency to worry, while also causing them to seek the kindness and attention readily available from a physician.

Patients may not readily connect their care-seeking with their psychological distress, nor is it necessarily important that the physician get them to see such a relationship. However, the physician needs this perspective to treat the acute complaint reasonably and to address the underlying distress. Thus, when patients present with a sense of crisis about vague or relatively minor acute problems or about stable chronic problems, or they simply come repeatedly for such matters, the physician should ask, "Why now?" and explore interpersonal distress:

What else has been going on in your life?

Social Interference

A patient may tolerate symptoms until they hinder valued personal activities or otherwise jeopardize social function.

An older retired foreman had chronic obstructive lung disease and breathlessness for many years, but never sought medical aid. He just "slowed down." Only when he could no longer easily reach his local grocery (where he met daily with his friends) did he decide to seek care. Following medical evaluation, his physical limitations were assessed but no medical action was advised except for arranging transportation so he could continue meeting friends.

▲

Sanctioning

Sometimes, another person's suggestions to seek help will trigger a visit. Some patients only present with their complaints when another person has validated their need for medical attention or given "permission" for them to obtain help.

A factory manager, constantly complaining of fatigue, engaged in self-treatment with vitamins. Despite persistence of symptoms, he was reluctant to seek help. He finally came to the doctor at the urging of his wife (who reported she was exasperated with his complaints). In the interview with both husband and wife, this sanctioning was recognized; the patient's difficulty in seeking help was also acknowledged in eliciting his cooperation for going through a medical workup. In view of the joint decision-making, future communication of information about the patient's illness was addressed to both patient and wife.

A 62-year-old woman presented with a breast lump that she had noticed a number of months ago. She had just seen a television program about a woman who had bravely faced mastectomy, and thus found the courage to seek attention.

▲

Perceived Threat

Patients often present to the doctor because they are anxious about the implications of a symptom. A variety of events may alter the patients' interpretation of the seriousness of an illness.

A 24-year-old college student with intermittent frontal tension headaches, customarily managed with rest and aspirin, presented to the doctor. His father had recently died of a brain tumor. In the interview and treatment, the patient's fear of a brain tumor was acknowledged. A detailed neurological examination was provided to address his concerns, but he was also helped to grieve his father's death.

A 72-year-old man presented with a long-standing, easily reducible right inguinal hernia. He had sought medical consultation after mentioning the matter to a friend, who had warned him about the dangers of strangulated hernias. The swelling was not bothering the patient, and he was not interested in an operation unless he was in danger. He was reassured.

▲

Reduction of Barriers

A variety of obstacles hinder patients from consulting with physicians. Among these barriers are the accessibility of the physician (distance from the patient's home or work, availability and ease of transportation, difficulty in speaking to the physician over the phone or getting an appointment, expense, and so forth) and a variety of personal factors that are social, economic, and psychological (ability to take time off from work, need for "permission" to allocate time and money for personal needs, conflicting demands on time and resources, readiness to recognize the potential seriousness of the problem, willingness to accept help).

Well, I had to come in with my daughter today for her school physical, so I figured I'd get this rash checked.

I just got my Medicaid card back, so I can afford to have some tests and more asthma medicine.

My husband is on vacation, so I was able to leave the kids at home with him.

I wanted to get it checked last week, but I knew you were away. Then the phone was busy when I called yesterday. Today I got right through to the secretary, and she gave me this appointment.

The Nature of the Symptom

Finally, the quality of the bodily distress may trigger a visit, particularly when discomfort becomes intolerable.

A 50-year-old carpenter had such sudden, severe back pain that he could not move. He quickly sought emergency care because he "could not take it." In treatment, the patient was quickly medicated to obtain relief.

▲

Eliciting Information About Triggers

More often than not, if one listens carefully, the patient's narrative of the illness will bring up the trigger elements, and the interviewer may simply ask for elaboration upon or confirmation of what was heard:

Do I understand that you felt this pain had just lasted too long?

Do I understand it was your wife who was concerned about your condition?

When the trigger is not evident, some of the following questions can be tried:

How did you decide to see us for this trouble?

What made you decide to get help for your pain?

Was anyone else involved in your coming for medical advice? I see, it was your husband. What did he think?

Did you discuss it with anyone else? What did they think?

NONVERBAL COMMUNICATION

The body says what words cannot.

Attributed to Martha Graham

The physician, listening from day to day, catches a hint of it [the poem] in his preoccupation. By listening to the minutest variations of the speech we begin to detect that today, as always, the essence is also to be found, hidden under the verbiage, seeking to be realized.

William Carlos Williams
The Autobiography (1951)

Communication occurs along two channels, verbal and nonverbal. The verbal transmits information as words and conveys most of the overt meaning of the interview, as would be captured in a verbatim transcript. The nonverbal includes communication through appearance, body language, touch, smell, and those qualities of speech that give spoken words meaning beyond what would be imparted by reading them silently.

Verbal information alone does not account for the richness of interpersonal communication; nonverbal channels do. Nuance and emotional meaning are particularly conveyed through nonverbal means. Expert interviewers "intuit" their patients' feelings, using nonverbal clues, and they use this information to guide the interview. Furthermore, the affective relationship of doctor and patient is primarily established through nonverbal communication. The satisfaction that patients derive from their medical encounters is evinced in greatest part from the personal regard, interest, and friendliness conveyed by the doctor in his or her nonverbal manner.

Every individual shares in a large stock of biologically determined nonverbal behaviors such as crying or smiling, but also develops his or her own personal ones. Both doctor and patient bring their behaviors to every encounter, for instance, in the way they greet each other, sit, walk, speak, dress, gesture, talk, and so on. Moreover, both parties are constantly "decoding" each other's nonverbal behaviors, reading meaning into them. This process of conveying and interpreting signals is nonverbal communication. For example, a patient decodes a doctor as "not very friendly" because he does not smile or his voice sounds gruff, while the doctor notes that the patient seems angry because she raises her voice and blushes while answering.

Nonverbal communication is important, yet it most often is carried out without self-awareness or conscious control. Furthermore, nonverbal messages are often difficult to interpret reliably or to use. Some are quite difficult to recognize, while others may be beyond conscious recognition, requiring specialized techniques for demonstration. Our own nonverbal behaviors, even when we see and hear them, are not easy to change. Indeed, the practical benefits of teaching how to use nonverbal communication are currently unclear. We suspect that clinicians can benefit from special training in recognizing and responding to "body language" and to other nonverbal behaviors of patients; they are likely to alter only a few of their own behaviors. Therefore in this chapter, we remind you about appreciating your patient's, and perhaps your own, nonverbal cues, while suggesting a few practical clinical applications.

How Does Nonverbal Communication Work?

The two major sources of nonverbal communication in the interview are observable behaviors, or "body language" (such as appearance, gestures, facial expression, and how closely one chooses to sit or stand near the other person) and qualities of speech, or paralinguistics (such as tone, pace, emphasis, and pauses). Except in the physical examination, the physician's physical contact generally plays a lesser part, although it should be noted that forms of touch—the handshake, a supporting arm, an embrace, placing a hand on the patient's arm or shoulder—can convey interpersonal messages that are therapeutic.

In general, nonverbal channels qualify verbal information. They give emphasis or otherwise clarify what is being said. For instance, a raised voice, tightly pursed lips, and a clenched fist convey the immediacy and severity of anger. Intonation or gestures can even tell us that the intended meaning of speech is the opposite from the verbal content, as when a patient uses an ironic tone, shakes his head slowly as if to be saying "Yes," and rolls his eyes upward while saying "That's great" or "I'm glad to hear that."

Nonverbal messages may be redundant, conveying meanings that are evident from the verbal channel or other nonverbal communication. For instance, a young man may say he is depressed or report a sense of sadness and hopelessness, while we also notice that he moves slowly, has a slumped or defeated posture, maintains a morose facial expression, and looks like he is about to cry, while speaking slowly in a sad tone, punctuated by long pauses and sights. Any one of these behaviors may be an early clue to the patient's depressive feelings or may confirm the interviewer's final impressions.

Nonverbal messages are often ambiguous. An isolated nonverbal behavior may be read with multiple meanings, depending on its context. In the case of the sad patient, for instance, the slowness may reflect physical problems, such as muscular stiffness, pain, or fatigue. The monotonous voice may be indicative of a variety of emotional and physical disorders or simply be this patient's normal speech pattern. Even a readily recognized behavior such as crying can be associated with such diverse emotions as sadness, anger, and joy, or with neurological deficits. Therefore we must often rely on other clinical information to validate our impressions of the meaning of specific nonverbal behaviors.

The ambiguity of nonverbal messages may lead to misinterpretations. For instance, some physicians always (and unconsciously) raise their voice for non-English-speaking persons and the elderly, and thus are sometimes perceived as impatient or gruff by such patients. Cultural differences can also lead to misinterpretations. For example, there are distinct ethnic and racial differences in the "rules" for normal physical closeness and for eye contact and patterns of gaze in daily conversation. A physician who talks while standing close or maintaining direct eye contact may seem intrusive or hostile to some patients, normal to others. Similarly, certain dress and body language may convey cheerfulness, kindness, and openness in some contexts, while suggesting sloppiness or seductiveness in others. A man's beard may seem, on first impression, to signify friendliness and being "laid back" to some persons, while indicating hostility and stiffness to others, at least until the visual message is modified by other verbal or nonverbal communication.

Nonverbal clues may also be discrepant from each other or from verbal communication. This typically occurs when the patient is trying to cover up feelings or dissemble. While most patients can adjust the verbal meaning of their speech intentionally to deliver a false message, the nonverbal channels are less under conscious control. Even when a person is not aware of an emotion or is trying to conceal it, the affect can express itself: nonverbal information may "leak out." For instance, an interviewer may tell a patient, "Take all the time you need," but be noticed glancing at his watch, fidgeting with his pen, moving his feet restlessly, and making so little eye contact that observers (such as the patient) correctly presume that he is feeling rushed and impatient. Only very skilled actors are able to consciously choose a message and then convey it consistently through both verbal and nonverbal channels. Less skilled actors, such as most patients and doctors, leak discrepant or incongruous messages. Of course, such clues may not be detected.

Decoding Nonverbal Communication

Recognition of nonverbal messages can facilitate a better understanding of the patient. Students of nonverbal communication note that this channel particularly conveys affects (anger, sadness, joy), interpersonal behaviors (deception, attraction, intimacy), and personality attributes (friendliness, suspiciousness, hostility).

Some further examples of nonverbal messages that may be recognized and potentially useful are described below.

Sources of Nonverbal Communication

Posture
Note particularly whether the patient is leaning toward or away from you and how this sign of interest, involvement, and interpersonal comfort changes over the course of the interview. Body language may suggest openness (sitting back comfortably in the chair, arms resting comfortably at the sides, legs uncrossed) or tension, defensiveness, or disagreement (sitting erect and pushed back against the chair or slightly turned away from the interviewer, arms crossed and held over the chest, legs tightly crossed). Tension is often evident in the hands as fidgeting, drumming, wringing, or intermittent clenching of a fist.

Proxemics (closeness)
How far from you the patient chooses to sit may reflect cultural patterns, but might also suggest defensiveness or suspiciousness (indicated by a preference for increased distance) or a desire for more intimacy (when sitting closer). As patients become more comfortable and "feel closer" (and sometimes when they are acting manipulatively), they tend to move closer. Of course, patients often have no choice about seating.

Touching
Touching may convey empathy, affiliation, or attraction, though this gesture may also be decoded as intrusive, sexist, or patronizing.

Gaze and eye contact
Pay particular attention to instances when patients avoid your gaze, perhaps signaling shame, shyness, submission, avoidance, or deception.

Facial expression
The face is rich in expression; the interviewer's attention to the patient's face is well rewarded. Facial expression reveals the patient's momentary feelings about you and the interview. A subtle smile or smirk or a twinkle in the eyes may suggest a sense of pleasure about matters that are overtly described as undesirable. A tense, rigid expression may indicate a need to hold back or control feelings. A slight flush suggests embarrassment or the emergence of strong feelings.

Intonation
When patients are feeling sad, they tend to speak quietly and slowly. The voice may become deeper or gravelly, and they often look down. Anger tends to raise voice pitch, while attempts to control emotions may lower pitch.

Speech rate and pauses

Anxiety is often signaled in the rapidity of speech. When patients pause slightly longer than expected after an interviewer's question, they may be weighing what to say rather than giving a spontaneous (and perhaps more truthful) thought.

Using the Patient's Nonverbal Communication

Most of the time, nonverbal messages are taken in by the clinician with little self-awareness and are used to clarify verbal meaning. Since the patient usually does not consciously intend to convey meaning through nonverbal behaviors and since such nonverbal messages may be ambiguous or unclear, the interviewer must be cautious about treating such data as recognized facts without making sure the patient accepts their validity. Occasionally, nonverbal messages can be "fed back" to the patient to elicit more information. For instance, when a patient's nonverbal messages suggest more affect than the patient is reporting directly or when otherwise unappreciated (or even denied) affect is leaked, the clinician may acknowledge or interpret these messages:

> You seem hurt. How come?
>
> You act depressed to me.
>
> You look scared.

Attempts at concealing feelings may be confronted directly:

> You say everything is fine, but you seem upset.
>
> Somehow, you don't look like you really mean it when you say that.

Using Your Own Nonverbal Communications: Can You Change Yourself?

Observing oneself and becoming aware of one's own nonverbal messages is difficult, especially when those messages are discrepant from what one is thinking and feeling or are different from what one intends to convey to others. However, self-monitoring is aided by the use of videotapes or audiotapes, by obtaining direct supervision of interviewing, and by attending to how you affect your patients.

Changing your nonverbal habits is also difficult and often comes off as simply being manipulative. Mimicking friendly or empathic behavior, for instance, is rarely convincing. Nonverbal behaviors are instinctive and part of your personality and thus are more often factors to be recognized and reckoned with than features that can be readily changed. However, you may consider modifying some behaviors that are problematic in the clinical encounter (e.g., nervous habits) or that trouble particular patients (e.g., restraining your exuberance or limiting physical contact). You may also practice and try to be more expressive of facilitative behaviors that come naturally, such as broad smiles, greeting with a warm handshake, nodding your head to encourage the patient, sitting near the patient's bedside, and keeping your head at the same height as the patient's while talking—all of which might be considered "good manners."

Finally, your nonverbal messages are more likely to convey interest and concern if you clear your mind of distractions so that you can listen attentively and if you make a conscious effort to find something you like about patients and to try to appreciate their suffering.

ASKING ABOUT ALCOHOL

> *"Your patients are abusing drugs whether you see it or not."*
>
> Advertisement to Physicians

> *Sixty-five percent of Americans report drinking alcoholic beverages. Seven percent—over 13 million persons—are alcoholic, and 10% or more of adult office patients are likely to be.*

> *Five percent of physicians personally engage in substance abuse, chiefly alcohol; significant abuse among medical students has also been described.*

Substance abuse is the chronic excessive use of alcohol or other drugs despite known adverse effects on social, psychological, and physical functioning. Medical practitioners commonly miss this diagnosis. In working up every patient, careful inquiry about alcohol and other drugs will help identify those who misuse these substances.

Blocks to Recognizing Alcohol Abuse: The Patient's and the Doctor's

Patients rarely complain directly about substance abuse or seek help for it. Indeed, accurate information about drug and alcohol habits is often difficult to obtain from patients who are abusing these substances. One reason is that patients consciously conceal such problems because of shame and guilt. They avoid disclosing painful facts about their lack of control and the negative consequences of their habits, and they shun situations in which they may be rebuked about their behavior.

A second, related reason for the difficulty of eliciting accurate information is the strong tendency for substance abusers to deny their own habit. They *unconsciously* keep their behavior from clear self-awareness. Alcoholics regularly fail to recognize the adverse effects of their drinking. Even when confronted with seemingly incontrovertible signs (e.g., "the shakes," gastritis, cirrhosis, accidents, and injuries), they minimize, rationalize, or frankly ignore the facts. Such denial is an unconscious process—not a willful "cover-up"—and may partially reflect the effect of chronic intoxication upon memory. Denial allows the psychological contortion whereby drinking may be alternately perceived as a source of problems and as a solution to them.

Nondisclosure and denial make substance abusers "difficult" patients. The doctor's goals for the interview—to obtain accurate information about substance abuse, to achieve consensus about what behavior requires attention, and to arrive at a mutually acceptable plan for treatment—conflict with the patient's pattern of avoiding acknowledgment of the problem. Indeed, in few other interview situations are clinicians so regularly subject to being misled and even to perceiving the patient as an adversary. Moreover, when patients are confronted with their behaviors, potentially difficult emotions (anger, shame, and guilt) are evoked, and the interviewer may be perceived as antagonistic.

Another block to the diagnosis of alcoholism arises from the clinician's attitude. Ambivalence about drinking is common. On the one hand, popular culture tends to associate alcohol use with relaxation and sociability and to look upon drunkenness with amusement, even tacit approval. On the other hand, alcohol abuse is often viewed with marked disdain—as evidence of a terrible personal failing and of psychological or moral weakness. Rather than being a victim of a disease, the alcoholic is seen as willfully self-destructive. The clinician's disapproval colors the care of the patient and interferes with the development of a therapeutic alliance.

Furthermore, for clinicians who come into frequent contact with patients in advanced stages of substance abuse, particularly in the general hospital where relapse and serious complications are the rule, a pessimistic, hopeless feeling about alcoholics often prevails, perhaps reinforced by the helplessness expressed by patients. Physicians with unrealistic expectations about the course of alcoholism may repeatedly find themselves let down by the patients they try to help and thus come to view alcoholics as uncooperative, self-destructive, dishonest, and unable to carry through with medical advice. The clinician's pessimism hinders effective therapy with such advanced alcoholics, while also leading to a lack of enthusiasm and diligence in identifying and treating earlier, more treatable stages of the disease.

A clinician may feel particularly awkward labeling patients as alcoholics or substance abusers when their behavior does not seem grossly different from that of friends (or perhaps oneself). Labeling may be easier when the patient is a skid row bum, but many alcoholics are young and come from social and educational backgrounds similar to those of the clinician. Moreover, there is no laboratory test or "gold standard" criterion for identifying alcoholism. The diagnosis is based on the history. The clinician often lacks rigorous guidelines about what should be considered alcoholism or problem drinking (vs. heavy drinking or "normal" use), while the patient is unlikely to help the physician by concurring that substance abuse is occurring. Laboratory tests rarely can help one make the diagnosis. Therefore the clinician must be willing to use a potentially stigmatizing label and to make a clear, independent judgment of substance abuse.

Getting Around the Difficulty: Effective Screening for Alcohol Abuse

The clinician who expects to identify alcoholics by asking patients directly about the quantity of drinks they consume will detect only a small proportion of persons for whom alcohol is already a problem, mostly those with a far-advanced condition. Recognition of the early signs of problem drinking (and hence the ability to intervene before the habit becomes more intractable) requires a careful, skilled interview.

Earlier portions of this text describe the basic interviewing techniques (such as establishing trust and rapport, being empathic and nonjudgmental, and ensuring confidentiality, and so forth) that help patients talk about matters they ordinarily would keep private. Remember that most alcoholics feel quite guilty or ashamed about their behavior and their lack of control, and that they may have already encountered harsh, scolding, punitive physicians.

A valuable initial technique in obtaining a history of alcohol use is to avoid direct inquiry about the amount of alcohol consumed or any discussion that requires the patient to acknowledge directly that alcohol is a problem. Problem drinkers tend to give misleading answers about the quantity of alcohol used or may engage the interviewer in what often proves to be a useless discussion about how much other people drink and what is "normal." Instead, seek information about the adverse consequences of substance abuse, particularly about impaired control, physical and psychological dependence, and various medical, psychological, occupational, social, and legal outcomes of problem drinking. Nonjudgmental questions, such as those included in two batteries of screening questions discussed later—the CAGE test and the MAST test—will generally be answered accurately enough for the interviewer to obtain a fair picture of the impairment from substance abuse, if not the quantity consumed.

Specific Approaches to Identifying Alcohol Use

Screen Everyone

In view of the prevalence of alcoholism in the medical population, obtain at least a basic screening history for alcoholism on all patients.

Be Alert to Clues

Alcoholic patients may complain of a variety of physical or psychosocial problems that are consequences of substance abuse—seizures and blackouts (not remembering what happened while drinking); pancreatitis, gastritis, hepatitis, cirrhosis, and a number of other gastrointestinal disturbances; peripheral neuropathy; hypertension (often poorly responsive to treatment); accidents and fights; fatigue; sleep disturbances and depression; marital and work problems; and other drug problems—yet not connect these problems to drinking. Indeed, "problems of daily living" may be the most common early signs of disease. The alert interviewer will particularly want to explore the possibility of alcohol abuse when such complaints are noted. Other clues include poor compliance and the chronic use of minor tranquilizers. A family history of alcoholism also makes substance abuse much more likely to be a problem or concern for the patient (see Quick Tips: Clues to Identifying Alcohol Abuse).

QUICK TIPS

Clues to Identifying Alcohol Abuse

- Seizures
- Blackouts
- Gastrointestinal disturbances
- Peripheral neuropathy
- Hypertension
- Accidents and fights

- Violent behaviors
- Fatigue
- Sleep disorders
- Depression

The CAGE Test

The CAGE test consists of four questions on effects of drinking (Table 10-1). We encourage you to use the CAGE test or a similar brief screening instrument with all patients who give a positive answer to the basic screening question, "Do you drink alcohol?" These four subtle, well-tested questions (with very good sensitivity and specificity, a positive predictive value around 62%, and a negative predictive value around 98%) help the interviewer gain access to essential data for identifying substance abuse while avoiding direct confrontation with denial. The first CAGE question, "Have you ever felt the need to *Cut* down on drinking?" teases out concerns about controlling the drinking behavior, and, if answered affirmatively, can be followed by questions about when and why the patient wanted to cut down and why it might be difficult. The second question—"Have you ever felt *Annoyed* by criticism of drinking?"—helps identify whether others have been adversely affected by the patient's habit and, if answered affirmatively, leads to questions about who has been bothered and why. The third question—"Have you ever had *Guilty* feelings about drinking?"—may elicit the ubiquitous sense of guilt of those who cannot control their substance abuse, or may be followed with a

---

Table 10-1   The CAGE Questionnaire
Have you ever felt the need to *Cut* down on drinking?
Have you ever felt *Annoyed* by criticism of drinking?
Have you ever had *Guilty* feelings about drinking?
Have you ever taken a morning *Eye* opener?

From Mayfield D, McLead G, Hall P: *Am J Psychiatry* 131:1121, 1974.

question—"Ever done things you regretted?"—leading to a discussion of undesirable behaviors attributed to intoxication (rowdiness, getting in accidents or fights, family problems, losing a job, getting arrested). Finally, the fourth question—"Have you ever taken a morning Eye Opener?"—identifies one of the common signs of serious physical dependence and may be followed by further inquiry about the alcohol withdrawal syndrome (e.g., "Did you need to steady your nerves? Treat a hangover?" "Do you ever get the shakes when you stop drinking?"). One positive answer to the CAGE test should lead to further inquiry about problem drinking; two positive answers can be considered as strong evidence of alcoholism. Defensiveness in response to the questions should also support the interviewer's concerns about a drinking problem.

Among patients who *never* use alcohol are recovered alcoholics. Thus, if a patient reports not drinking, you should inquire if he or she ever drank regularly or had a problem with alcohol.

The MAST Questionnaire

The MAST questionnaire (Table 10-2) addresses in detail a variety of medical and psychosocial disorders that are regularly associated with substance abuse, as well as some specific questions about the medical and legal consequences of alcohol abuse. Review it as a useful guide to further inquiry.

Other Sources of History

Additionally, whenever you suspect alcoholism but the diagnosis is not confirmed by the patient, seek information from family, friends, and others in the patient's network.

Characterizing Drinking Behavior

While the approaches described above are directed at identifying problem drinking and at avoiding being misled, further characterization of the patient's drinking behavior is useful for individualizing counseling and referral.

Characterizing the Patient's Drinking Behavior _____

Development of the habit
> When did you start drinking?
>
> When did you start drinking regularly?
>
> How has your drinking changed?
>
> Do you use any other drugs? Prescription or other?

Drinking Pattern
> Where and when do you drink?
>
> Who provides the alcohol?
>
> Who are the people you drink with?

Table 10-2	The MAST Questionnaire		

1. Do you feel you are a normal drinker? — (No 2) Yes
2. Have you ever awakened in the morning after some drinking the night before and found that you could not remember part of the evening? — (Yes 2) No
3. Does your wife (or husband or parents) ever worry or complain about your drinking? — (Yes 1) No
4. Can you stop drinking without a struggle after one or two drinks? — (No 2) Yes
5. Do you ever feel bad about your drinking? — (Yes 2) No
6. Do you ever try to limit your drinking to certain times of day or to certain places? — (Yes 0) No
7. Do your friends or relatives think that you are a normal drinker? — (No 2) Yes
8. Are you always able to stop when you want to? — (No 2) Yes
9. Have you ever attended a meeting of Alcoholics Anonymous? — (Yes 5) No
10. Have you gotten into fights when drinking? — (Yes 1) No
11. Has drinking ever created problems with you and your wife (husband)? — (Yes 2) No
12. Has your wife (husband or other family member) ever gone to anyone for help about your drinking? — (Yes 2) No
13. Have you ever lost friends or girlfriends/boyfriends because of drinking? — (Yes 2) No
14. Have you ever gotten into trouble at work because of drinking? — (Yes 2) No
15. Have you ever lost a job because of drinking? — (Yes 2) No
16. Have you ever neglected your obligations, your family, or your work for two days or more in a row because of drinking? — (Yes 2) No
17. Do you ever drink before noon? — (Yes 1) No
18. Have you ever been told you have liver trouble? — (Yes 2) No
19. Have you ever had DTs (delerium tremens), severe shaking, heard voices or seen things that weren't there after heavy drinking? — (Yes 2) No
20. Have you ever gone to anyone for help about your drinking? — (Yes 5) No
21. Have you ever been in a hospital because of drinking? — (Yes 5) No
22. Have you ever been a patient in a psychiatric hospital or on a psychiatric ward of a general hospital where drinking was part of the problem? — (Yes 2) No
23. Have you ever been seen at a psychiatric or mental health clinic, or gone to a doctor or clergyman for help with an emotional problem in which drinking has played a part? — (Yes 2) No
24. Have you ever been arrested, even for a few hours, because of drunken behavior? — (Yes 2) No
25. Have you ever been arrested for drunk driving or driving after drinking? — (Yes 2) No

A score of three points or less is considered nonalcoholic; a score of four points is suggestive, and a score of five points or more indicates alcoholism.

*From Selzer ML: The Michigan alcoholism screening test, *Am J Psychiatry* 127:1653, 1971.

Do you have close friends who are heavy drinkers?

Do you have nondrinking friends?

Do you drink alone?

Motivation

What do you think leads you to drink?

What beneficial effects do you note with drinking?

What problems?

How do you feel about your drinking?

Have you ever seen it as a problem?

Consumption

When was your last drink?

What kind of alcohol do you drink?

How much do you drink? How often?

How rapidly is it consumed?

Management of the Alcoholic Patient

Alcoholism is a long-term health problem, a chronic illness. It rarely admits to a simple, quick cure. Treatment goals must often be modest, yet many patients eventually make significant progress. Patients may be slow to recognize their problem or to seek help. Improvement is often followed by relapse, so ongoing follow-up is essential.

Once you make the diagnosis of alcoholism from the interview and perhaps further characterize the patient's drinking behavior, the next step is to ascertain whether the patient accepts the diagnosis. Some patients have made a correct self-diagnosis before the interview, but often the clinician's conclusion is rejected, or, if accepted, is not acted on.

While the acquisition of a good history of alcohol abuse requires a supportive, empathic approach, the interviewer who wishes to counsel alcoholics must also learn to be direct and gently confrontational with patients who deny their drinking problems. Confrontation may begin with a nonjudgmental but firm report on specific evidence of addictive behavior, loss of control, and various adverse consequences of the habit and with statements that indicate the clinician's serious concern. Patients should not be pushed beyond their limits; the clinician's presentation should focus calmly on the concrete evidence of problem drinking, but need not alienate the patient by seeming to label the patient as deceptive or bad. Patients generally benefit from clear, nonjudgmental statements about the nature of their problem and its seriousness and from firm, repeated suggestions about making changes and obtaining help.

Many alcoholic patients are, at heart, despondent and will benefit from a hopeful, encouraging approach. Remember that they feel powerless and will appreciate your acceptance.

Patients and family members regularly need basic education about the disease of alcoholism and about the medical and psychosocial effects of problem drinking. Involvement of the family, friends, or employers may also help patients recognize the seriousness of their problem.

When patients do accept the diagnosis or at least recognize a problem and are willing to consider measures to examine or change their behavior, then the clinician is faced with decisions about the best mode of treatment for that individual, including whether the patient should be managed solely by the primary care physician or should be referred to a psychotherapist, a community agency, Alcoholics Anonymous, or an inpatient facility. Patients who do best with primary care physicians often have major medical problems (cirrhosis, cardiomyopathy), are aided by strong, stable social networks, and enjoy confidence in their physician. Additionally, a variety of pharmacological interventions may help manage drug withdrawal or promote abstinence. Regardless, keeping contact with patients and families during counseling is important for supporting their efforts to abstain. The references at the end of the chapter explain more about dealing with patients who deny their problem and about helping patients with counseling and referral.

THE SEXUAL HISTORY AND OTHER PERSONAL TOPICS

A 14-year-old girl comes to your office for the first time and requests a pregnancy test. How will you find out what she knows about sexual anatomy and physiology? What is her actual sexual practice? Does she need information about contraception? Does she need a pelvic exam? Should you involve her family? How will you discuss these topics?

A 35-year-old single male hospital administrator presents with "jock itch." As you conclude your evaluation and prescribe antifungal lotion, he asks if the rash is contagious. You suspect he is concerned about sexually transmitted disease. How will you inquire about his sexual activity? Does he have one or more partners? Of what sex? Is he concerned about AIDS? How should confidentiality be addressed?

A 56-year-old man is leaving the hospital 10 days after a heart attack. You assume he is concerned about resuming sexual activity, but what should you tell him? What kind of specific, clear advice can you offer?

Everyone has a sexual life—thoughts, feelings, and behaviors that usually play an important role in one's well-being. Sexuality is a common concern for patients in adapting to medical and psychological disorders and their treatment. Yet the topic of sexuality is often overlooked in clinical work.

The discussion of sexuality in the medical interview—bringing up the topic, getting an appropriately detailed history, addressing concerns, and, when necessary, providing counseling, referral, or other treatment—is influenced by a number of inhibitions that both doctor and patient bring to the encounter: social taboos, shame, and guilt about sexuality, intolerance to some of the diverse attitudes and values on this topic or to particular practices, and concerns about seeming to be intrusive, voyeuristic, or seductive. The sexual history might be easy in a more open culture in which we all were comfortable with every sort of attitude, feeling, and behavior in the private sexual life of consenting adults, and if patients sensed neither guilt nor shame about fantasies, wishes, or practices, nor expected disapproval from their physician. However, despite the "sexual revolution," patients cannot disclose sexual fantasies and such practices as masturbation or anal intercourse as easily as they discuss a sore shoulder or a cold. Thus a sexual history requires special attention.

Four general principles of interviewing about sexuality deserve mention. (Similar principles apply to interviewing about such other "personal" topics as marital discord, family violence, substance abuse, and even talking about professional fees.)

First, if you don't ask about sexuality, you probably won't find out about it. Patients regularly avoid the topic or refer to it with vague innuendos and faint clues. Topics such as rape, sexual abuse, or incest are rarely introduced at office visits without the initiative or encouragement of the physician. The clinician has the responsibility to broach the discussion of sexuality—to "open the door." A sensitive introduction of the topic is often greeted by patients with a sense of profound relief. Of course, not everyone will want to talk about the subject, even after appropriate preparation, and, in such circumstances, patients are generally quite adept at avoiding discussion by being reticent or evasive, giving nonverbal clues that the interviewer is being intrusive, or explicitly rejecting the topic.

At the end of this section, strategies are noted for introducing sexuality into the routine interview and for raising this topic in conjunction with specific physical or psychosocial problems or for the purpose of health education and disease prevention.

Second, if you don't ask about sexuality, you won't learn how to talk about it. Discussing sexuality with patients helps you become more comfortable with asking about it and with responding to the answers you get. The student who wants to learn to provide basic sexual counseling must make a conscientious effort to discuss sexuality with patients.

Third, effective interviewing about sexuality requires a knowledge base. Just as clinical knowledge about heart and lung disease is necessary for effectively interviewing a patient with chest pain, a background knowledge about human sexuality is needed to take a sexual history. Patients may assume that their doctors have expertise on sexuality, but many physicians are poorly informed and may be reluctant to introduce and pursue a subject about which they have not been trained. A few references that can provide the required knowledge have been listed at the end of the chapter (see Suggested Readings).

A solid intellectual grounding in human sexuality, of course, does not automatically enable the interviewer to deal with this topic in the clinical interview. Opportunities for practicing the sexual interview, observing role models, and being supervised will help beginners use their background knowledge to communicate effectively with patients. A good knowledge base (and a bit of clinical experience) also helps answer two questions that students often ask: "Why should I bring up sexuality?" and "When should I bring it up?" (Table 10-3).

Table 10-3   Why Discuss Sex?

1. Sexual activity is related to the etiology, pathophysiology, and presentation of common illnesses, such as:
   Sexually transmitted diseases
   Urinary tract infections
   Atrophic vaginitis
2. Fertility and family planning are major health concerns for some patients
3. Many medical conditions and their management directly affect sexual function:
   Congenital abnormalities of the genitourinary tract
   Endocrinological and genetic disorders
   Neurological dysfunction
   Vascular diseases
   Genitourinary diseases
   Pelvic surgery
   Arthritis
   Diabetes
   Physical handicaps
   Debilitating chronic illness (e.g., advanced heart or lung disease)
   Medications
   Pregnancy
4. Many psychosocial problems and their management affect sexual function:
   Depression, anxiety
   Marital or other interpersonal discord
   Altered self-image (e.g., following mastectomy)
   Substance abuse
   Psychotropic medication
5. For comprehensive counseling on rehabilitation (e.g., after myocardial infarction or surgery of the breast or pelvis)
6. For health promotion and disease prevention—counseling on topics such as:
   Sexually transmitted diseases
   Contraception
   Physical and emotional well-being
7. For health education—misinformation and ignorance are common, and physicians are important sources of knowledge and advice
8. "To open the door"—introduce the topic to define the scope of communication and of the doctor-patient relationship

Finally, once the interviewer learns about sexuality and becomes comfortable with the topic, most difficulties in obtaining a sexual history (and with investigating other "personal matters") represent problems with the basic interviewing principles that have already been described in Part I of this text. Therefore some elementary interviewing principles are recapitulated in the next section of this chapter to identify common problems encountered in discussing sexuality. Later, a few special techniques are described that are useful for interviewing about sexuality and other emotionally charged topics.

Basic Interviewing Techniques for the Sexual History and Other Personal Topics

Trust

Establish rapport before pursuing difficult topics. If an initial inquiry about sexuality is rebuffed, try again later (but don't defer the discussion indefinitely). Many difficult topics do not need to be explored fully in a single interview, especially in the initial encounter, and are best handled over time as the doctor-patient relationship develops.

Setting

Choose a conducive setting. Sexuality is difficult to discuss without privacy. Don't expect the patient to respond openly to questions about sexuality while lying in stirrups for a pelvic examination or while standing naked for a hernia check.

Manner

A relaxed, matter-of-fact manner eases communication. A degree of formality in discussing sexuality helps patients appreciate that the topic is being introduced for professional medical reasons, yet excessive formality can make the physician seem too distant. On the other hand, extremely casual inquiry about sexuality, which does not reflect some delicacy in discussing the topic, may make the patient feel awkward, threatened, or intruded upon and hence unwilling to disclose personal information.

Language

Pay attention to words. You will often need to define clinical terms and also provide basic sexual education about anatomy and physiology. An important step for students is to become comfortable introducing such words as "vagina" or "penis" in the clinical interview. Beware of resorting to sexual euphemisms ("your privates") and vague terms ("down below"); such terminology may seem condescending, will sustain the patient's lack of technical knowledge, and will reinforce a sense that the topic is off bounds.

Unfamiliar technical words, however, may bewilder the patient or make the discussion seem sanitized and awkward. At times, lay terms—"getting my friend," "gay," "going down," and even "down below"—may be the patient's easiest way of referring, respectively, to menstruation, homosexuality, oral-genital sex, and the genital area. If you are comfortable with such words, you may facilitate discussion by initially adopting the patient's vocabulary, while also introducing more formal terminology. However, slang or vulgar terms should be used reluctantly, since they may embarrass the patient and cause confusion about whether the clinician is maintaining a professional role.

Facilitation

Patients often introduce sexual issues obliquely, and the interviewer must be prepared to pick up on subtle leads. Be ready to listen, facilitate, and clarify with a nonjudgmental attitude. Open-ended questioning and the physician's willingness to ease the conversation toward sexual topics will often be sufficient to produce an initial sexual history.

Allow enough time for the topic. When you do not have time, acknowledge the importance of the topic and arrange for later discussion. If you introduce sexuality during routine questioning, make sure the patient appreciates that you are ready to discuss the matter more fully. Beware of introducing sexuality during a rapidly administered review of systems during which you mostly expect "no" as an answer.

Sexuality is a topic that makes patients and interviewers anxious. Anxiety often leads to premature closure on a topic: incomplete histories, failure to acknowledge concerns, facile advice, inappropriate reassurance, and so on. Listen and explore before responding.

Responding to Affect

Acknowledge discomfort about the topic. Attend to the patient's verbal and nonverbal expressions of difficulty in discussing sexuality and respond empathically. Where appropriate, offer reassurance.

> I suspect you are not used to talking much about these matters.

> I'm glad you've brought up this personal concern. I know it's rather personal and may be difficult to discuss, but I also see it as an important health issue.

You may also explore the discomfort itself:

> Why is that difficult to talk about?

The answer here often leads to a useful discussion.

Beware of Assumptions, Stereotypes, and Intrusive Values

Do not assume that your patients are well informed on sexual topics or that an eagerness to talk about one aspect of sexuality connotes willingness to discuss other aspects. Remember that patients vary widely in their knowledge about sexual anatomy and physiology and in their attitudes and understanding about such topics as premarital and extramarital intercourse, birth control, abortion, sexual education for children, gender identity and role, masturbation, homosexuality, the menstrual cycle, menopause, and impotence. Beware of ageism. Many elderly persons are sexually active. If they are not sexually active, they may be distressed by impaired sexual function and its effects on relationships. Many have concerns.

The admonition to avoid assumptions is particularly important in interviewing about sexual orientation and practices. A wide range of sexual preferences may be expressed in fantasies, attitudes, and behaviors. Do not make assumptions about whether a patient is sexually active or is heterosexual, homosexual, or bisexual. Patients may not be married to their sexual partners, nor are they necessarily sexually active with their spouses. Marriage or heterosexual relationships do not exclude a homosexual orientation.

When a patient has not made his or her sexual activity and preferences clear, but you need to pursue this matter, do not simply ask, "Are you married?" Better questions include:

> Who are the most important people in your life?
>
> What is your relationship like?

Follow up, if necessary, with more specific questions about sexuality:

> Are you sexually active?
>
> Do you relate sexually to men, or women, or both?

Similarly, until you know about a patient's sexual practices, consider using terms like "partner" rather than "boyfriend" or "wife."

Confidentiality

Maintain and assure confidentiality. (See the section Difficult Questions and Confidentiality in Chapter 3 and Confidentiality: What to Include in the Record in Chapter 17.)

Educate the Patient

Ignorance and misinformation about sexuality are widespread. The interview provides many opportunities to offer basic sexual education (including about anatomy and physiology), discuss common sexual concerns, advise on family planning, and dispel myths and confusion. Education often begins by clarifying terms:

> Are you familiar with some of these words, like vagina? Would you like to learn about these parts of your body and these words the doctors use?
>
> Have you had any sex education that taught you such words as clitoris or uterus?

Counseling on Health Concerns

Addressing sexuality is important in the tasks of promoting health and preventing disease. Family planning and sexually transmitted diseases are health issues for many patients. AIDS is a serious risk for some patients and a concern for many others. General satisfaction with sexual functioning should be a topic of *routine* clinical inquiry. Questions that open lines of communication include:

> Are you satisfied with your sexual life?
>
> Do you have any questions or concerns related to sex that you would like to discuss today?

Sexuality also plays an important role in many common clinical settings (see Table 10-3). In such circumstances, if the patient does not initiate discussion of sexuality, bring up the subject.

Self-Awareness

Students and physicians must find ways of discussing sexuality that best fit their attitudes, values, personality, and clinical competence and that also suit the particular patient and clinical setting. An awareness of one's own difficulties with taking a sexual history can guide one to appropriate remedial actions, such as taking steps to assure the topic is regularly addressed, seeking further training, or referring personally troublesome problems to consultants.

The too-frequent omission of pelvic and rectal examinations in both routine and nonroutine care serves as an example of the importance of self-awareness and of professional integrity. Many patients will be happy to avoid these examinations (as might the physician, especially late at night on the wards or when the emergency ward or office is rushed and busy). Physicians and patients find ingenious ways to collude in not performing a complete examination (as well as in avoiding talk about sexuality). The performance of the examination can be delegated (e.g., to a nurse-practitioner, who might also handle portions of the sexual history and counseling), but the responsibility for assuring appropriate care rests on the doctor. Physicians should similarly be aware of personal tendencies to omit examination of the breast or male genitalia.

Methods for Introducing Difficult Topics
Using Introductory Statements

As in all phases of the interview, you should inquire about a topic only when there is reason for you to know—when your understanding about these matters is relevant to the care of the patient. You cannot assume, however, that the patient will appreciate the appropriateness of your inquiry. Therefore, when you introduce the topic of sexuality, special efforts may be required so that the patient is not taken aback. Similarly, even if the patient introduces the topic, the interviewer often will want to explore well beyond the patient's initial presentation—clarifying details about current sexual functioning, obtaining a history of past sexual behaviors, and extending the range of sexual topics that are being addressed. The physician must explain the relevance of the discussion, obtain the patient's cooperation, alleviate embarrassment, and attend to concerns about confidentiality. Statements to introduce the topic can be helpful.

Introducing Difficult Topics

Statements of relevance or importance

We've talked about holding off on heavy exertion for a while and about an exercise schedule as you recuperate from the heart attack. I think it is important that we now also talk about your sexual relationship and about when you can exert yourself in sexual activity.

You've reached an age when I think it is important for you to have regular checkups, including a vaginal or pelvic examination that allows us to check you for the earliest signs of cancer. Have you been getting "Pap" smears?

Many young women your age have gotten a little information about the changes that occur in your body around age 11 to 14, in particular about the beginning of periods or monthly bleeding or menstruation. You will want to understand these matters. What have you been told to expect?

Statement of assumptions

I suspect you have had some questions in your mind about how this operation will affect your sexual life.

I wonder if you haven't had some concerns about your femininity and your ability to have regular sexual relationships after this surgery.

Statements of reassurance or empathy

Many of the subjects we are talking about are very personal, and you may have some concerns about other people learning about them from me. I want you to know that I am not writing this in your record.

I know you may not be used to discussing such matters and might find some of this a touch embarrassing at first.

Statements of ubiquity

Just about everyone has concerns about sexuality and has some difficulties with sexual function at some time or another. What about you?

Even though sexual feelings and sexual activities are normal and common at your age, most adolescents feel awkward talking about these matters. You may have been told that it is bad or unusual to have such feelings or to act upon such feelings.

Many couples find that their sexual life is not as satisfying at times as they wish. Difficulties with sexual function are very common. What has your experience been?

Highly Directive Questions

When asking about universal behaviors or feelings that are not commonly discussed, you may sometimes want to form questions that strongly direct the patient into further elaboration. For example, rather than saying, "Do you ever masturbate?" you ask, "Do you recall how old you were when you started to masturbate?" These highly directive questions may best be introduced with a statement:

> Sexual experiences with persons of the same sex are common for men and women at some time in their lives. Tell me about your own experience.

> When children become teenagers, their parents are often concerned about sexual experimentation, pregnancy, and venereal disease. Which of these areas has concerned you about your kids?

Directing the Flow of the Interview

The flow of the interview can be directed by the physician so that it gradually approaches topics of increasing emotional sensitivity. For instance, the interviewer who finds the patient stumbling over questions about current sexual attitudes or practices may turn the discussion to topics that are usually much easier to discuss, such as early sexual learning or attitudes:

> When did you first learn about sex? Who taught you? What were some of your earliest feelings about sexual relationships? [rather than asking how the patient now feels about sex]

> What were your family's attitudes about sexuality? How was nakedness handled in your home? Was sexual education given at home? [rather than talking about current practices]

Discussion about the past is often easier than about the present, and inquiries that focus on knowledge are often less charged than inquiries about attitudes or behaviors. For instance, in talking to a woman who is disappointed that she has not gotten pregnant after a year of marriage but who is shying away from providing the necessary information about her sexual activity (especially the pattern of coitus), you might begin by asking,

> What have you read or heard about why you have not gotten pregnant?
> What is your understanding about how you can improve your chances?

Such questions usually lead the patient to bring up the very topics that concern the physician and may better facilitate the interview than such direct questions as "How often are you having sexual relations?" or "Does your partner ejaculate inside your vagina?"

■ CONCLUSION

Few novice clinicians are comfortable introducing and discussing highly personal matters. Yet many emotionally charged, value-laden topics have a direct bearing on the patient's physical condition, emotional well-being, and future health. If you make a personal commitment to developing your skills in interviewing, you have the opportunity to create for your patients and yourself a relationship in which these topics can be raised and addressed.

THE OCCUPATIONAL HISTORY: STRESS, SATISFACTION, HAZARDS

Nearly everyone works or has worked. While the industrial "working man" has been the traditional focus of occupational medicine, any job can have an impact on a patient's health (Fig. 10-1). Thus, no work should be exempt from inquiry about stress, satisfaction, and hazardous exposures. For instance, numerous accounts of the lives of medical students, resident physicians, practitioners, and other health professionals have reported psychological stress, as well as sleep deprivation and exposure to infectious agents.

Why Learn About a Patient's Work?

The reasons are several and include seeking essential social history, assessing stress, recognizing workplace health hazards, and appreciating the significance of a disability and the potential for rehabilitation.

Essential Social History

The work history gives you an invaluable perspective on the patient. By asking "What's your work?" or "What has your work been?" you find out how a person may spend (or has spent) much of his or her life. With the "graying" of the population, chairs in doctors' offices and beds in hospitals are increasingly occupied by retired, nonworking persons who are often unfortunately identified in the medical record and in clinical communications primarily by the chronic disease they carry ("This 75-year-old male with metastatic lung disease ...") rather than by their previous occupation or current activities and

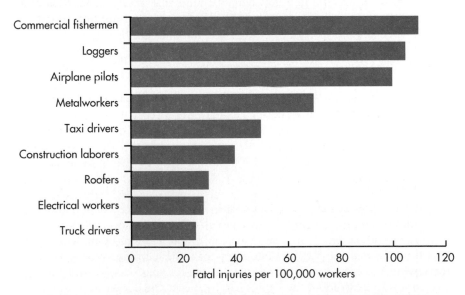

Fig. 10-1   Most dangerous jobs. (Data from Bureau of Labor Statistics, 1995.)

other important biographical information. Occupation can also provide a quick reference to income, education, social status, and the patient's sense of self, while work may be an important source of life satisfaction.

> The job is OK, but the main thing is seeing my friends at work.
>
> I like being able to support myself and my family.
>
> I hate hanging around the house, not being able to work. I like to be active.
>
> I can't retire. I love my medical practice.

Stress

Information about a patient's job may suggest sources of physical and psychological stress. "Job stress" accounts for considerable illness, medical consultations, and exacerbations of existing disease—even more work-related problems than caused by exposures to hazardous substances.

> Night shift really screws up my life.
>
> Working in this cold weather makes me sick.
>
> I can't stand this supervision hassle.
>
> I'm burned out.
>
> I can't lift; it pains my back.

Jobs most commonly considered physically stressful are those in manufacturing involving repetitive motion (machine operations) or lifting that produces musculoskeletal strain (although back strain is often associated with less strenuous occupations, including office work). Jobs considered psychologically stressful are those in service industries with high interpersonal demands of "meeting the public" or where management exerts close supervision.

Hazards and Exposures

The work history may reveal on-the-job hazards and toxic exposures. Occupations may be associated with such hazards as burns, falls, injury to limbs or eyes, or acoustic trauma. Exposures include a variety of etiological agents, some of which cause acute disorders (such as asthma induced by cotton dust or plastics, neurological poisoning from insecticides, or contact dermatitis from numerous substances), chronic diseases (such as pneumoconiosis from coal mining or acquired immune deficiency syndrome from an accidental needle stick), or hazards to a fetus (hydrocarbons, including anesthetic gases). Many patients are unaware of such exposures, and many substances produce disability only after a long latent period, even after the patient has left the job. The recognition of occupational hazards and exposures is not only important for the care of sick persons; the elimination or reduction of risks may also prevent disease. Five percent to 10 percent of deaths and of morbidity from cancer, cardiovascular, and cerebrovascular disease and chronic respiratory disease can be attributed to occupational injury and illness.

Of course, hazards are not always confined to the workplace. Industrial by-products may contaminate a home, neighborhood, or community, thus exposing nonworking patients, as has happened where factories extracting beryllium or processing asbestos have polluted the atmosphere or where soil has been contaminated with polychlorinated biphenyls and hydrocarbons. Moreover, hobbies and other nonwork activities may be associated with significant health risks, such as sports injuries. Commuting to work in heavy traffic may lead to significant exposure to carbon monoxide. Burns, falls, and self-poisoning are important hazards in the home for children.

The recognition of an occupational exposure as the cause of an illness, as with all medical diagnoses, depends on the traditional steps of the clinical method—history, physical examination, and laboratory tests—but particularly requires a careful lifetime history of the patient's job, searching for potentially hazardous exposures. Common symptoms or signs of work-related disease are, by themselves, often not specific for the diagnosis of any single occupational disorder. For instance, the constellation of dyspnea, cough, restrictive lung function, and opacities on a chest x-ray can be a manifestation of a variety of illnesses, including occupational respiratory disease. The history of the patient's work provides essential "clues" that connect common symptoms and signs to a specific job hazard and to a disease. The history should also include habits, because a toxic agent from work may not act alone to produce disease. In many instances, occupational disease is multifactorial, developing by exposure to injurious agents acting addictively or synergistically, as for example, when smoking contributes to the development of carcinoma of the lungs in a patient who has been exposed to asbestos.

Assessing Disability and Planning Rehabilitation

Finally, in assessing the effects of an illness or injury on a patient's life, a knowledge of the patient's occupation is often essential. The disability that results from a medical condition is a reflection, in part, of the way the patient uses his or her body at work. A minor tendon injury to the hand may be of little importance to most people, yet have disastrous consequences for a violinist. Similarly, the process of rehabilitation after a heart attack or major abdominal surgery may be quite different for a heavy laborer than for an office worker.

Taking the History

For a routine history, three types of data are collected: job description, job satisfaction, and exposure.

Job Description

Seek a full description of the patient's job duties.

> What kind of work do you do?
>
> What's it like?

Job Satisfaction

> How do you like the work (e.g., the hours, co-workers, your supervisor, the pay, the work conditions)?
>
> Do you want to stick with this job?
>
> Where do you see yourself working in the next 5 or 10 years?

Seek out stresses, or what is now commonly called "burnout." Also, remember that the patient's account of his or her work often deserves comment:

> Sounds like an interesting job.
>
> Sounds strenuous.

Exposure

A history of exposures has three specific informational goals: (1) the relationship of the patient's symptoms to work, past or present, (2) the quality and the quantity of any hazardous exposure, and (3) the presence of similar illnesses in persons with similar exposures.

1. *Relation of symptoms to work or other activities.* For many complaints, routine questions should be:

> Does this problem seem to be related to any activities at work or at home?

When you suspect an exposure, additionally useful questions include:

> Do you notice any difference in symptoms on weekends or vacations?
>
> Has the condition changed when your work changed?

2. *Surveying for hazardous exposures.* The review of systems or the subsection on *exposures* in the past medical history should routinely include, whenever relevant:

> Are your work conditions safe?
>   Are there risks of accidents or injury?
>
> In your job or leisure-time activities, do you work with or around any hazardous materials—substances that might make you sick?
>
> How about in your past jobs or hobbies?
>   Chemicals, dusts, or fumes?
>   Radiation?
>   Lead?
>   Solvents?
>   Asbestos?
>
> Do your job or hobbies involve:
>   Prolonged sun exposure?
>   Loud noises?
>   Physical stress?
>   Emotional stress?
>   What about tension on the job?

Do you know what to do to protect yourself from hazardous exposures?
What do you actually do?

3. *Patient's account of co-workers' health.*

Have your co-workers had similar problems? Family? Neighbors?

A history of similar illnesses among a patient's co-workers is a significant epidemiological observation that suggests an etiological relation to work. Indeed, the identification of disease agents at work often follows the recognition of clusters of illness, disabilities, or deaths in industry. Similar observations about illnesses among family or neighbors may also suggest common hazardous exposures.

Detailed History of Occupational Exposures

In patients whose health problems are suspected to be related to occupational exposure, a more detailed history is often required, usually entailing a lifetime history of jobs and a careful assessment of the quality and quantity of exposure. Additional sources of information are also commonly utilized.

Chronological Account of Jobs

A chronological lifetime work history—the career—should be sought in addition to the patient's current job description. The necessity for a chronological history is based on the fact that hazardous exposures occurring early in a worker's life may have a long latency before symptoms are produced or the worker seeks medical help. Occupation-related malignancies may be detected many years after the last exposure to the etiological agent. For example, in 1986 a salesman was found to have a pleural mesothelioma; in World War II he had been exposed to asbestos for 6 months as a shipyard worker.

Such a job history is often complicated and difficult to compile. The worker may have forgotten dates of employment and of brief, but critical, jobs. The average worker often holds several jobs in a lifetime, particularly in the United States, where workers frequently move from place to place and from job to job. Thus carefully review all the patient's employment, beginning with after-school work and moving forward chronologically to the present.

Quality and Quantity

What are the quality and quantity of exposure? The patient may know the trade name of a metal or chemical with which he or she worked, but it is necessary to learn about the material's physical state and concentration when the exposure took place. For example, at high temperatures a relatively harmless chlorinated hydrocarbon, trichloroethylene, which is widely used as an industrial solvent, is converted to phosgene, a well-recognized lung irritant.

Similarly, freshly generated cadmium oxide fumes cause acute chemical pneumonia, whereas "old" cadmium compounds may not have such effect. Although materials may be very alike in chemical structure, they may differ completely in toxic effect.

Factors governing total dose or quantity of an occupational exposure are many. Duration of work is of obvious first importance. So too is whether or not the job was done with protection or in close proximity to the hazard. Were the exposures intermittent or steady? The levels high or low? Work conditions are also significant. If the work took place in a hot climate with great physical effort, the increased respiratory demands can result in a greater dose of inhaled material. If drilling work was done in a wet atmosphere, less dust would be airborne than if, for example, dry drilling or surface grinding had been done.

Additional Sources for the History

In the past, workers often did not know about hazardous materials at work. In today's workplace they generally have the right to know about such exposures. Laws mandate that employees be informed about what materials are toxic and be trained to handle them safely. Material Safety Data Sheets are prepared that identify the chemicals, handling precautions, and hazards. A first step in clarifying exposures, therefore, is to request Material Safety Data Sheets.

When such data are not available, the physician may seek out other sources of information: the patient's foreman, employer, or plant physician; the state agency responsible for occupational disease; a university laboratory concerned with toxicology; or the insurance carrier of the employer. Occupational hygienists and doctors in large companies (such as the utilities, oil refineries, automobile makers, and chemical manufacturers) may provide help in identifying a toxic exposure. If employers are not cooperative on a voluntary basis, the state agency for occupational disease is empowered to enter factories to examine working environments where potential hazards are reported.

PSYCHOSOCIAL ASSESSMENT*

> *Amid an eternal heritage of sorrow and suffering our work is laid, and this eternal note of sadness would be insupportable if the daily tragedies were not relieved by the spectacle of the heroism and devotion displayed by the actors. Nothing will sustain you more potently than the power to recognize in your humdrum routine, as perhaps it may be thought, the true poetry of life—the poetry of the commonplace, of the ordinary man,*

*Portions of this section are adapted from unpublished course material developed by Byron Good, Mary Jo Delvecchio Good, and Mark Herrera at the University of California in Sacramento Medical Center, and later used by the Goods at Harvard College and Harvard Medical School.

of the plain toil-worn woman, with their loves and their joys, their sorrows and their griefs. The comedy, too, of life will be spread before you, and nobody laughs more often than the doctor at the pranks Puck plays upon the Titanias and the Bottoms among his patients.

> *William Osler*
> *The Student Life (1905)*

Most people have a furious itch to talk about themselves and are restrained only by the disinclination of others to listen. Reserve is an artificial quality that is developed in most of us but as a result of innumerable rebuffs. The doctor is discrete. It is his business to listen, and no details are too intimate for his ears.

> *W. Somerset Maugham*

Earlier chapters of this text provide guidelines for a brief psychosocial assessment, such as would be acquired while characterizing the present illness (especially by encouraging elaboration on personal information, affect, adaptation, and the patient's perspective) and obtaining a basic social history. The following section of this chapter suggests additional themes to explore for a more comprehensive and systematic assessment.

No simple outline will encompass the wealth of psychosocial issues that you eventually will want to be able to explore with your patients. However, to organize your initial approach to psychosocial assessment, we offer here a general framework of four broad topics: (1) the meaning of illness, (2) stress, (3) coping and support, and (4) personal development. These topics overlap considerably, so questions about one will naturally lead to discussion of others.

A list of helpful questions is provided for each topic. The questions can be used early in your training to learn about psychosocial assessment, even though you may still be unfamiliar with the basic concepts in behavioral science or clinical knowledge that you ultimately need to guide your inquiry and make sense of the data you collect. Your studies eventually should address such matters as how culture and personal experience influence the meaning of illness; personality, emotions, defenses, interpersonal relationships, psychological stress, coping, psychopathology, and the mental status; social function, networks, and support; and human development from birth through death. The suggested questions serve as a bridge between fundamental psychosocial concepts taught in the classroom and the specific methods of inquiry that are used in clinical practice.

Because each of these four topics is complex, we suggest that you *not* try to learn all of them at once. Instead, in your earlier interviews, practice exploring one topic at a time, while later attempting more complete assessments.

Who Needs More Psychosocial Assessment?

Before going on to describe the four assessment topics, consider some common clinical situations that call for a more elaborate psychosocial evaluation:

First, many patients have obvious psychosocial problems that require thorough exploration. Such problems may be the patient's reason for visit or may appear to be the underlying cause or a major contributor to the presenting complaints. Additionally, significant problems, unrelated to the reason for visit, may be suggested in the course of obtaining a standard history: a problem with work, home life, or leisure time is mentioned in the present illness; a patient bursts out crying or expresses sadness while you explore the social history; or a recent death of a close relative is reported in the family history.

Second, you may hypothesize that unacknowledged psychosocial factors bear on a patient's medical disorders and on their management. Your suspicion about important underlying psychosocial problems might be raised in the following settings: a patient's somatic symptoms are not

---

QUICK TIPS

Identifying Depression

Depression is a common and often overlooked condition in clinical medicine. It should be considered in patients who appear or complain of being sad or depressed, but also when patients note physical or psychological symptoms such as insomnia, fatigue, lack of pleasure, change in usual mood (including anxiety or irritability), chronic pain, and sexual dysfunction. We use the following mnemonic, SIG: E-CAPs, roughly translated as Prescribe Energy Capsules:

S   **S**leep disorder: trouble sleeping or sleeping too much
I   Loss of **I**nterest or markedly diminished interest or pleasure in daily activities, especially previously enjoyed activities
G   Feelings of worthlessness or **G**uilt
:   **[Colon]**—constipation
E   Loss of **E**nergy, feeling tired, fatigue
C   Impaired **C**oncentration, indecisiveness, trouble remembering or thinking
A   Change in **A**ppetite with significant weight loss or gain
P   **P**sychomotor retardation or agitation
S   **S**uicidality or recurrent thoughts of suicide and death

Among persons who are particularly prone to significant depression are those with a personal or family history of depression or suicide, general medical illness, substance abuse, and stressful life events with a lack of social supports.

readily explained by a physical disease; the doctor-patient relationship is perceived as "difficult"; the patient's emotional response seems inappropriate; or compliance with treatment is erratic. In these situations, a little extra time spent on evaluating the patient can effectively avert misunderstanding and clinical error. For instance, you might pursue questions about life stresses in order to account for one patient's unexpected level of pain or disability or for another's frequent visits, medication requests, and phone calls. Does the patient's illness have a special meaning that hinders openness with the physician or makes the patient unexpectedly anxious or depressed? Has loss of social supports affected the patient's ability to deal with the illness? Does the patient's coping style help explain unanticipated behavior? Is this a lifelong pattern of maladaptation or a new problem?

Third, you may consider a more elaborate assessment simply to know more about a patient, a process which, in turn, may foster a closer therapeutic alliance. A deeper appreciation of psychosocial background is particularly important when you are therapeutically responsible for patients with serious conditions. Periods of major stress—anticipating surgery, the onset of major illnesses, a significant deterioration of functional status—suggest the need for such assessment.

Fourth, for preventive health purposes, you may want to incorporate some screening psychosocial questions into your standard interview. For instance, while providing an annual checkup for a 55-year-old hypertensive man, you might briefly ask about the personal meaning of high blood pressure, the onset of major life changes in family or work (e.g., children leaving home, death of a parent), how he has coped with such stress, and his anticipation of retirement.

Finally, as a learning practitioner, you will simply want to carry out a detailed psychosocial assessment in order to practice your interviewing skills. Your patients will appreciate this extra attention.

Assessing the Meaning of Illness

Questions about the personal meaning of illness will help you appreciate what being sick and obtaining help signify to the patient. You seek out the patient's perspectives, in particular the meanings that may not be completely congruent with your own, that might help you understand the patient's behavior and that might be used in providing reassurance or improving compliance. For instance, do discrepancies between the patient's attributions and your own lead to differences in how the illness is viewed (e.g., as a loss, threat, or gain)? Are there disparities between your professional view and the personal meaning for the patient of diagnostic and treatment efforts (e.g., a "routine" medical procedure is perceived as excessively dangerous, therapeutically useless, or otherwise unreasonable)?

Questions About Meaning of Illness

Onset of illness

When did your illness first begin?

What do you believe made It begin at that time?

Were there other important things going on in your life at that time? Do you think your illness may be related to these matters?

Etiology or underlying cause

What do you believe is causing your symptoms?
>   What disease do you have?

Why do you think you got it?
>   For example, does it run in your family?
>   Were you worn down or under a lot of stress?
>   Was it something you caught?
>   A reaction to something?

Have you discussed it with others?
>   What did they say?

Pathophysiology

Can you tell me how you believe this illness works? What image do you have about it?

[You may need to probe, for example]
>   Most people have some idea of how an illness works and It may be different from the doctor's. I would like to know how you think about your illness working.

Course and severity

What do you see happening to you with this illness?
>   Do you think it will get better or worse?
>   Will it clear up soon?
>   Is it permanent?
>   Progressive?
>   Debilitating?
>   Do you think you might die from it?

Are there any things you are worried about or that you fear from this illness?
>   What do you fear the most?

What do you think might happen if you don't come to the doctor?
>   If you don't get diagnostic tests or treatment?
>   How bad do you think it might become?

Treatment

How have you treated this problem so far?
>   What kind of help or advice have you gotten from family, neighbors, or other people?
>   Have you consulted anyone else [healers, doctors]?

What do you think needs to be done for your problem now?
>   What made you come to the doctor now?
>   What do you hope the doctor can do for you?

What did you hope to learn from the doctor?
  Are there any other things you hoped to talk about?

What do you make of the treatment so far?
  Has it helped?
  Made things worse?
  How?

Formulations Based on the Assessment of Meaning

Having elicited the patient's personal meanings, formulations that use this data might be recorded as follows.

Example 1: Despite her respect for her physician and her faith in modern medicine, Mrs. Olsen tends to view the onset of this illness as a punishment for her past behavior, not as an unfortunate but inexplicable biological event. While complying fully with her prescribed regimen (indeed, she seems extremely eager to portray herself as a cooperative patient), she sees her future as largely determined by her own ability to be "good" and by God's grace. We will try to address some of these issues through the chaplain.

Example 2: This patient's notion of the etiology and pathophysiology of his illness is coherent and essentially consonant with our medical views, but he has unrealistic expectations of both the side effects and the value of chemotherapy for his condition. Based on his aunt's experience with pancreatic cancer, he sees treatment as causing pain, nausea, vomiting, weight loss, and a rapid demise. While he has heard of excellent responses and even cures of some forms of cancer, he doubts that he could obtain such results. He would benefit from more discussion about the proposed management plan.

Assessing Stress

Stress may lead to distress. A foremost task in psychosocial assessment is to learn about personally important life changes and to appreciate how the patient is affected. The patient should be encouraged to discuss what he or she feels to be major stresses, including possible precipitants of illness and the sequelae of illness itself, as well as events not apparently related to illness. Any major change in the patient's life may constitute a significant stress, including events that are generally perceived as desirable (e.g., being promoted, having a child, buying a new home, going to medical school). Seemingly minor events—death of a pet, a move within the same neighborhood—may sometimes hold great personal meaning and constitute a significant stress. In general, stresses include: (1) loss; (2) unmet basic human needs, ranging from food and shelter to satisfying relationships or opportunities for creativity and fulfillment; (3) excess demands of various sorts (see the following topic: Assessing Coping and Support); and (4) threats to what is fundamentally important to the person.

To systematically explore potentially stressful events, see the following section.

Questions About Stressful Events

General

In general, how have things been for you during the past year or two?

Has it been a stressful time? Have you been under any pressures?
  During the past year, have you had any upsets in your life?
  How serious have these been for you?

What are the main problems you are facing now?

Family life and other close relationships

Who are the persons closest to you?
  How has your relationship been over the past year or two?
  Any difficulties?
    What have they been like?
    How serious do they seem?

How have your family relationships been over the past year?
  Your relationship with your wife (or husband)?
  With your children?
  With your parents?
  With other members of your family—brothers and sisters, in-laws?

Any difficulties?
  What have they been like?
  How serious do they seem?

Are there other important people in your life?

Work and finances

During the past year or two, how have things been at your work? [Similar questions may be used for homemakers about managing the home]

Have you had problems related to your work or career?
  Has your job been difficult?
  Do you like what you are doing?

Have you had money troubles?

How serious have these problems been?

Social life

How has your social life been?

Have you felt isolated?

Any difficulties meeting people?

Any conflicts with friends or neighbors?

Any changes in your leisure time?
  Hobbies?
  Sports

How serious have these difficulties seemed?

Sexual life

Have you been satisfied with your sexual relationships?

Any difficulties?

How serious have these seemed?

Habits

[Questions about habits and health are ordinarily asked in conjunction with the standard medical history.]

During the past year, have you had difficulties with drinking?
Smoking?
Drugs?
Your weight? Diet?

Health

During the past year, have you had difficulties in your life that resulted from illness?
What are the problems your sickness has caused for you?
How has it affected your work?
Has it affected your personal relationships?
Has it caused financial problems?
Are you applying for a disability?

What are the problems your sickness has caused for your family?

Has your health affected your ability to enjoy yourself?
From being able to move around or exercise as usual?
From being able to drive or get to places you usually go?
From seeing people?

How serious have these been?

What would your life be like now if your illness went away?

Formulations Based on Assessment of Life Stresses

Example 1:   While Mrs. Williams has tolerated well a number of previous moves necessitated by her husband's business, the recent dislocation has been troublesome. She has been unable to make friends readily, her husband has been less available, and, for the first time in her life, she is not near enough to her sisters to visit frequently. However, she has a number of hobbies that may allow her greater social contact here, and she is planning to return to Ohio soon for a long family visit.

Example 2:   Mr. Bellow has recently been severely dysphoric (but not truly depressed) because of his worsening chronic illness, his need to quit work (which had provided an important sense of personal worth and was the focus of his social life), and the more immediate disappointment about his children leaving home. His wife remains supportive and their marital-sexual relationship is fulfilling, but he would benefit from an opportunity for more ventilation of his frustration and sadness.

Assessing Coping and Support

All persons face stress in their lives, but their experience of distress reflects both the personal meaning of the stress and their resources for coping. In this section of the psychosocial assessment, you explore how the patient is dealing with stress and investigate his or her support system. What resources does the individual have and how are they used for responding to particular kinds of stress? Are the resources adequate or are they seriously compromised? Does the pattern of coping lead the individual into additional conflicts and problems or is it generally adaptive?

Coping and support have both psychological and social dimensions. The psychological dimension includes the cognitive domain—how the patient obtains and uses information to deal with problems—and the affective domain—how the patient responds emotionally. Psychological resources may include information and advice, intrapsychic coping mechanisms, and emotional support and counseling. Social resources include the patient's social network and other providers of instrumental support—financial, housing, transportation, personal services, and so on.

Questions About Coping and Support

General
I wonder if you can tell me how you manage (or deal with) these difficulties?

Psychological Coping
How has your mood been?

Any difficulties with the way you feel?
For example, have you been feeling depressed or sad?
Anxious or fearful?
Do you get mad easily? Lose control of your temper?

How serious have these been?

How do these difficulties affect you?

How do you cope with these feelings?

How well do you feel you manage?

Do you feel you have as much support as you need?

Social Support
Whom do you turn to in a troubling situation? Whom can you go to for help?
What is your relationship like? Are you close?
Are they readily available?
Are they supportive?
Are you satisfied with this relationship?

[For information:]
Who helps answer your questions about those problems?
Who helps you figure out what you should do? Who advises you?

[For emotional support:]
Whom can you turn to for emotional support?
Whom can you let know about a matter that is seriously troubling you?

[For instrumental help:]
Who helps you out with a financial problem?
Getting transportation? Help around the house and so forth?

[The social network and its supportiveness:]
> Who are the most important people in your life?
>> What is your relationship like? Are you close?
>> Are you satisfied with the relationships?
>> Are they supportive? In what way?
>
> With whom are you living?
>> What is your relationships like?
>
> Do you have other close friends—people with whom you feel at ease and can talk things out?
>> Are you satisfied with these relationships?
>> What about your family members? What kind of help can you count on from them? Where do they live? What kind of contact do you have with them?
>
> Do you have supportive relationships at work?
>
> Do you have persons you enjoy doing things with outside of home or work?
>
> What sorts of groups (religious, political, or social) do you belong to? Are there supportive people there?
>
> What professionals can you turn to—a social worker, nurse, physician?
>> What kinds of experience have you had with doctors and other medical professionals in the past?
>> What have you learned about how you work best with doctors? With other medical professionals?
>> How do you usually handle it when you have a problem with your health?
>
> Are you receiving any help from community agencies? The visiting nurse? Homemakers? Senior citizens? Others? From the state? Welfare? Social Security?
>
> How hard is it for you to go for help?

Formulations of Coping and Support

Example 1:   The patient has remained extremely active and almost oblivious to his considerable medical problems until this recent stress, which has resulted in a significant loss of function. He now seems unable to ignore his disability or to carry out many of the activities that previously kept his attention off being ill. He sees himself as worthless and has little sense that others value him as he is now. He has a large, concerned family and an extensive network of "buddies," but these relationships seem to support denial rather than allow ventilation of his frustration or even recognition of his considerable strengths. He would benefit from some regular counseling, either individual therapy or preferably a group that would allow him to see how others cope.

Example 2:   Because of her progressive dementia, Mrs. Harrel has become totally dependent on her landlord for shopping, cooking, and management of financial matters. Her family continues to provide some financial support, but lives away and will offer nothing else. She has now ejected two homemakers and refused a third. Her landlord has been increasingly upset about the messiness of her apartment, though he otherwise remains happy to look after her. The landlord's own health problems may also hinder his ability to help her. In the meantime, efforts need to be directed toward getting Mrs. Harrel to accept cleaning services. The visiting nurse has been a welcomed friend and may be able to persuade the patient to accept help.

Assessing Development

This final portion of the psychosocial assessment is primarily useful for providing a perspective on data gathered in the three previous areas. Three broad hypotheses are considered:

1. Can current troubles best be understood as new problems or are they manifestations of more long-standing, recurrent psychosocial difficulties?

2. How can an understanding of the patient's past—his or her upbringing and later development—help us appreciate present functioning?

3. Can the patient's current problems be characterized as a developmental crisis, as a dilemma reflecting the demands of various life stages and transitions?

The developmental assessment, even more than the previous areas of assessment, depends on a specialized background knowledge about normal and abnormal psychosocial development and must be tailored to the individual patient. On the one hand, specific issues need to be explored for each life stage. In your reading about adult development, for instance, you should become familiar with common crises associated with choosing a vocation, establishing intimate personal relationships, becoming a parent, being satisfied with a career, having children leave home, retiring, dealing with the illness and death of parents and friends, and accepting one's own aging and eventual death. Additionally, specific problems in current psychosocial function raise particular questions about past development. For example, the presence of chronic pain or other persistent psychosomatic complaints might lead to an investigation of the role of pain and sickness in the patient's earlier life, particularly of how physical complaints may have been a major source of attention. Similarly, the identification of a patient's violent or abusive behavior leads to an exploration of similar behavior in his or her family-of-origin.

The following questions, focusing on early development, are useful for many patients and will often lead the patient into discussing critical developmental issues. You are referred to the Suggested Readings for more guidance about assessing adult development.

Questions About Development _____

Where were you born?

What do you remember about your early childhood?
    With whom did you live?
    What was your family life like?

Tell me about your parents.
    What were they like?
    What was your relationship like?
    How did you get along with them?
    How did they get along with each other?

Did they seem satisfied with their lives? If not, why?
How did they support themselves?
  Were you economically comfortable?

What about brothers and sisters?
Older? Younger?
What was your relationship like?

Were there other important people in your life then?
Tell me more about them?
Others who helped raise you?

Was there ever any physical or sexual abuse?

What about school?
How far did you go in school?
What was it like for you?
What kinds of friendships did you have?
How did you do academically?
  Did you feel successful?

Was religion important in your upbringing?
How did it affect you?

What was your adolescence like?
How did you get along with your parents?
What were your relations like with kids your own age?
  Did you have good friends?
  Did you date?
What about sexual relationships?
  What were your early sexual relationships like?

When did you leave home?
Who have been the important people in your life since then?

How have you supported yourself? What kind of work have you done?

Have there been major losses in your life? Major setbacks?

Formulations Based on Assessment of Development

Example 1:   The patient describes her parents affectionately, but notes their strictness and "old-fashioned" ideas about child-rearing. Her father, whom she describes as stern and forbidding, insisted that his daughters spend long hours on household chores, socialize only with "good" families (which often meant not being able to play with neighborhood friends), and not attend any social activities except for a few organized by the church. Her mother was warm but submissive to the father's rule. The patient had little contact with her only sibling, who was 8 years older and whose eventual pregnancy out of wedlock and subsequent alienation from the family served to increase her parents' rigidity. The patient attended parochial schools and was a good student, but never talked with boys. She had a few close female friends, but in retrospect, she feels they also suffered from a very restricted upbringing.

At age 18, she finished school and began working as a clerk for an insurance company while continuing to live with her parents. At work, she met Bob, who was her first "date." He particularly impressed her because of his good humor and tolerance. He introduced her to movies, dancing, smoking, alcohol, and eventually to sex. They were married after about 6 months. After about 4 months of marriage, Bob began coming home drunk and was both verbally and physically abusive. He deserted her after about 6 months of marriage, soon after she discovered she was pregnant. The patient then returned to her family's home and her father's rule. For the past 2 years, she has continued to work as a clerk, while bringing up her daughter with the help of her mother and has generally shunned social activities outside the immediate family. She has become increasingly frustrated by her restricted life and has been eager to allow her daughter a more "modern" upbringing, yet feels unable to leave home.

She will be referred for long-term case work.

Example 2:   Mr. Percy describes a generally happy upbringing: warm family relationships, enjoyable and successful school life, and a full range of social and leisure activities. At age 18, he joined the Marines and was assigned to Vietnam. There, he says he "did his job, like everyone else," which included considerable combat duty, witnessing the death or mutilation of a number of friends, and his eventual leg injury and prolonged rehabilitation. Since discharge, he has drifted from job to job, has had no sustained close relationships with persons of either sex, and has been plagued by "nervousness," insomnia, and intrusive thoughts about war and violence.

While he has tried brief individual therapy, I think he might do well in either more long-term therapy or group work, and have asked Dr. Barsky to evaluate him for these possibilities.

Advanced Practice in Psychosocial Assessment

An essential step in a more advanced approach to clinical problem-solving is to generate psychosocial hypotheses. Each hypothesis is based on etiologic and pathophysiologic concepts that help explain the patient's condition, as well as on specific treatment options. Each hypothesis is also associated with a typical set of questions that generates the data necessary to assess whether such a condition is present or not.

For instance, when an elderly patient seems to be following a diet erratically, despite your emphatic instructions about the importance of careful adherence, you might wonder why. Clinical experience might lead you to ask:

- Is there an undiagnosed clinical disorder? For instance, is he becoming demented or is he losing interest in caring for himself because of being depressed?
- Are there underlying social problems? Perhaps he is unable to pay for the proper food. Has he been abandoned by his family, and thus lacks needed assistance in shopping and preparing food? Is the prescribed diet compatible with his need to take meals in a nearby restaurant or to eat primarily canned food?
- Do behavioral difficulties explain the problem? For instance, has he had long-standing difficulties modulating his eating habits? Are the proposed dietary changes reasonable for this patient, given his basic eating patterns?

- Does the noncompliance reflect psychodynamic issues? For instance, is the patient's frustration about his medical condition and his increasing dependence showing up as negativism toward the doctor and passive undermining of the prescribed regimen?
- Is the patient's viewpoint discordant with the physician's, such that the patient assigns different meanings to the illness and its management? What significance does the patient attach to eating, including his usual diet, favorite foods, and the proposed nutritional changes? Are there preferred religious or ethnic styles of preparing meals and eating them? How has the proposed diet been explained and negotiated? Perhaps the patient does not think any diet is "worth it," or he believes that he should eat lustily in order to feel better.

Similarly, when you suspect that a patient is depressed, you learn to search quickly for the seven criteria of a major depression (sleep disorder, loss of interest, guilt, lack of energy, difficulty with concentration, appetite disturbance, psychomotor retardation, and suicidal ideation or behavior) (see Quick Tips on p. 149). If the diagnosis is confirmed, a number of additional hypotheses might be entertained (e.g., Is this a recurrent psychobiological condition that may be associated with a manic-depressive illness or a family history of depressive disorder? Would it be relieved with psychotherapy, medication, or electroconvulsive treatment?).

■ CONCLUSION

In your earliest clinical experiences, we suggest that you simply set out to learn from the patient, using your own curiosity and common sense, aided by interviewing skills that help you facilitate patients' telling of the story of their illness. Remember that psychosocial problems, like other symptoms, have "dimensions" and thus should be characterized in terms of onset, duration, course, severity, adaptation, premorbid function, and so on. As you become more familiar with clinical interviewing, even if you have not yet had much training in the psychosocial basis of illness, the suggested questions in this chapter will let you deepen your assessment by exploring the interactions of the patient's life and illness.

SUGGESTED READINGS

Attributions

Kleinman A: Explanatory models in health-care relationships: a conceptual frame for research on family-based health care activities in relation to folk and professional forms of clinical care. In Stoeckle JD, editor: *Encounters between doctors and patients: an anthology,* Cambridge, Mass, 1987, MIT Press.

Mechanic D: Social psychologic factors affecting the presentation of bodily complaints, *N Engl J Med* 286:1132, 1972.

Stoeckle JD, Barsky AJ: Attribution: uses of social science knowledge in the "doctoring" of primary care. In Eisenberg L, Klcinman A, editors: *The relevance of social science to medicine,* Dordrecht, The Netherlands, 1980, D Reidel.

Young A: The anthropologies of illness and sickness, *Annu Rev Anthropol* 11:237, 1982.

Triggers

Barsky AJ: Hidden reasons some patients visit doctors, *Ann Intern Med* 94:492, 1981.

McKinlay JB: Social networks, lay consultation and help-seeking behavior, *Soc Forces* 51:275, 1973.

White KL, Williams TF, Greenberg BG: The ecology of medical care, *N Engl J Med* 265:885, 1961.

Zola IK: Pathways to the doctor—from person to patient, *Soc Sci Med* 78:677, 1973. Reprinted in Zola IK: *Socio-medical inquiries recollections, reflections, and reconsiderations,* Philadelphia, 1983, Temple University Press.

Nonverbal Communication

Bull P: *Body movement and intrapersonal communication,* Chichester, England, 1983, John Wiley & Sons.

Dimatteo MR: Nonverbal skill and the physician patient relationship. In Rosenthal R, editor: *Skill in nonverbal communication: individual differences,* Cambridge, England, 1979, Oelgeschlager, Gunn and Hain.

Ekman P: *Telling lies: clues to deceit in the marketplace, politics, and marriage,* New York, 1992, WW Norton.

Hall ET: *The silent language,* New York, 1973, Anchor.

Hall ET: *The hidden dimension,* New York, 1990, Anchor.

Roter DL, Hall JA: *Doctors talking with patients/patients talking with doctors: improving communication in medical visits,* Westport, Conn, 1993, Auburn House.

Asking About Alcohol

Barnes HN, Aronson MD, Delbanco TL, editors: *Alcoholism: a guide for the primary care physician,* New York, 1987, Springer-Verlag.

Bean MH: Denial and the psychological complications of alcoholism. In Bean MH, Zinberg NE, editors: *Dynamic approaches to the understanding and treatment of alcoholism,* New York, 1981, Free Press.

Clark WD: Alcoholism: blocks to diagnosis and treatment, *Am J Med* 71:275, 1981.

Prochaska JO, Norcross JC, DiClemente CC: *Changing for good: a revolutionary six-stage program for overcoming bad habits and moving your life forward,* New York, 1994, Avon Books.

Samet JH, Rollnick S, Barnes H: Beyond CAGE: a brief clinical approach after detection of substance abuse, *Arch Intern Med* 156:2287, 1996.

The Sexual History

Dickes R: Sexual myths and misinformation. In Simons RC, Pardes H, editors: *Understanding human behavior in health and illness,* ed 3, Baltimore, 1985, Williams & Wilkins.

Kaplan HS: *Illustrated manual of sex therapy,* ed 2, Bristol, Penn, 1988, Brunner/Mazel.

Katchadourian HA: *Fundamentals of human sexuality,* ed 5, New York, 1989, Holt, Rinehart & Winston.

Kolodny RC, Masters WH, Johnson WE: *Textbook of sexual medicine,* Boston, 1979, Little, Brown.

Owen WJ: The clinical approach to the male homosexual patient, *Med Clin North Am* 70:499, 1986.

White J, Levinson W: Primary care of lesbian patients, *J Gen Intern Med* 8:41, 1993.

The Occupational History

Callahan JP, editor: *The physician: a professional under stress,* Norwalk, Conn, 1983, Appleton-Century-Crofts.

Goldman RH, Peter JM: The occupational and environmental health history, *JAMA* 246:2831, 1981.

Levy BS, Wegman DH, editors: *Occupational health,* Boston, 1983, Little, Brown.

Muldary TW: *Burnout and health professionals: manifestations and management,* Norwalk, Conn, 1983, Appleton-Century-Crofts.

Newman LS: Occupational illness, *N Engl J Med* 333:1128, 1995.

The Occupational and Environmental Health Committee of the American Lung Association of San Diego and Imperial Counties: Taking the occupational history, *Ann Intern Med* 99:641, 1983.

Psychosocial Assessment

Erikson EH: *Childhood and society,* ed 2, New York, 1963, WW Norton.

Lazare A: Hidden conceptual models in clinical psychiatry, *N Engl J Med* 288:345, 1973.

Simons RC, Pardes H: *Understanding human behavior in health and illness,* ed 3, Baltimore, 1985, Williams & Wilkins.

LEARNING FROM HEARING AND SEEING YOURSELF

Student in a videotape review seminar: *My God, I didn't realize I missed that.*

Instructor: *Okay, but we all heard how much else you learned!*

When your clinical encounters are videotaped, you have an opportunity to learn by again seeing and listening to your patient and yourself. Even a brief segment of videotape will often reveal an enormous amount of verbal and nonverbal data about the interview, including material that was not recognized at the time of the actual encounter. Indeed, much of the "real life" clinical interview goes by too quickly to be thoroughly appreciated, especially by novice clinicians. Yet many important missed features will be readily evident and easily pointed out by instructors, fellow students, and yourself when studied in the reflective, and sometimes playful, atmosphere of a videotape review seminar.

Videotape review not only helps you sharpen your understanding of what happens in the encounter, but also lets you consider various strategies for responding to what has been observed. You will find few right or wrong answers about how to interview, but can gain a much better sense of how various approaches affect your patient and yourself, and you can consider incorporating new techniques into your clinical work. You may want to try role-playing a different approach. As you recognize more of the riches of the interview that are evident on videotapes and as you broaden your repertoire of interviewing approaches, you will find yourself better able to appreciate and respond to the complex events of your encounters with patients.

LEARNING IN A VIDEOTAPE REVIEW GROUP

Videotape review is carried out with a small group of your peers and supervisors. When reviewing your own interview, you will be both a teacher and a learner. You teach by providing the group with your interpretation of the events on videotape, including your rationale for and responses to what happened in the interview. Your recall will help you explicate your logic of questioning and listening and may evoke your feelings of the moment. For instance, the tape may be stopped at some point and you will reflect, along with the group, on questions such as:

What is happening here?
> What do you make of the situation?
> What do you notice?

What is the patient saying?
> What do you make of the patient's nonverbal behavior
> (posture, gestures, tone, and so forth)?

What were you thinking then?
> What were you feeling?

What did you do?
> How did it affect the interview?

You learn by hearing and seeing yourself and the patient interact and by the observations, interpretations, appreciation, and advice of your peers and supervisors. Your colleagues in the group will notice features of the interview that are not readily apparent to you. From the information you obtained, they may bring up new hypotheses about the patient's medical and psychological problems. They may affirm your response to the patient, while also offering alternative approaches. Common tactics for supervisors and peers include:

1. Making observations, for instance, about successful behaviors, nonverbal clues, the patient's mood or personality, and changes in the relationship as the interview progresses.
2. Offering hypotheses about the significance of statements or behaviors.
3. Seeking the interviewer's impressions.
4. Challenging the group: "What would you do here?"
5. Generalizing: "This situation is like another case when. . . ."
6. Empathizing (e.g., "This is a tough situation. Let's see what you did.").
7. Role-playing the situation posed by the videotaped interview. Such an exercise either allows others to try out the interviewer's role and demonstrate different approaches or gives the interviewer a chance to rehearse different behaviors ("Okay, now let's have Tim be the patient and Dave will take a crack at interviewing" or "How would you do it now? I'll be the patient").
8. Offering suggestions and a rationale for alternative strategies.
9. Reassuring a self-deprecating interviewer.
10. Complimenting.

GROUND RULES FOR GROUP REVIEW

1. "Warm-up" is essential in the early sessions. In the first meeting, participants should introduce themselves and say a few words about themselves. For instance, who has been videotaped before—"Is this your first time on TV?"—and what kind of interviewing and supervision experiences have participants had before. Later sessions might begin with an opportunity to pick up on topics from the previous discussion, raise is-

sues from recent clinical encounters, or propose topics for the day's session.

2. All participants, including the supervisors, should eventually have an interview taped and reviewed. Everyone feels that being exposed will result in shame. No! If possible, begin with the supervisor's tape, which will presumably demonstrate good technique but also show that everyone can be self-critical and use others' input to improve interviewing skills.

3. Everyone should participate as co-instructors. Any group member may request that the videotape be stopped or replayed and may ask questions or make observations. In general, the interviewer should have the first opportunity to comment on the tape.

4. Be critical but avoid the hazard of only citing errors or of being overly censorious of oneself or others. Be curious and welcome the opportunity to recognize lapses and improve yourself, but appreciate that all of the group are learning, including the supervisors. Point out what went well. Videotapes regularly demonstrate how a patient begins to respond warmly to the interviewer, how an initially anxious patient relaxes, and how a novice student looks and acts like a doctor. End the session with praise.

5. There are two "schools" of videotape review: the microanalysts (or "stop-button jockeys") and the macroanalysts (or "beholders of the big picture"). Microanalysts like to watch 5 to 10 seconds of the videotape at a time and then review each segment one or more times. They find too much to talk about in even a minute of recorded interview. The macroanalysts like to sit back and watch 5 to 10 minutes before commenting. Either school has its virtues, and participants in a videotape review seminar need to negotiate an approach that is mutually satisfactory.

SUGGESTED TOPICS

The following list offers some potential topics for beginning to reflect on the interview.

Starting Up

- How do the patient and doctor introduce themselves? Is the patient put at ease?
- What is the balance between "social chat" and "getting down to business?"
- Do the seating, posture, and eye contact affirm attention to the patient?

Process

- What kind of relationship is developing?
- What kinds of questions are being asked—open-ended vs. forced choice, unbiased vs. leading, one-at-a-time vs. complex, and so forth—and how did they influence the interview?

- How are facilitating comments or gestures used? Silences?
- Does the interviewer stick to medical "facts," or are psychosocial leads followed up?
- Is the patient allowed to tell his or her story or does the interviewer determine the agenda?
- Is affect recognized, elicited, and responded to?
- Does the physician communicate empathy or positive regard?
- Is the patient interrupted, and how is this explained to the patient?
- How are transitions handled?
- Does the interview follow a logical flow?

Medical and Psychological Diagnosis

- Is a complete, accurate account of the reason for the visit obtained, including all the dimensions of the symptoms and the relevant positive and negative features? What is the medical diagnosis?
- Have the relevant psychosocial data (e.g., social history, current stresses, emotional reactions, sources of support) been elicited?
- Who is this patient? How is the patient understood in terms of personality, social background, ethnicity, mood, and other characteristics?
- What kind of historian is this patient? Does the patient amplify, deny, and so forth?
- Has the patient's perspective (attributions, concerns, expectations, requests, triggers) been appreciated? What is the personal meaning of the symptoms?

Exposition Phase and Health Education

The portion of the interview that comes after the physical examination is seldom videotaped but deserves considerable attention. Most interview instruction focuses on eliciting information from patients, but examination of the exposition phase is a modern necessity in an age where the doctor's teaching is so important for patients' participation in treatment and decision making. Put the videotape camera on again after the physical examination.

- Is understandable language used, and are unfamiliar terms explained?
- Are opportunities for patient education recognized and utilized? Are questions sought?
- Does the interviewer negotiate over the goals and methods of treatment, recognizing the possibility of conflict?
- Are instructions clear, brief, simple? What educational strategies are employed? How is learning reinforced?
- Is the patient's feedback sought on the information transmitted, and is the patient asked to rehearse the treatment plan?
- How does the interviewer handle topics about which he or she lacks adequate information? Is uncertainty acknowledged?

- How did the interviewer attempt to motivate the patient? How were the patient's anxieties, strengths, and limits on changing recognized, and what supports were mobilized?

The Interviewer's Experience

- How did it feel being the doctor?
- How did this patient affect you? What did you like or dislike? How did you respond?
- How did various difficult topics (e.g., sexuality, loss) or affects (e.g., anger, sadness) affect you? How did you respond?

SCORING THE INTERVIEW

Videotaped interviews, especially interviews with simulated patients, are increasingly being used to provide practice, feedback, and skill ratings for students and residents. Checklists or similar instruments provide a rating form for your performance and can also be used by you and your observers— fellow students, preceptors, and the simulated patient—to evaluate your interviewing skills and guide further learning.

CONCLUSION

By observing and discussing videotaped clinical encounters, you acquire skills, but you also develop habits of self-reflection, the hallmark of the learning practitioner.

SUGGESTED READINGS

Ende J: Feedback in clinical medical education, *JAMA* 250:777, 1983.
Stoeckle JD, Lazare A, Weingarten C, et al: Learning medicine by videotaped recordings, *J Med Educ* 56:518, 1971.

CHAPTER 12

THE MENTAL STATUS EXAMINATION

Alzheimer's disease afflicts 4 million Americans:
- *10% of people over 65*
- *47% of people over 85*

One third of general medical inpatients have cognitive disorders, and only two thirds of them are recognized.

Students often find the mental status examination to be intimidating and perplexing. Although formal, detailed mental status testing does require considerable study and practice for mastery, many elements of this examination are already familiar to you. The purpose of this chapter is to help you recognize these familiar aspects and to describe a systematic approach for initially assessing and recording the patient's mental status, providing a basic framework you can use for expanding the proficiency and complexity of your exam.

MENTAL STATUS TESTING IN EVERYDAY CLINICAL LIFE

The mental status examination can be thought of as a method for systematizing observations that we usually make when meeting new acquaintances. While conversing with people for the first time, we try to establish rapport and get them to talk about themselves and their interests. We commonly ask questions that help us "get to know" them. We find out what they are like: how they appear, how they talk and act, what their mood and thinking are like, and so on. Indeed, some of the more subtle abnormalities of the mental status examination—blunted intellect, lack of humor, poor enterprise—are often paid little attention in evaluating patients, yet are readily recognized "findings" in our everyday social encounters.

The clinical interview provides similar opportunities to assess a patient's mental functioning. After a few minutes of a routine interview, you should be able to say whether your patient:
- Appeared and acted appropriately for the setting
- Was alert and attentive
- Understood normal conversational language and used it in such a way as to provide clear answers
- Recalled recent and remote events clearly
- Exhibited normal affect
- Demonstrated reasonable thought processes and content (i.e., made sense, seemed reasonably well informed, and had a realistic, coherent appreciation of his or her situation)

Later in the interview, as you explore the present illness and past medical history and learn about how the patient lives, you refine your appreciation of the patient's intelligence, reasoning, judgment, fund of information, and memory. You become informed about mood and affect as you characterize a person's adaptation to an illness, listen for and encourage expressions of feelings, and inquire about relationships, work, and leisure. You notice whether the patient appropriately expresses humor or gravity, or perhaps seems particularly sad, anxious, irritable, suspicious, or euphoric. You may observe that the patient has preoccupations or unusual thoughts. Additional history from family members or acquaintances may indicate that the patient is having trouble carrying out his or her usual daily tasks in the home or otherwise is thinking or behaving differently.

Thus, in the process of performing a standard history and physical examination, the attentive clinician can carry out the bulk of the basic mental status review. Only a few additional screening questions are required to ensure that important disorders have not been overlooked or that more detailed testing is not needed.

THE CLINICIAN'S FEELINGS AS A CLUE TO MENTAL STATUS DISORDERS

Neuropsychiatric disturbances may first become apparent to the clinician as a vague sense of discomfort in the interview, as a feeling that the patient is eccentric, vague, strange, evasive, boring, unfriendly, or threatening. When you (or other caretakers) avoid, dislike, or feel uncomfortable with a patient, try to figure out why. The explanation may sometimes be an unrecognized mental status disorder. For instance, when you find yourself irritated with a patient who seems uncooperative, further exploration of the mental status might indicate that the patient's problem is difficulty with attention, slowed mental or motor processes, tangential thinking, a negativistic attitude, or an inability to relax or stay still.

THE FORMAL MENTAL STATUS EXAMINATION

A thorough and systematic examination of mental function is indicated when you encounter a patient with disturbances in behavior, thought, or emotions, when the family or others report such disturbances, or when the patient's medical condition otherwise suggests the need to investigate neuropsychiatric functioning. Present your findings in an organized fashion, using the categories shown in Table 12-1.

An additional useful (though rarely recorded) category is personality style, as based on psychoanalytic concepts about "defenses" and described in Kahana and Bibring's classic paper "Personality Types in Medical Management." The box on p. 171 lists major personality styles. These seven styles (and others) typify how *normal* people cope with anxiety, and their

Table 12-1	Categories for Organizing the Formal Mental Status Examination
Category	**Sample Observations**
Appearance	Elderly, agitated, disheveled, muscular, well dressed
Behavior	Polite, cooperative, avoids direct eye contact, restless, moves slowly and rigidly
Level of consciousness	Alert, drowsy, unresponsive to loud noises or painful stimuli
Attention	Readily distracted, neglects right side, concentrates successfully on serial tasks
Speech and language	Rapid, hesitant, incoherent, garbled, uses nonsense words, mute
Mood	Sad, anxious, agitated, euphoric
Affect	Demonstrates wide range of appropriate affect, including anger, sadness, crying, laughter
Orientation	Knows person, place, date
Memory	Recalls recent and remote events
Thought content	Suicidal ideas, preoccupied with loss of job, says commentator on TV is talking about him
Thought processes	Logical, loose associations, unclear reasoning, sluggish
Insight	Has little appreciation of what's wrong, saying he has a liver condition that will improve soon without treatment
Judgment	Says, "If I reject dialysis, I'll probably die in a few weeks."
Higher cognitive functioning	Bright, dull
Fund of knowledge	Knows last five presidents, describes recent events in Nicaragua
Calculation	Serial subtraction of 7s: 100, 93, 86, 79, 72
Assessment	Overall impression is that his depression and suicidality have resolved, and that he currently shows moderate sadness but an otherwise normal range of affect and no significant cognitive deficits or disorders of sleep, appetite, or energy.

Typology in Personality Style

- Dependent and demanding (passive-aggressive)
- Controlled and orderly (obsessive-compulsive)
- Dramatizing, emotionally involved, and captivating (hysterical)
- Long-suffering and self-sacrificing (masochistic)
- Guarded and querulous (paranoid)
- Aloof and uninvolved (schizoid)
- Feeling of superiority (narcissistic)

recognition by the physician can be extremely helpful in facilitating clinical management. Barsky has also described how some patients tend to amplify or minimize bodily complaints, and this personality trait is regularly important in evaluating the presentation of physical symptoms. Additional helpful schemes for appreciating personality include "hateful patients" (Groves) and "neurotic styles" (Shapiro). Ethnic styles (Zola, Zborowski) also influence communication patterns.

The categories for a relatively complete mental status examination are described more fully in the discussions that follow, along with more sample observations. Unfortunately, the neurological, psychiatric, and general medical literatures do not use a common scheme for conceptualizing the mental status, so when reading about this examination, you may encounter a host of overlapping and inconsistently applied terms.

Appearance and Behavior

- How old does the patient appear to be? Does the patient appear much younger or older than his or her actual age?
- General health
- Cleanliness and self-care (shaven, use of makeup, condition of hair and nails)
- Dress: Care in dressing (neatness, cleanliness vs. disheveled, dirty, stained, neglecting one side of the body). Type of clothing (appropriateness to social setting and season; highly stylized, eccentric, muted)
- Facial expression (tense vs. relaxed, blank, fixed, smiling, staring)
- Posture (erect, slumped, bizarre stance)
- Motor activity: Amount and character (overactive, restless, fidgety, frenzied; motionless, underactive, slow). Abnormal movements (rigid, tremulous, repetitive movements, mannerisms, posturing)
- Attitude and cooperation (friendly, interested, flirtatious, belligerent, combative, preoccupied, restless, withdrawn, suspicious)
- Eye contact
- Response to environment and appropriateness of behavior (talking to self, becoming hostile when certain subjects are broached, startles when phone rings)

Level of Consciousness and Attention

Performance of the entire history and portions of the physical examination, including most of the mental status examination, presupposes that the patient has a fairly normal level of consciousness (i.e., the patient is alert rather than lethargic, somnolent, stuporous, or comatose) and exhibits normal arousability (responds to usual speech rather than requiring special maneuvers to gain and maintain attention). The patient's attention, concentration, and cooperation are also required. Significant disturbances in these functions would normally be mentioned at the beginning of the history under *reliability.*

- Level of consciousness (alert, drowsy, stuporous, hypervigilant). Rather than using vague labels (e.g., semicomatose) for patients with depressed consciousness, describe the patient's response—verbal and physical—to verbal, visual, and tactile (including, at times, painful) stimuli (e.g., "No response to commands, calling his name, or being touched firmly, but moves all four extremities when shaken or pinched").
- Attention is the ability to focus on specific stimuli and screen out irrelevant stimuli, rather than being distracted or attending only to one portion of the body. Apprehensive patients will often have trouble attending to complex tasks, although they have no cognitive deficit when more relaxed.

    Tests: (1) spell "world" backwards; (2) repeat five digits; (3) calculate serial subtractions of 3 or 7 from 100.

- Concentration (ability to persist with tasks vs. distractability in many tests in the mental status examination).

Speech and Language

Spontaneous speech and conversation during the history can be characterized as follows:
- Quality or quantity, including fluency, clarity, speed (e.g., slurred, garbled, stuttering, slowed, rapid, pressured)
- Content and organization: coherence, logic, relevance, redundancy, precision; spontaneity; disordered syntax, loose associations; circumstantial, evasive, perseverating; periods of prolonged silence or seeming distraction (also see Thought Content and Process)

The characterization of speech problems also requires testing for neuromuscular events involved in speaking; this aspect of the examination is not presented here.

When you notice abnormalities of language or want to provide a detailed evaluation of this neurological function, you can systematically evaluate input, processing, and output. Language input or reception includes listening and reading, while output or expression includes speaking and writing. Processing or understanding is evaluated by observing both input and output; nonverbal inputs (such as recognizing an object by sight or touch) and nonverbal outputs (such as motor acts) can be studied. Basic tests evaluate listening, reading, comprehension, naming, and writing:

- Listening (with verbal response)—"Repeat this phrase: 'No ifs, ands, or buts.'"
- Reading (with nonverbal response)—"Read and obey the following: 'Close your eyes.'"
- Comprehension (verbal instructions, nonverbal response)—"Take this paper and fold it in half and place it on the floor."
  Comprehension with minimal reliance on either verbal or nonverbal expression can be tested with "yes-no" questions—"Is your name Robert?"
- Naming (test for visual recognition and verbal expression)—Point at a common object (c.g., a watch or pen) and ask the patient to identify it.
- Writing—"Write a sentence."

Abnormalities in speech and language are often best characterized by including a verbatim sample.

Mood and Affect (Emotional State)

The term *mood* is used to describe a prevailing emotional tone; the term *affect* refers to moment-to-moment expression of emotion and the range of observable emotion. Mood and affect have qualities such as range, intensity, changeability, and appropriateness. A common and important clinical finding is discordance between patients' stated feelings and their nonverbal communication.

Both inquiry and observation are used to examine mood and affect. Pay attention to the four basic affective states: sadness (including grief and depression), happiness (including elation and mania), anxiety (including panic), and anger. See the following questions:

Questions About Mood and Affect _____

How are your spirits? How is your mood?
  In general?
  This moment?
  How are you feeling about the way your life is going?
    Your future?

Have you had any change of feelings come over you?

Are you nervous?
  Anxious? Irritable? Frightened?
  Are there specific situations that make you feel panicked?
    Are you afraid of crowded places?
    Going out alone?

Have you been angry?
   Out of control?

Have you been sad?
   Felt like crying?
   Cried a lot?
   Felt discouraged?
   Felt like you cannot go on?
      That life is not worth living? [see Suicidality under "Thought Content and Process" later in this section]

What do you do for fun?
   Have you been able to enjoy yourself?

How is your energy?
   Ambition?

Are you able to concentrate?
   To think clearly?
   Has your memory changed?

How is your sleep?
   Appetite?
   Sexual drive?

How do these feelings affect you?

Patients may describe themselves or appear in some of the following ways: sad, depressed, lacking energy, apathetic, unable to enjoy life; energetic, happy, euphoric, irritable, angry, furious; anxious, fearful, panicked; or "feeling fine" (perhaps despite events that would lead one to expect differently). The observer may note the following: the affect and its quality and appropriateness; the ability of the patient to describe his emotional life; such behaviors as retardation, agitation, lability, irritability, suspiciousness, defensiveness, impulsiveness; the communication of guilt, shame, worry, self-deprecation, or suspiciousness (see also Thought Content and Process); and how the patient affects the examiner (e.g., producing fright, boredom, sadness, hopelessness, or anxiety).

Orientation and Memory

Testing for orientation and memory may require specific questions, rather than reliance on observations made during routine history-taking. Some of the questioning can be handled unobtrusively by focusing on data that can be easily verified and that normally are a topic of conversation during interviewing:

What day did you get admitted?

Can you give me your address and phone number?

If you test the patient more openly and formally, explain why you are asking such questions. Encourage and reassure the patient as you go along, and let the patient guide you to testing at the appropriate levels of difficulty.

> Now I would like to ask you some routine questions to test your memory. Some of these questions may seem a little silly, but being sick can affect your ability to think clearly, and it's important that I check you.

> Let me first ask you some simple questions. Do you know today's date?

Orientation

Orientation is a complex phenomenon, primarily reflecting memory and perceptual abilities, and is impaired by a variety of common neuropsychiatric disorders. The most frequently employed formal tests of the mental status involve examination for the ability to identify person (the patient's name, age, and birth date, or the name and occupation or function of the examiner or another familiar person), place (the name of the institution or type of building the patient is in and where it is located), and time (date, day of week, hour, and season). A normal response is often abbreviated "oriented × 3."

Person
> What is my name?

> What is my occupation?

[Alternatively, ask for the name of a relative or a familiar person or request that the patient identify the occupation of a person with a readily recognized uniform (e.g., a nurse). Many physicians ask for the patient's name, but an inability to recall one's own name is rare for an alert person and usually indicates a psychiatric rather than neurological disorder. A more useful inquiry about the patient would be to ask about age and date of birth.]

Place
> Where are we right now?

> What is the name of this place?

> What kind of place is this?

> What city are we in? What state?

Time
> What is today's date (year, month, date)?

> What day of the week is it?

> About what time is it?

> What season of the year is it now?

Memory

In testing memory, ask about confirmable data, since confabulators may give accounts of the past that are convincing but incorrect. A variety of overlapping and inconsistent terms are used to describe memory, but the following categories are useful:

- **Long-term, or remote, memory** is tested by obtaining either verifiable personal information or widely known historical facts.

  Birth date, address, phone number, names and birthdays of children or relatives.

  Name the last four U.S. Presidents or describe major historical events (e.g., Kennedy assassination).

This aspect of memory overlaps with *fund of information* (see Higher Cognitive Function later in this section).

- **Recent memory** is tested by inquiring about orientation or asking the patient to recall verifiable events of the past few days.

  How long have you been in the hospital?

  Who is your doctor here?

  Did you get any tests today? What tests were done yesterday?

  Can you recall any recent news?

- **Immediate recall** (sometimes called registration, short-term memory, or immediate retention) is tested by digit or phrase repetition, and overlaps with attention.

  Repeat a sentence: "No ifs, ands, or buts."

  Repeat a six-digit number forward or a four-digit number backward

- **New-learning ability** is similar to recent memory, but also tests immediate recall. The examiner says, "I am going to name three objects. I want you to try to repeat them after me and to remember them." The examiner then slowly names three objects ("car, house, dress" or "red car, brown house, green dress") and asks the patient to repeat them. If the patient can repeat the three objects immediately, the examiner says, "I'm going to ask you about these objects in a few minutes." After 3 to 5 minutes of further discussion or physical examination, the patient is asked "Now repeat those objects I mentioned." In the record, note, for instance, "$\frac{2}{3}$ objects remembered over 5 minutes."

Thought Content and Process

The content of thought includes major concerns (worries, conflicts, interests, feelings of inadequacy, longings, ambitions, somatic preoccupations), obsessions, phobias, perseverations, strange experiences, suicidal or homicidal ideation, and various distortions of perception such as disturbances in the sense of self (depersonalization, derealization) or of the control of thinking.

Testing thought process means observing the patient's ability to make sense and grasp relationships. The process of thought has qualities of flow (speed, efficiency) and coherence or logic. You may identify some of the following disorders of thought process and content.

Questions About Thought Content and Process

Delusions

Delusions are fixed, false beliefs that are not in keeping with the patient's culture and that often contain misinterpretations or a finding of special meaning in events (e.g., a sense of being singled out or being paid special attention, or of being persecuted or influenced).

Have you felt that people have been taking special notice of you?

Have you noticed that the television or newspapers have had messages especially for you?

Have other people been able to control your thoughts or read your mind?

Hallucinations

Hallucinations are false sensory impressions, cither auditory, gustatory, olfactory, or tactile.

Have you heard voices?

Have you heard your thoughts out loud, as if they were spoken?

Have you seen anything unusual, perhaps things that do not really exist?

Illusions

Illusions are misinterpretations of real experiences, (e.g., a delirious patient thinks the doctor in the white coat is an ice cream vendor).

Bizarre, paranoid, or grandiose thinking

Are there thoughts that continually run through your mind?
   Thoughts that frighten you?

Do you ever have a feeling that people are talking about you or watching you?

Homicidality and suicidality

Have you had thoughts about harming others?

Have you had any thoughts about harming yourself?
   About taking your life?
   [No]: Have you ever considered suicide in the past?
      Attempted suicide?
   [Yes]: Tell me more.
      How serious are you?
      How would you do it?
      Do you have any plans for doing it?
      Do you have the means (pills, gun, other) to hurt yourself?
         Could you stop yourself?
         What keeps you from doing it?
         Would you be able to call for help before you did anything serious?

Thought is generally evaluated through open-ended questioning. Directed questions may help identify delusions, hallucinations, and suicidality:

Sometimes people who are upset [or very ill] have unusual [or frightening] thoughts. Has this happened to you?

Have you heard or seen things that turned out not to really be there or that others could not hear or see?

Insight and Judgment

Two aspects of thought occasionally require separate attention. The term *insight* refers to the patient's ability to understand that he or she is suffering from an illness. Does the patient appreciate his or her situation in a manner similar to that of the examiner? Useful questions include:

Why are you here today? Did you want to come?

Do you think anything is wrong with you? Why?
  Do you have a physical illness?
  Trouble with your thinking?
  With your emotions?
  Have you changed?

What do the doctors [or family, or others] make of it?

What do the tests show?

Do you believe you are thinking clearly?

Do you think you need any help?
  What kind?

Do you think you will get better?

What are your plans for the future?

More sophisticated concepts of insight—an awareness of how feelings affect behavior or of how past experiences influence current perceptions—are used in psychiatric evaluations.

Judgment is best described in medicolegal terms:

Does the patient appreciate the consequences of various actions? For example, what if treatment were foregone?

Further questions include:

Is the patient able to reason about actions and their consequences?
Does the patient act impulsively?
Would the patient act on the basis of delusional beliefs or hallucinatory perceptions? On wishful thinking?
What is his or her capacity for homicidal or suicidal behavior?
What is the basis for the patient's reasoning? Is such judgment appropriate to the patient's age and cultural background?

A less useful but commonly employed notion of judgment is to conceive of it as a higher intellectual function, characterized by a person's responses to hypothetical questions such as:

> What would you do if you found a stamped, addressed envelope on the street?
>
> What would you do if you were in a movie theater and saw a fire?

Higher Cognitive Function

Cognitive or intellectual function may be conceptualized as involving either basic levels, such as consciousness, attention, concentration, orientation, and memory (and, in some schemes, language and thought) or higher functions, such as fund of information, calculations, and abstraction (and, in some schemes, insight and judgment). Tests of visual perception and constructional ability may also be included under higher cognitive function or higher intellectual function.

For patients with intact basic cognitive abilities, you should learn to characterize the higher-level functions, especially fund of information and calculation. Tests of such higher intellectual functions can also be used to screen for defects of basic cognitive function, since, for instance, calculations are dependent on attention as well as arithmetic ability.

You need to inquire about the patient's level of education, type of employment, and cultural background in order to estimate his or her optimal level of cognitive functioning. Waitresses should be able to make change, while a migrant farm laborer might be expected to have only rudimentary arithmetic abilities. A recent immigrant would not be expected to know U.S. history or current affairs, but might have detailed information on other topics of personal interest, such as car repair, foreign affairs, or cooking. Similarly, you cannot interpret patients' responses to questions about current events without knowing their habits of reading or listening to the radio or television.

The examination of higher cognitive function includes some formal questioning:

> How are you at figures? . . . Not so good . . . How would you do in subtracting 7 from 100? . . . Try it.
>
> In order to test your concentration, I would like to ask you to try the following: Repeat this number, 1 6 7 4 3 . . . That's fine. Now let's try a longer number.

Higher cognitive function includes the following categories.

Fund of Information

> Who is the President? Who was President before him?
>
> [Alternatively]: Do you recall any recent, important news?
>   What have you read in the paper or heard on the news?
>   Do you know anything about what is going on in Northern Ireland? With the Red Sox?

Name four large cities in the United States.

Why are these people famous: George Washington, Shakespeare, Christopher Columbus, Einstein?

Calculation

"Serial 7's" (or "serial 3's")
Subtract 7 from 100 . . . Now subtract 7 from that . . . and 7 from that. . . .

Simple addition, subtraction, multiplication:
What would you get in change if you bought a 35-cent candy bar with a dollar bill?

Patients may also be questioned unobtrusively in the course of the interview, for example:

Patient: We moved to Chelsea in 1938.
Interviewer: So about how many years have you been living there?

Abstraction

Similarities:
What is the similarity between a plum and a peach?
A plane and a boat?
Red and blue are colors. A chair and a table are both what?

Proverb interpretation:
Tell me what people mean when they say:
People in glass houses shouldn't throw stones.
Don't cry over spilled milk.
A rolling stone gathers no moss.

Perception and Constructional Ability

Write your name

Draw a clock with the correct time

Copy this figure:

LEARNING AND PRACTICING THE MENTAL STATUS EXAMINATION

Incorporate a basic mental status examination into your routine history and physical examination, learning to pay attention to data that are evident in the course of the encounter, as well as including a few formal tests when the situation warrants. Beware of a common pitfall: beginning medical students tend to interpret mild disorders as "normal"—"I have a friend [or relative] that sometimes does that," or "At 85 years of age, what do you expect?"—thus dismissing significant mental status findings. Hone your skills in doing a basic examination by carefully recording your findings and practice a relatively elaborate examination and specialized tests on appropriate patients. Moreover, as soon as you suspect mental status problems, institute formal testing, as outlined earlier. Don't wait until the neurological portion of the physical examination to discover that your careful history was provided by a confabulator.

Introductory training in interviewing should sharpen your basic observational skills and provide a vocabulary and framework for systematically evaluating a patient's mental status. By reviewing videotaped or live medical interviews and comparing your observations with those of other clinicians, you can become more aware of the vast amount of mental status data available in a few moments of such encounters and of how to quickly appreciate this valuable information (see Quick Tips: Performing the Mental Status Examination).

QUICK TIPS

Performing the Mental Status Examination

- The components of the mental status examination will vary tremendously depending on the clinical situation.
- For most relatively well patients who have had a complete history and physical examination, you will not need to do a formal mental status examination.
- For most other patients, focus on orientation, recent and remote memory, new learning ability, and calculation.
- In cognitive testing, performance on any higher-level testing requires satisfactory performance on lower functions.
- Remember that the validity of a *single test* is often questionable.
- Record any abnormal findings from the mental status examination in the *neurological* area in the Physical Examination.

COMMON QUESTIONS ABOUT THE MENTAL STATUS EXAMINATION

How Complete a Mental Status Examination Should I Do?

The components of an appropriate mental status examination vary tremendously from patient to patient, depending on the clinical setting, the purpose of the evaluation, and the expertise of the examiner. No brief, clear-cut answer to this question can be provided, but some examples may be helpful.

For instance, when a young and generally healthy person presents with a cold, you may rely entirely on mental status information obtained during a brief, focused history and physical examination. For an older patient who has congestive heart failure and is getting an annual checkup, you acquire most of the mental status data in the course of a comprehensive history and physical examination, but you might also include a few formal screening questions for disturbances in orientation, memory, concentration, and higher cognitive function.

In ambulatory general medical practice, simple screening techniques are favored, particularly for the gross recognition of depression and confusional states (including dementia). Your primary job is to recognize whether any significant abnormality is present. A more comprehensive mental status examination should be used whenever the patient has neuropsychiatric complaints, such as difficulty with memory or concentration, or when the examiner suspects or detects a central nervous system disorder, a systemic illness with potential central nervous system manifestations, or a psychiatric or behavioral problem.

What Formal Tests of Mental Status Should I Apply to All Patients?

None need be applied universally, but a few are used regularly and should become quite familiar to you. For most relatively well patients who undergo a complete history and physical, you should be able to describe the major categories of the examination adequately without formal testing. For the majority of inpatients, as well as for many outpatients who, because of age, illness, or treatment, are at significant risk of having a mental status disorder, beginning students should use the following formal tests, unless these portions of the examination are clearly covered during the course of the routine history and physical:

1. Orientation
2. Recent and remote memory
3. New learning ability
4. Calculation

In elderly patients, a "mini-mental status" (Fig. 12-1) or a similar brief, formal psychometric instrument can be useful.

The Significance of Abnormal Findings In the Mental Status Examination Seems Less Clear Than for Other Parts of the Physical Examination. Once I Have Identified and Reported a Finding, What Do I Make of It?

The interpretation of a single mental status test usually depends on the relation of that finding to many other mental status observations, as well as to other data from the history and physical examination. Dissimilar conditions produce identical or similar results on individual mental status tests. Unintelligible speech, for instance, might be the primary manifestation of such varied disorders as a paralysis of the muscles used for speaking, lack of coordination of speech acts, aphasia (a specific central nervous system disorder in the reception, comprehension, or expression of language), delirium, dementia, or acute psychosis. Similarly, in cognitive testing, a hierarchy of mental functions exists such that the performance on any higher-level testing re-

MAXIMUM SCORE	SCORE	
		ORIENTATION:
5	( )	What is the (year) (season) (date) (day) (month)?
5	( )	Where are we (state) (county) (town) (hospital) (floor)?
		REGISTRATION:
3	( )	Name 3 objects: 1 second to say each. Then ask the patient all 3 after you have said them. Give 1 point for each correct answer. Then repeat them until he learns all 3. Count trials and record.
		TRIALS
5	( )	**ATTENTION AND CALCULATION:** Serial 7's: 1 point for each correct. Stop after 5 answers. Alternatively spell "world" backwards.
3	( )	**RECALL:** Ask for 3 objects repeated above. Give 1 point for each correct answer.
		LANGUAGE:
2	( )	Name a pencil and watch (2 points)
1	( )	Repeat the following: "no ifs, ands or buts" (1 point)
3	( )	Follow a 3-stage command: "Take paper in your right hand, fold it in half, and put it on the floor" (3 points)
1	( )	Read and obey the following: "Close your eyes." (1 point)
1	( )	Write a sentence. Must contain subject and verb and be sensible). (1 point)
		VISUAL-MOTOR INTEGRITY
1	( )	Copy design (2 intersecting pentagons. All 10 angles must be present and 2 must intersect). (1 point)

_____
30

TOTAL SCORE _____

Assess level of consciousness along a continuum.

| Alert | Drowsy | Stupor | Coma |

Fig. 12-1   "Mini–mental status" form for formal testing of mental status disorders. (Adapted from Folstein et al.) Scores of 20 or less suggest organic impairment (dementia or delirium) or, less commonly, severe schizophrenia or depression; further evaluation is required.

quires satisfactory performance of lower functions. For instance, a typical test of calculation requires that the patient first have a satisfactory level of arousal, be able to attend to the examiner's questioning for a suitable length of time, be cooperative, understand the language and be able to express answers in that language, remember the question and retain the results of previous calculations, as well as having been trained to make such calculations. Thus an error in serial subtractions of 7 from 100 could represent a disorder in many facets of cognitive function or perhaps merely reflect physical limitations (e.g., inability to talk) or premorbid level of functioning (e.g., lack of education) or lack of effort. The interpretation of the test result would depend on the results of the history, physical examination, and the characterization of related and more basic cognitive functions.

An appreciation of the patient's socioeconomic class, cultural background, education, and other psychosocial factors is often required to determine the significance of findings, including minor errors in orientation, long-term memory, or fund of knowledge. What was the patient's previous daily function, and how has it changed? Has the patient deteriorated from baseline? Is this dress and behavior consistent with the patient's background? What events—medical and psychosocial—might be invoked to explain such alterations in mental status?

Furthermore, the validity of a single test is often questionable. The clinician may wish to do the following:

1. Verify impressions through alternate tests (e.g., "Patient gave serial 7's: 100, 92, 95, 87, 80; serial 3's: 100, 97, 94, 92, 95, 92; "world" spelled backward: 'dlrow'")
2. Reproduce results, often relying on the highest level of functioning in repeated tests (e.g., "In three attempts at testing over 6 hours, remembered no more than one object after 3 minutes")
3. Quantify test results (c.g., use a standardized, scored, or timed test)
4. Describe the setting of the testing, if relevant (e.g., "Examined in a noisy EW room when his temperature was 102.0° po" or "Did not appear to be trying hard" or "Brought in by police and examined while in restraints")
5. Describe the quality of the performance, as well as the results (e.g., "Did correct serial 7's from 100 to 65, but very slowly and labored" vs. "Serial 7's: 100, 93, 84, 77, 70, 63, 59—done rapidly and without apparent concern for accuracy")
6. Present results in an objective fashion that can be interpreted by others (e.g., include actual responses, such as drawings or verbatim speech samples)

If a Large Part of the Mental Status Examination Is Acquired During History-Taking, How Can It Be Recorded Under Physical Examination?

The data for the mental status examination are obtained during the course of both the history and the physical examination. Some evidence is "subjective" (i.e., patient report—"I feel terrible") and some is "objective" (i.e., physician observation—"Looks forlorn, cries readily"), while some could fall into either category (i.e., as data from inquiry or from observation). When the mental status is normal, minimal mental status descriptions may be scattered throughout various portions of the write-up: in the statement of reliability, the present illness and past medical history, the statement of general appearance, as well as the mental status portion of the neurological examination. However, when abnormalities are present and a more elaborate description of the mental status is required, it is largely gathered and recorded, by convention, under the neurological section of the physical examination. Here, patient reports that could be included in the history might be treated as "objective" data (e.g., "Says she is sad and hopeless"). Analysis of how the patient presents the history is included under the neurological section (e.g., "Gave inconsistent responses"). Narrative data that bear on the mental status examination (e.g., the story of the evolution of a paranoid psychosis, provided by a source other than the patient) is presented in the history, but may be referred to, summarized, or partially restated in appropriate form in the neurological examination. Also, as described earlier, most reports or observations of disturbed emotion, behavior, and intellect are only interpretable when correlated with a characterization of the patient's usual status; such a description of "premorbid" function is provided by a note in the history.

SUGGESTED READINGS

Barsky A: Patients who amplify bodily sensations, *Ann Intern Med* 91:63, 1979.

Cassell EJ: An everyday language of description. In *Talking with patients,* vol 1, *The theory of doctor-patient communication,* Cambridge, Mass, 1985, MIT Press.

Folstein MF, Folstein SE, McHugh PR: "Mini-mental state": A practical method for grading the cognitive state of patients for the clinician, *J Psychiatr Res* 12:189, 1975.

Glick TH: *The process of neurologic care in medical practice,* Cambridge, Mass, 1984, Harvard University Press.

Groves J: Taking care of the hateful patient, *N Engl J Med* 298:883, 1978.

Kahana RJ, Bibring GL: Personality types in medical management. In Zinberg NE, editor: *Psychiatry and medical practice in a general hospital,* New York, 1964, International Universities Press.

Shapiro D: *Neurotic styles,* New York, 1965, Basic Books.

Strub RL, Black FW: *The Mental Status Examination in Neurology,* ed 3, Philadelphia, 1993, FA Davis.

Zborowski M: Cultural components in response to pain, *J Soc Issues* 8:16, 1952.

Zola IK: Culture and symptoms: an analysis of patients' presenting complaints, *Am Sociol Rev* 31:615, 1966. Reprinted in Zola IK: *Socio-medical inquiries: recollections, reflections, and reconsiderations,* Philadelphia, 1983, Temple University Press.

CHAPTER 13

DIFFICULT RELATIONSHIPS

A difficult patient is one who in some way frustrates a physician's need to control the relationship

L. P. WHITE

AN INTRODUCTION TO "DIFFICULT DYADS"

In working with people in any setting, you may like some better than others, and you may dislike at least a few. In the work of doctoring, clinicians find profound gratifications in their relationships with some patients, but find others difficult and a few persistently troubling. Even the best doctor-patient relationships have rocky moments, since few patients unfailingly behave as we might hope. Indeed much of the demanding and sometimes draining quality of a vocation of clinical service arises not from the long hours and intellectual demands or the inevitable uncertainties that must be tolerated, but from the hard work, often in stressful circumstances, of getting along with other people.

The notion of difficult relationships has been around for a long time, even though such terms as "problem patients," "crocks," or "difficult dyads" only became common in the 1950s. Clinicians in the past have acknowledged their trouble with some patients and tried to improve their relationships through understanding the patient and altering their own attitudes and behaviors. For instance, as early as 1904, Richard C. Cabot, Physician to Outpatients at the Massachusetts General Hospital wrote:

To improve practice requires more science and more Christianity ... We need for efficient treatment a fund of patience, cheerfulness, or readiness to be interested in each least promising and most unattractive individual in the clinic that in my experience comes out of the spirit of Christianity.

Nowadays, we formulate the challenge of difficult patients in psychological, behavioral, and secular terms. We try to understand why some patients behave as they do; why we experience their behavior as difficult; what kind of relationship has developed; and how, calling on various intellectual and emotional resources (including a fundamental regard for fellow human beings), we can best carry out our professional calling to serve the patient.

Whose Problem Is It?

Unfortunately, patients are often called "difficult" as if the fault were all their own. The problem lies not simply with the patient, but with the doctor-patient relationship, in which the doctor has a major part. Difficult to whom? Patients only become difficult when they evoke in the clinician such uncomfortable feelings as frustration, confusion, anxiety, sadness, anger, or disgust, and then are labeled as "problems." Difficult patients mean difficult relationships.

At one extreme in the spectrum of difficult relationships are the patients who tend to irritate even the kindest, most tolerant, understanding, and well-trained physician. Attempts to analyze problems with these unruly characters invariably focus on qualities of the patient, but the clinician profits from a better appreciation of his or her vulnerability to such people and of how and why these patients disturb us.

At the other extreme are the patients whose behavior may ultimately be viewed as quite appropriate to their condition and who, ideally, should not be difficult. Yet, they trouble the clinician. In this category of difficult relationships fall many patients for whom we simply lack a framework to make sense of their behavior (including perhaps an appropriate diagnosis) or for whom we lack appropriate management skills. For instance, persons with unrecognized cognitive deficits or psychiatric disorders often are annoying to clinicians, as may be patients who simply do not respond to our treatment. Other difficult relationships may be provoked by stressful situations (e.g., being overworked and sleep deprived) or may reflect the clinician's personal vulnerabilities or identifications ("She reminds me of a patient who really made me miserable"; "My father has this same problem"; "He's my age, and it could happen to me").

Between these extremes are a great number of patients whose behavior at certain times may be recognized as less than exemplary and for whom clinicians have variable tolerance as well as variable skill and ease in management. Attention must be focused on both parties and on how they relate to each other. Yet the final common pathway for labeling a patient as difficult is that he or she is difficult to the clinician. *All problematic relationships reflect a vulnerability of the clinician.* Ultimately, these difficult relationships can be better understood and often improved through further training and clinical experience.

Recognizing a Difficult Relationship

Patients may provoke anger, guilt, frustration, dread, confusion, hopelessness, withdrawal, and so on, yet we may not readily realize how we are being affected. We may simply avoid the patient. Disagreeable feelings may be suppressed, especially when they seem improper or incongruent with our preferred self-image as the accepting, unruffled, or beloved doctor. We may also resort to such labels as "gomer," "complainer," "nervous Nellie," "turkey," or "clinger"—opprobriums that thrust blame on the patient but should also alert us that the relationship is problematic.

As usual in clinical medicine, the first step to solving a problem is to see it clearly. A rational, analytic approach to difficult dyads cannot begin until the clinician consciously identifies the relationship as problematic. A key skill is self-reflection. One needs to recognize when a relationship is troubling, rather than simply reacting to one's own irritation. Then, by reflecting on the relationship, perhaps aided by a colleague or supervisor, the clinician has the opportunity to understand the patient better, to see more clearly his or her reaction to the patient, and often to find ways of improving this relationship and others like it.

A Typology of Difficult Relationships

Patients and doctors find myriad ways of not getting along well, and the varieties of difficult relationships do not admit to an easy classification scheme. However, the typology presented in the following sections is useful for introducing this complex subject. These typological categories are not mutually exclusive; more than one may be fruitfully used to help unravel the complex reasons that a particular patient is perceived as difficult (see Quick Tips: Types of Difficult Relationships).

QUICK TIPS

Types of Difficult Relationships

- Vexatious characters
- Patients with disconcerting medical conditions
- Patients with troublesome emotional reactions
- Patients whose somatic complaints have no physical basis
- Situations in which barriers to communication exist
- Discordant expectations
- Conflicted roles and ethical problems
- The distressed clinician

Vexatious Characters

For some patients, difficult relationships—with clinicians and with other people—are a regular feature of their lives. Many of these patients have personality or other serious psychiatric or behavioral problems, manifested in such conduct as being unruly, demeaning, nasty, demanding, or manipulative, and they seem to drive almost every doctor a little crazy. Groves has labeled one such group as "hateful patients," and, indeed, a peculiar mark of certain character disorders is an uncanny ability to excite antipathy. They may "collect injustices" done to them by their doctors, making their physicians feel inadequate. Similarly, some chronic alcoholics vex clinicians by denying their drinking or its seriousness, while presenting with flagrant, recurrent complications of substance abuse. Other character types seem skilled at promoting relationships in which an authoritarian figure (such as the physician) acts punitively toward the "bad" patient.

A variety of patient personality styles will be perceived as difficult only in particular circumstances. For example, certain flamboyant, dramatizing, emotionally involving persons tend to be seen as charming and entertaining most of the time. Yet they may be considered problematic when they pay too little attention to a medical treatment that the clinician feels is important or when they focus too much attention on appearances and on being admired rather than on clinical issues of greater concern to the physician. Highly orderly, controlled patients tend to take an active role in caring for themselves and are generally appreciated by the doctor for being very compliant, but they may be irritating when the busy clinician perceives them as overly concerned with the minutiae of care (e.g., bringing in long lists of questions and reporting multiple minor symptoms).

Many other patient characteristics, such as physical appearance, emotional responses, and psychological defenses, will similarly affect, in various ways, the relationship with the doctor. Potentially troubling examples include patients who are dirty, obstreperous, seductive, manipulative, deceitful, or suspicious; patients who greatly amplify or minimize symptoms; patients who demand medicines, reassurance, or frequent attention; patients who are noncompliant, including persons who reject important diagnostic and therapeutic interventions or leave the hospital against medical advice; and patients who are chronically anxious or depressed.

Disconcerting Medical Conditions

The process of medical training involves a progressive desensitization to situations that many students find troubling, as well as a growing ability to act therapeutically in these situations. A variety of taboos are overcome about touching other people, examining bodily orifices, causing discomfort, and even cutting into the body. The clinician gradually gets used to working with patients with such potentially disconcerting medical conditions as facial disfigurements, skeletal deformities, malodorous wounds, fungating tumors, extreme frailty, dementia, psychosis, and terminal illness. Most important for interviewing, students learn how to ask "personal questions," exploring the intimate lives of patients and opening up discussion of such topics as sexuality, substance abuse, and dying. Additionally, for many students, medical school confers a first close experience with such potentially upsetting phenomena as violence, drug abuse, homosexuality, socially deviant behavior, or poverty.

The desensitization, however, is incomplete. Even experienced clinicians want to avoid certain clinical situations, and may choose a career partly on the basis of such preferences (e.g., not wanting to work with very sick children or emotionally disturbed persons). Students, moreover, are necessarily thrust into clinical work without having fully undergone the dramatic socialization process of developing a degree of detachment. New and stressful settings—the trauma service, the intensive care unit, a terminal care facility, a burn unit, a venereal disease clinic, or a psychiatric ward—are often upsetting, as may be individual patients.

Why do some conditions bother us more than others? Elements of personality and background help explain feelings of distress around patients. Sometimes, clinicians are simply troubled by their lack of knowledge and skill in managing these problems. Some "cases" are too complicated (and, eventually, some may seem too simple). Patients with progressive neurological deficits or terminal disease may frustrate us if we are bothered by our limited ability to restore health. Each disconcerting condition requires self-analysis.

Troublesome Emotional Reactions

Students frequently have difficulties when they find themselves in emotionally charged situations that are common to medical practice yet uncommon in daily life and for which they may have had little clinical preparation. For instance, many patients are encountered who display intense emotions such as fear, anxiety, sadness, or anger. Even when these affects are normal responses to stressful situations, they may be unsettling to the novice interviewer. The student may not know how to help patients deal with these emotions. Similarly, patients who exhibit strong denial in the face of serious illness may be perceived as difficult. Some troubling emotional reactions are described in later chapters.

Patients may develop strong feelings about their physicians. One of the most troubling of patients' emotional reactions is when they dislike us.

> *Many a time a man must watch the patient's mind as it watches him, distrusting him, ready to fly off at a tangent at the first opportunity; sees himself distrusted, sees the patient turn to someone else, rejecting him. More than once we have all seen ourselves rejected, seen some hard-pressed mother or husband go to some other adviser when we know that the advice we have given . . . has been correct. That too is part of the game.*
>
> *William Carlos Williams*
> *The Autobiography (1951)*

Despite our best efforts, patients do not invariably appreciate us. As surely as the physician is viewed at times as a hero, he or she will also encounter rejection and scorn—maybe even from the same patient who recently was so grateful!

Likewise, patients may develop a strong attachment to a physician, sometimes independent of any feelings the physician harbors for the patient. Such patients may make us uncomfortable because of the intimacy they search for or seem to find in the relationship or the seemingly excessive power and wisdom they assign the physician. They may want to treat us as children, parents, closest friends, or lovers.

Somatic Complaints Without a Physical Basis

The "positive review of systems" and the consternating problem of persons who seem to be physically well yet have persistent bodily concerns or complaints are discussed in the portion of this chapter titled The Doctor and the Somatizing Patient.

Communication Barriers

Problems in communication typically occur when patients have deficits in hearing, language, or intelligence or when they are overtalkative, excessively reticent, or vague. Some "different" patients are difficult because they do not speak English well or come from other cultural backgrounds. When communication barriers exist, the clinician may be uncertain about the patient's understanding and expectations. Feeling "unconnected" to the patient, the physician finds the process of care less gratifying, even if overt difficulties do not arise. Moreover, interviewing may require considerable extra effort; the clinician, especially when pressed for time, may resent the additional work (and the patient). (See Communication Styles and Communication Barriers later in this chapter.)

Discordant Expectations

Both patients and doctors harbor notions of how each other should behave and may be intolerant of deviations from this norm. Failure to recognize and address such conflicts is often responsible for a difficult relationship. As discussed in Chapter 14 ("Conflict" section), discordant expectations need to be negotiated.

Many patients seem difficult because they do not behave in the way we expect of a "good" patient. Their so-called difficulty may simply be that they are unlike us. They may not exhibit what the physician considers common courtesy or respectful behavior. Some "different" patients speak English well and even seem to share the same cultural background as the clinician, but nonetheless have their own perspective about illness, the appropriate behaviors for patient and doctor, and the right approach to diagnosis and treatment. They may not accept our diagnosis, follow our recommendations, or otherwise meet our expectations for the patient in the sick role. A simple example are those patients whose previous practitioner let them drop into the office whenever they wished and was accustomed to receiving telephone inquiries at all times. Such patients may be considered unreasonably demanding by a new physician who only offers visits "by appointment" and wants after-hour phone calls reserved for emergencies. More subtle conflicts poison many relationships.

Power is an omnipresent issue in human relationships. The doctor and patient may have discordant expectations about control in the clinical encounter. How much authority should either exert over the process of the interview? About management decisions? How should information and decisions be shared? Either party may be rankled when the other person seems to prefer too great or too little a role in decision-making or does not respect the other's expertise.

Clinicians are not always fully aware of the many expectations they have of patients. Insofar as we apply our notions of the "good" patient unselfconsciously (i.e., with assurance that our personal standards have some absolute value and that all patients have the capability of behaving as we wish), many persons will be disliked rather than tolerated as different. Balint has written about the "apostolic function" of doctors:

> *Apostolic mission or function means in the first place that every doctor has a vague, but almost unshakably firm idea of how a patient ought to behave when ill. Although this idea is anything but explicit and concrete, it is immensely powerful, and influences, as we have found, practically every detail of the doctor's work with his patients. It was almost as if every doctor had revealed knowledge of what was right and what was wrong for patients to expect and to endure, and further, as if he had a sacred duty to convert to his faith all the ignorant and unbelieving among his patients.*

Conflicted Roles and Ethical Problems

Clinical situations may arise in which physicians have difficulty maintaining their traditional professional role with the patient or in which ethical concerns arise. The customary neutrality of the doctor, for instance, is distorted in caring for patients for whom one has a personal attachment outside of the clinical encounter (e.g., relatives, close social acquaintances, or fellow physicians); "detached concern" may be hard to maintain. A strong personal or sexual attraction to a patient can corrupt professional goals and make for a troubling relationship. The doctor-patient exchange may also be warped when patients are celebrities or otherwise popular or notorious figures, since the behaviors of both doctor and patient may be affected by status differential, concerns about publicity, and demands of the patient's public family.

Ethical dilemmas are posed when the doctor seeks to serve the patient while also addressing potentially conflicting personal, professional, or societal goals. For instance, physicians (and students) in clinical research or training may find themselves enthusiastically promoting their research or pedagogy, but note a conflict between soliciting patients' participation and the obligation to serve the best interests of the patient. In other settings, being helpful, pleasing the patient, and maintaining the relationship may clash with such standards of conduct as honesty and protecting the common good. For instance, clinicians may develop a somewhat adversarial role toward persons who seek narcotics, disability certification, and excuses from work, school, or jury duty, especially when the patient's medical disorder does not clearly justify these requests.

Indeed, the loyalties of the doctor may often be divided between the patient and intermediaries. Physicians commonly provide care under "contract" with third parties, such as the welfare department, immigration services, courts, or other government agencies, insurance companies, prepaid health plans, a hospital or group practice, or the parents or relatives of a patient. A Public Health Service physician will test an immigration applicant for HIV antibodies—not for the benefit of the patient but with the purpose of excluding persons with this condition from residence in this country. In such situations, the patient may view the physician as someone who needs to be convinced or pleaded with, rather than as an objective, sympathetic helper; the physician, in turn, may wonder if the patient is being manipulative or deceitful.

Increasingly, physicians act as "gatekeepers," providing patients with personal medical care while also having the responsibility of deciding who has access to limited health resources. Pressure to reduce resource utilization may be subtle and minor (e.g., emanating from a vague personal sense of social responsibility or from casual comments of colleagues) but can also be overt and compelling (e.g., arising from a strong sense of personal mission, from directions of a supervisor, or from significant financial incentives). A patient who seems to overutilize services may be perceived as undesirable, especially if the physician or the practice organization directly experiences a monetary loss each time a patient goes to the emergency ward, visits the office, is admitted to the hospital, stays an extra inpatient day, or requires a consultation or procedure. Even in representing the government, the physician, by virtue of being a taxpayer, may feel that benefits for welfare recipients are a burden on his or her livelihood.

These situations raise serious ethical questions that deserve not only reflection but also action that maintains a proper relationship between physicians and patients. At times, patients should be warned about the physician's dual obligations. For instance, a military psychiatrist might need to advise certain patients that their report of particular behaviors (e.g., homosexuality), even though considered normal by professional medical standards, would be transmitted to superior officers and perhaps considered improper. Similarly, the physician's potential for personal gain or loss from clinical decisions should be made evident to patients.

The Distressed Clinician

The doctor may come to a relationship already feeling distressed. A tired, upset, or otherwise unhappy interviewer may find even relatively routine clinical encounters difficult. No patient is a "good patient" to the admitting resident who is feeling barely able to care for his or her workload. A well-justified phone call in the middle of the night may be greeted with irritation when one feels desperate for sleep. When life is not going well for the interviewer, the doctor-patient relationship may be difficult.

Resolving Difficult Relationships

An excellent general rule when a patient seems difficult is to put more energy into trying to understand that person better. When we know more about our patients—what they are thinking, how they perceive their illness, why they are behaving the way they do—we usually appreciate them and like them better. Our sense of the difficulty may even take on a different perspective, so our discomfort may lessen or even resolve or turn into respect and appreciation. Understanding often helps us be more accepting, less critical: "Yes, he's furious, but only because he's so desperate for approval; his hurt and anger come quick." We may also recognize tactics for improving the relationship, including ample apologies.

Unfortunately, with many difficult patients who seem to be acting badly, our tendency is to disparage, dismiss, or otherwise avoid them. When you find yourself in this frame of mind, try to reflect on why a patient is bothering you. Why are you having trouble being nonjudgmental and accepting? Why does this particular person get you upset?

A further strategy for dealing with difficult relationships is to talk about them and get help. Share your frustration with a colleague, consultant, or understanding friend. Blow off a little steam. Complain bitterly. You do not need to mince your words. There is no harm in having these feelings toward your patient or in expressing them in the right setting. Often a little ventilation to a sympathetic listener will help you bear with the uncomfortable feelings. You may come away feeling better and ready to approach the problem freshly. Additionally, seek appropriate supervision or consultation. Mental health consultants may be particularly able to steer you toward better understanding and practical solutions. Some training programs offer group sessions—Balint groups—in which students, residents, and staff can bring up problematic cases for discussion.

Some difficulties may indicate poorly negotiated conflicts in the doctor-patient relationship, reflecting differences between the participants in knowledge, attitudes, or values. (See Conflict: Negotiation and Management in Chapter 14.) To deal with such conflicts, a fairly straightforward, cognitively oriented strategy for negotiation and limit-setting can be tried:

Negotiating Conflicts

1. Establish an atmosphere of trust and open communication
2. Identify and clarify the conflict

> We seem to have a clash here. You have been calling as often as once or twice a night. From my point of view, many calls were not emergencies and could have waited until regular calling hours.

3. Acknowledge the needs of the patient

> I understand that you have lots of concerns that you want to talk to me about. I realize that you often have a sense of urgency about calling.

4. Define rights and duties

> I have agreed to be accessible and I will always return your call. At the same time, I expect you to use evening calls only for urgent matters. You can bring up other concerns at office visits and during regular calling hours.

5. Negotiate a plan. Seek a mutually agreeable arrangement, perhaps reflecting some concessions or newly generated alternatives.

> I need your help. How about an agreement about when you will reach us? Would you be willing to call at night only if you have an emergency?

6. Monitor the agreement

> If that's okay, let's try it for a few weeks and then sit down and go over how the arrangement is working.

Finally, the topic of difficult relationships leads into a consideration of an extensive body of knowledge about psychosocial aspects of medicine. Clinical training on such topics as normal emotional responses, personality, coping, defenses, psychopathology, and cultural influences on health behavior may be useful in understanding problematic relationships and in enabling the interviewer to deal better with patients. Many difficulties are manifestations of recognized clinical disorders—psychiatric, behavioral, or social—and of common responses of clinicians to such disorders. For instance, training about substance abuse or suicidal behavior should facilitate recognition of these disorders and ease of management. Such matters are the subject of psychiatric texts. Subsequent chapters, however, explore some common themes in difficult relationships: troubling patient emotions, barriers to interpersonal communications, bodily complaints that cannot be explained on a physical basis, and the dying patient. We also encourage you to consult the texts cited in the Suggested Readings.

■ CONCLUSION

One of medicine's greatest challenges and also one of its greatest rewards is learning to get along well with people of all backgrounds and personalities. In a life of service to the needs of others, the physician encounters abundant stresses. A discussion of difficult relationships should remind you of the many ways clinicians struggle to understand and work with diverse persons and of how efforts to be tolerant and appreciative of others may help you be a more effective, humane, and happy clinician.

Difficult relationships can be exasperating, but they often prove to be fascinating. Eventually, you may look with great fondness on so-called difficult patients as you realize how deeply they once troubled you, how much energy you put into improving the relationship, and how much you learned from them. The difficulty lies, at least partly, in you, so your ability to understand problematic relationships and to achieve some resolution often marks significant personal and professional growth.

THE DOCTOR AND THE SAD OR CRYING PATIENT

Give sorrow words; the grief that does not speak
Whispers the o'er fraught heart and bids it break.

William Shakespeare
Macbeth

Emotions are part of being ill. While patients may come to the doctor expecting to talk mostly about medical "facts," they also bring along feelings about their sickness and their lives. Eliciting these affects is necessary for understanding patients' illnesses; responding to emotions can be therapeutic. Moreover, the affective exchange—verbal and nonverbal—between you and your patient is a major determinant of the quality of your relationship and of patient satisfaction.

This section and the two that follow discuss those common emotions that patients bring to the encounter and that interviewers may find difficult. The first is sadness.

The Interviewer's Response to Sadness

Sadness is distressing for the patient experiencing it and often for the clinician attending that person. The interviewer may feel bad for the patient or even responsible for provoking the sorrow, although the source of the sadness is the personal world of the patient. Perhaps being uncomfortable about intruding into the patient's emotional life or aggravating the distress, the interviewer will be reluctant to explore the sadness further.

A natural response when someone is unhappy is to do something quickly to make that person feel better—to console or brighten up the patient. Affects, however, rarely admit to such facile manipulation. Another tactic is to try to dismiss the sadness with such instructions as "Don't take it so seriously" or advice that "it will all be okay." But this approach is rarely helpful; you merely communicate that you are not interested in the patient's feelings or that you disapprove of displays of emotion.

Another natural response to sorrow is to change the topic, steering away from charged matters while hoping that the affect will go away. Patients will often cooperate with this approach, since most persons are uncomfortable about displaying distressing emotions and do try to suppress them. However, by avoiding the sadness, the clinician misses an excellent opportunity to learn about the patient. Moreover, the relationship gets narrowly defined as medical "business only," rather than including the ill person's emotional experience. The affect, of course, persists, but is left for the patient to handle alone.

A Clinical Approach to Sadness

A basic tactic in responding to sadness (and other affects) is to try to understand the patient's feelings and the circumstances that brought them about. Your task when confronted with a patient who expresses important emotions should be to listen, encourage the expression of affect, and learn more about what led to those feelings.

For patients who are crying or overtly expressing sadness, you may simply respond with facilitative gestures or attentive silence. Allow the patient to let out the feelings. You may also explicitly encourage "the tears."

> It's good to get it out.

Crying, of course, should not be equated with sadness. Some people cry when they are angry, frustrated, relieved, or joyful. You may need to ask why the patient is crying.

If the patient's words or nonverbal behavior merely hint at sadness, seek further expression:

> Patient: . . . When that happens, it really gets to me.
> Interviewer: Say more about how it affects you.
>
> Patient: . . . and that can be kind of depressing.
> Interviewer: I can see how you might feel. Tell me more.
>
> Interviewer [to patient who has a sad facial expression or moist eyes]: You look like you are feeling sad. What are the tears about?

Some patients will respond to such prompting with more tears and by telling the story of their sadness. Others, even if sadness is suggested by their story or their nonverbal behaviors, will contain their thoughts and feelings. Try further gentle encouragement. If patients still do not elaborate, you may conclude that you have misunderstood them or that they prefer for now to suppress the feelings. You cannot force a patient to disclose more, and your firm pressure to express emotions may heighten the patient's anxiety and defensiveness. However, you may still want to acknowledge the affect and open the door to future discussion:

> I sense that this is really troubling you, and I see that it is quite hard for you to talk about it now. Perhaps we will want to bring it up again later.

Clinical experience will help you appreciate when to encourage expression of affect and when to support the patient's defenses against the feelings, perhaps waiting for further trust and comfort to develop.

Offer empathic comments that validate the patient's emotional distress and show your understanding of the patient's suffering.

> You certainly have gone through a lot.

Patients will often apologize for revealing their sadness, and should be reassured that you accept their feelings and behavior:

> Patient: I'm sorry, doctor. I really shouldn't act this way.
> Interviewer: That's okay. I can see that this has been troubling you a great deal.

For most sad patients, you accomplish a major therapeutic act by simply allowing the patient to release feelings. Do not shy away from tears. Patients and clinicians may worry about "opening Pandora's box" or may fear that crying, once begun, will never stop. In reality, a brief sharing of the affect is usually followed by the patient becoming composed, feeling better, and being grateful for the clinician's concern. While a sympathetic interviewer may seek to assume the patient's burden of sadness and to make everything better, you fulfill your professional role better by simply providing a setting in which the patient can comfortably express and reflect on emotional problems. On occasion, you may be able to suggest some specific actions to alleviate the sadness. Only rarely do patients need help maintaining control of their feelings or more sophisticated psychological interventions for coping with sadness.

When Is Sadness More of a Problem?

In selected circumstances, sadness deserves further evaluation. Additional training in psychosocial assessment will help you recognize how sadness and normal grief differ from depression and pathological (unresolved or chronic) grief. You must learn how to assess suicidality, which may accompany these affects. You will also want to learn about "chronic depression" or dysthymic disorder, a condition in which a person may appear sad or depressed as a reflection of a long-standing personality trait; these patients cannot be expected to get over their sadness or to stop complaining, though they can be helped to feel better.

THE DOCTOR AND THE ANGRY PATIENT

Anger is a common and often healthy, adaptive response to life's stresses. It mobilizes patients to defend themselves against threats to their well-being; it can also command the attention and helping action of others.

Nonetheless, most of us are uncomfortable around angry people. We worry that the upset person might get out of control or that the hostility might be redirected toward us. Thus a common response to another's anger is to ignore or avoid it, hoping it will go away on its own, or to try to defuse or deflect it. And should we feel personally attacked, we tend to fight back, often provoking further anger.

How Anger Arises and Is Expressed

Anger is usually provoked by a painful experience, typically a loss or a threat of injury. A loss may be quite concrete—death of a friend, financial setbacks, physical disability—or more symbolic—a wound to one's self-esteem from being treated disrespectfully; feeling that others dislike you or are angry at you; a sense of helplessness, shame, or diminished future prospects; or a fear of illness.

Anger, like other emotions, can diffuse from the situation in which it arose to other settings. A common response to being humiliated is to try to restore one's self-importance by humiliating others. An angry person may let hostility out on whomever is a convenient target. Thus a patient who is frustrated by an appointment delay, denial of welfare assistance, or the expense of medication may direct anger at the doctor. The doctor, even if not responsible for these problems, somehow seems part of the overall victimization felt by the patient. Also, when patients feel stressed by illness, they may become angry over matters that ordinarily would incite little response.

Another characteristic of anger is that it often is suppressed. Getting mad is considered impolite, especially around such figures of authority as physicians. Students, nurses, secretaries, and the hospital's public relations offices are more acceptable targets (and also often have the privilege of hearing the patient's complaint about "the older medical doctors"). Some persons hide their hostile feelings, afraid that even a little expression will lead them to erupt into frank rage. Another reason to suppress hostility is the fear, sometimes realistic, that others will reject you for being angry.

Patients often imply anger without stating it overtly. The clinician may read the concealed emotion in the patient's demeanor, for instance, when patients raise their voice, tense their jaws, or clench their hands.

Responding to the Patient's Anger (see Quick Tips: Dealing with Anger)

An initial task when encountering anger is to help the patient feel safe enough to share the hostile tension. Suppressed feelings are more likely to be shared when trust has developed. The clinician gives the patient permission to express anger by acknowledging the emotion openly and by indicating that such feelings are acceptable:

> You seem upset. Could you tell me what's bothering you?
>
> I gather that you are angry. Tell me about it.

Some patients deny being "mad," "furious," or even "upset," but define their anger as being "a little irritated," "aggravated," "impatient," "annoyed," or "pissed off"; your language may have to be chosen to suit the individual patient.

QUICK TIPS

Dealing with Anger

- Help the patient feel safe to share his or her anger.
- Understand why the patient is upset and respond empathetically.
- Help the patient better understand his or her feelings and encourage reflection on various options.
- Don't take sides. Appreciate that the anger represents data about the patient. Acknowledge and validate your patient's distress.
- Avoid trying to defuse anger quickly by making excuses or attempting to mollify the patient.
- When patients are angry at you, hear them out and don't argue back.
- Consider approaches that empower the patient.

Most of the clinical situations in which anger arises represent transient responses to acute stresses and can be addressed quickly and satisfyingly for both the patient and clinician. The interviewer should simply try to understand why the patient is upset. Clarify how the patient is feeling and explore the events that led to the anger.

What happened?

What got you upset?

Your concerned inquiry about the anger will already be helping the patient. "Doing something" about anger rarely means correcting the perceived assault. But basic acts of clinical interviewing—giving patients permission to tell their story, allowing ventilation, bearing with uncomfortable feelings, and just listening seriously to complaints and suggestions—will empower patients ("Finally, someone is listening to me") and serve as an antidote to their frustration. Help the patient identify the underlying hurt. Try to respond empathically. Make summary statements that reflect back to patients your understanding of what they have undergone and felt and that indicate how you value their feelings. Your acknowledgment of their distress facilitates the telling of their account, while also supporting them.

It sounds like you have been kept waiting for quite a while and that it's gotten you quite upset. Apologies from all of us. But what happened?

That sounds miserable. You must be aggravated.

I can see why you're boiling. They've got you up against the wall.

Seeing this from your viewpoint, I understand why you are so out of sorts.

Occasionally, you will be able to assist the patient by suggesting remedial action or even offering advice. In general, your contribution to practical action comes from helping the patient to better understand his or her feelings and from encouraging reflection on various options, rather than from offering solutions to the problem.

In exploring patients' reasons for being upset, you may notice that a minor annoyance for one person is a major assault for another. For instance, some people give no thought to a 40-minute wait for their appointment; others become irritable at even the thought of a delay and are enraged after a 10-minute wait. Such differences between peoples' sensitivities may be a reflection of their current state of stress or of lifelong patterns. As a corollary to this observation, it is useless to "take sides" on whether anger is justifiable. Certainly, be wary of trying to minimize the significance of an insult (e.g., "That's not worth getting bothered about" or "I'm sure he didn't mean it that way"). Rather, appreciate that the anger represents data about the patient—his or her level of stress or sensitivity. While remaining neutral on whether patients are entitled to be so angry, you can acknowledge and validate their distress.

Avoid the temptation to try to defuse anger quickly by making excuses or otherwise trying to mollify the patient. You can seldom placate feelings or remove the aggravation. Do not suggest that the patient should calm down or take matters less seriously. Rather, listen and validate the patient's uncomfortable feelings.

Finally, not all angry patients should be approached in this exploratory fashion. Some patients are habitually angry, demanding, demeaning, and accusatory and require sophisticated management approaches. Other patients need help gaining control of their anger rather than ventilating it. For instance, anger may be a manifestation of psychosis, confusional states, or other major derangements of thinking and behavior. In such instances, the hostility needs to be interpreted and treated differently than previously described. Verbal threats, and especially physical threats, require special handling. Psychiatric textbooks and training will help you appreciate these less common and more problematic instances of anger.

When Patients Are Angry at You

If patients are mad at something you did, hear them out. You do not immediately need to defend yourself, apologize, or conciliate. Even if you are unjustly made the object of wrath, try to listen to the patient's viewpoint without responding to your own sense of personal affront. Join with the patient so that you are not merely the object of attack but a person who shares with the patient a sense of injury. Don't argue back. Remain neutral about blame, while acknowledging the legitimacy of the patient's feelings. The patient who has been allowed to ventilate and has had his or her feelings validated will generally find the anger dissipating quickly. Displacement of the anger will also tend to abate, and the patient may quickly be ready to move on with you to other matters, perhaps feeling an even greater sense of trust and solidarity.

Beware of cowering or of inappropriately trying to appease, but consider approaches that empower the patient:

> We've taken a tactic you dislike. Would it be alright with you if we tried this instead?
>
> Now that I see how you feel about the way we are treating this problem, I would be inclined to try something like you suggest.
>
> You're the boss.

Certainly, apologize for any affronts you recognize.

> I am sorry about this.
>
> I see how upset this has made you, and I apologize sincerely. It's our mistake.

You may choose to explain your behavior and invite the patient to see your view of the problem, but do not do so in such a way as to deny the patient justification for being angry:

> I had an emergency this morning that got me way behind schedule. I am sorry for the inconvenience I caused you.
>
> I don't think I realized how important it was for you to get these papers by today. I regret that my oversight has caused you this much trouble, and I'll make sure now that everything gets straightened out.

When the patient remains somewhat angry toward you even after you have allowed for ventilation and provided support, good questions are:

> What can I do for you?
>
> How can I help you with this?

The answer is often that there is nothing more you can do. The patient may even acknowledge that your listening has been helpful. Regardless, this sort of question helps the patient focus on the source of the anger and an appropriate role for you in dealing with it.

Similar principles apply when a patient is angry at another doctor or health care worker. Be quick to listen and empathize, but slow to judge or side with either party.

You will find your relationships with patients much more satisfying and successful if you allow them to express their anger toward you. Indeed, invite criticism. The alternative is for patients to complain to others, not allowing you to take corrective action, or for anger to infect the relationship in such forms as passive aggression, lack of trust, and noncompliance.

THE DOCTOR AND THE ANXIOUS PATIENT

Patients are inevitably anxious about going to the doctor. They are concerned about the meaning of their symptoms, how they will be perceived and treated by the office staff, how the physician will respond to their story, what kinds of questions they may be asked, how the examination might hurt or embarrass them, what will be found, what they will be told to do, and a variety of other uncertainties that lurk in the encounter. Anxiety is such a pervasive feature in medical work that most practitioners develop rather automatic, unselfconscious methods for dealing with it or perhaps ignoring it. Awareness of the role of anxiety in patient's lives, however, is essential for providing humane care and for understanding patient behaviors that may seem difficult.

What Is Anxiety and What Does It Do to the Patient?

Anxiety is an affect that signals a threat to the person's well-being. It is a response to danger. Overt physical dangers, such as facing a ferocious dog or losing control of a speeding car, are uncommon in everyday life, though in the medical world, patients regularly face bodily distress and risk of disability or death. Moreover, anxiety is not only a reaction to physical threats but also to perceived assaults on social and psychological well-being: the loss of a friend, job insecurity, financial pressures, and particularly injuries to self-esteem (disapproval, school failure, rejections and separations, helplessness, loss of control over anger, and so on). Anxiety may also be a response to intrapsychic conflicts that are outside of conscious awareness.

Anxiety can be helpful. The fight-or-flight response is mobilized; the alerted person is energized to respond to threats (e.g., to study for an upcoming test). With moderate degrees of arousal, coping may be enhanced— the patient thinks more clearly and quickly, focuses more energy on the immediate problem, and feels less need for food or rest. When anxiety is excessive, however, it can impair coping, as when a person freezes before an oncoming car or feels so frantic and overwhelmed as to become incapable of thinking straight and taking appropriate action. Severely anxious patients may feel that they are going crazy.

In assessing anxious patients, distinguish between acute anxiety and more chronic manifestations. While a brief arousal to danger is generally beneficial, a persistent response may be physically and emotionally exhausting and may interfere with work, concentration, and sleep. Some persons develop prolonged reactions to an acute threat, perhaps from some inner disposition to overreact. Others continue to be anxious because they are confronted with a situation for which they cannot find relief. Still others are chronically anxious regardless of acute events; they may fix their attention on some recent problem, but always feel themselves uncomfortably aroused.

How Patients Experience and Communicate Anxiety

Some patients experience anxiety primarily as somatic rather than psychological distress. They note (and may present with complaints about) tachycardia, sweatiness, restlessness, insomnia, and perhaps other vague physical sensations. Distinctive somatic patterns of anxiety are the hyperventilation syndrome and panic states.

Still other patients can recognize anxiety in their psychological selves but have a restricted vocabulary for describing it. For instance, some patients never say they are afraid or scared, but will admit to being worried. Others think that being "nervous" or "having trouble with your nerves" is acceptable, but shun descriptions of anxiety that they feel imply a mental disorder.

Anxiety, like other emotional states, can spill over from the specific situation in which it arose to other settings. Thus a person who is apprehensive about an upcoming operation may be unusually troubled by a host of minor annoyances. A patient who is worried about his teenage son's truancy may become fearful about his own health. Moreover, anxiety regularly spills over from one person to another. A common reaction to interviewing uneasy or fearful patients is to become anxious oneself. Similarly, anxious interviewers can unwittingly upset patients.

Denial: When Anxiety Is Missing

Denial is a common response to anxiety. It is an unconscious reaction whereby a threat and its attendant anxiety are minimized or excluded from awareness. Denial ranges from such commonly recognized feelings as "It can't be true" or "It hasn't really hit me yet" to such major interference with rational thinking as a failure to acknowledge significant events ("I'm sure this will go away" or "Nobody told me about needing an operation") and gross distortions of reality ("I don't really have cancer" or "There's nothing wrong with my [gangrenous] foot"). Also note that patients may consciously suppress upsetting facts ("I'm just trying not to think about it now"), rather than exhibiting the unconscious defense of denial.

The degree of denial reflects the patient's personality but also is usually commensurate with the severity of the anxiety-provoking threat. Thus denial is commonly seen in patients with life-threatening conditions. Denial, however, is not a fixed reaction; it tends to fluctuate, depending on the patient's emotional state, the setting in which the threatening topic is discussed, and the interviewer. For example, clinicians experienced in working with denying patients are often able to elicit realistic perceptions from a person who presents staunch denial to other interviewers. Sometimes patients seem to speak as if they had two minds—one realistic, one denying—and the interviewer may take the tactic of addressing the more realistic portion of the patient's self:

> I wonder if a part of you isn't feeling a little concerned about how things have been going.
>
> Most people in your situation would find this sort of situation troubling at times.
>
> I wonder if there haven't been moments when you, too, had some worries.

A clue to denial is often a discrepancy between what the patient says and what the clinician expects. Thus, patients in denial report feeling better than the clinical situation warrants or they find no distress where the interviewer believes some suffering is inevitable. Statements that reflect denial may be incorrectly interpreted as misunderstanding or ignorance; conversely, uninformed patients are sometimes mistakenly labeled as exhibiting denial.

Rather than causing difficulty, denial often makes patient management easier, since anxiety and its attendant problems are repressed. The patient is protected from overwhelming threats until he or she is better able to face the facts. However, denial can also cause problems. For example, a patient's unrealistic view about illness may lead to decisions to refuse beneficial treatment or to undertake activities that are harmful. Clinicians may also be irritated simply because the patient is not facing the clinical reality.

Denial is an unconscious protective process, not a rational behavior that can be challenged by argument or "broken through." Approach this psychological phenomenon with respect. The denying patient is generally helped by acts of psychological support, attempts to lessen the threat, and other efforts to improve the patient's coping, not by directly addressing the defensive denial itself.

How Anxiety Makes Patients Difficult

Anxious patients are difficult when, to the physician, they do not seem to be acting like "good patients." Anxious patients often have trouble concentrating and remembering and thus may not follow medical advice. Some seem difficult to evaluate because they amplify their symptoms or overreact to them, while others are stoical and underreact. Some become overtalkative, others reticent; some become aggressive, others withdrawn. Excessive use of alcohol, tobacco, and other psychoactive substances is common in face of anxiety, as are a variety of impulsive behaviors that may interfere with treatment. Some anxious patients may resort to extreme intellectualization and become obsessively involved with every detail of their care, demanding excessive attention from their physician. Other patients become suspicious, perhaps attributing their misfortune to other persons. Patients may become arrogant, asserting their self-importance and causing difficulty by demeaning the medical staff. Regression is also a common response—the patient becomes childish, less self-assured, passive, needy, demanding, and, for the physician and other caretakers, a difficult burden of care.

In general, excess anxiety tends to exaggerate the patient's usual personality style and to make coping mechanisms more rigid and thus less adaptive. How various persons respond to anxiety (a topic generally described under such titles as defensive styles, personality styles, or coping patterns) and how these traits influence both patients' response to illness and the doctor-patient relationship are described in detail in other writings (see especially the article by Kahana and Bibring in the Suggested Readings).

The Clinical Approach to Anxiety

Commonplace anxiety—a disturbing feeling that is mild, appropriate to the patient's situation, and of such a duration and intensity as not to impair the patient's ability to function—is usually easily managed by the patient, but sometimes is brought to the doctor's attention. Clinicians learn, often with little self-awareness, to maintain an outwardly unruffled appearance and to respond calmly, unhurriedly, and self-assuredly to patient's stories of distress. Basic strategies for responding to any emotion apply: elicit the feelings, try to understand what caused them, help patients make sense of the situation and their emotional response, listen empathically and be accepting and supportive, assist patients in sorting out options, and perhaps suggest new modes of coping. In general, resist the temptation to avoid anxiety and do not feel that you need to control it or make it go away; face it calmly and assuredly with the patient. Additional tactics that deserve special attention with anxious patients include the following:

- Take extra care to appreciate and respond to the patient's attributions, which often lie at the heart of the fright.
- Attend to issues of interpersonal closeness. Some anxious patients respond well to a directive, supportive, and intimate relationship that diminishes their uncertainty and isolation; others are made more anxious by such an approach and require a more distanced, less intrusive stance that helps them maintain a sense of autonomy and separateness.
- Be more specific and concrete than usual. Discussions, and particularly instructions, should be kept simple. Explain with extra care, attending especially to reassurance.

More severe anxiety may require vigorous action. The clinician must learn to recognize pathological forms of anxiety, including phobic reactions and panic disorders that may admit to specific treatment. Also, depression and psychosis may present with an agitated state, and are treated differently than anxiety states. Standard texts on psychiatry and psychiatric aspects of general medicine provide further detailed information on the topics of anxiety and denial, personality styles, defenses and coping, the management of severe anxiety, and the diagnosis and treatment of phobias and panic states.

COMMUNICATION STYLES AND COMMUNICATION BARRIERS

You will quickly learn that all patients will not allow themselves to be measured with the same rule. If you wish to learn anything useful from your patients, you must take each in his own particular way. A patient is lively, talkative, imaginative, and speaks fast and loose of all sorts of things at full speed, but seldom remembers to mention that upon which everything depends. Here you must apply the brake as quickly as possible, and ask short precise questions, while insisting upon short precise answers; else he breaks away from your examination, and all his remarks become immaterial. Another patient may be reticent and distrustful so that his evidence has to be hauled forth.

Thorkild Rovsing

Interviewing that initially relies on open-ended, nondirective questioning is ideal for the usual patient. However, for persons with unusual communication styles—for example, the talkative and the reticent—you will need to tailor your interviewing technique to the particular patient.

Most patients seem to quickly catch on to how the doctor wants them to provide a history. The unspoken rules include: speak freely but do not talk too much, give relevant facts and avoid digressions, allow the doctor to direct the exchange, and to interrupt when he or she wants to ask questions or change topics. The assumption that patients know exactly how we want them to behave in the encounter, including the appropriate style of communication, is common but unfounded. No one has instructed patients on behaving in these ways. However, most patients have learned tactics of politeness and deference between persons of different status and may have mastered the usual form of medical discourse from previous visits with doctors. Patients are able to pick up on the clues (largely nonverbal and unintentional) that the physician gives about his or her expectations. Clinicians become so used to this compliant behavior in doctor-patient relationships that they may quickly become impatient with a patient who acts otherwise. You should recognize, however, that many patients need instruction on how best to communicate and that interviewing techniques should be accommodated to patients' communication styles.

Common problematic styles are described below, along with suggestions for altering your interviewing approach when you encounter such styles.

The Talkative Style

Some patients talk too much. They take control of the interview when given the opportunity or, despite our attempts to restrain them, offer information that is largely irrelevant. The open-ended, nondirective interview can be disastrous. Garrulous patients may be colorful, skilled storytellers whom we would enjoy in another circumstance, but not when we feel pressed to get an accurate history in a limited time. They may launch into long-winded stories about themselves, their lives, and their illnesses, rambling from topic to topic, offering information that seems tangential or unimportant, and repeating themselves. They get to the essential point only slowly, if ever. Similarly, obsessive patients are often appreciated for their carefulness and precision in giving a history, but may flood us with endless minute details about their illness, perhaps coming to the interview armed with pages of notes from daily monitoring of their bodily sensations. Other patients become overtalkative when they are anxious or are eager to maintain control of a situation, such as the medical interview. Still others are chronically disorganized in their thinking. Occasionally, overtalkativeness is the first clue to a significant abnormality in the mental status, such as euphoria or confusion.

Many talkative patients, if given a few extra minutes, will settle into a more acceptable communication style. However, if patients do not get to the point and provide the facts you need after you have given them free rein, you may gently interrupt and explain what you would like from them.

> I am eager to hear about your exercise program, but I am not sure you are getting to the facts that I need most now. Could you tell me what happens when you have the chest pain?

> I appreciate that you have kept such careful track of your sweatiness, but I think it would be useful to hear about some other matters first. Would you go back to your heart pains?

Next, you can obtain control of the interview by asking focused, direct questions.

> I've heard what you've said about the pain. Now I would like to quiz you about it. What day did it begin?

Try to guide the patient toward brief, clear responses without offering leading questions. Avoid the usual facilitative comments and gestures, and, if needed, courteously interrupt and redirect the conversation. Avoid showing impatience, and remember that your interruption can be a humiliation or an affront. There is no perfect remedy for the overtalkative patient, but you can gain some control, using the above tactics.

The Silent or Reticent Style

At the other extreme, some patients volunteer very little information. They answer open-ended questions with a few words and give very limited responses. They prefer to say "Yes" or "No" rather than explaining or elaborating.

Reticence may have many causes. Some patients simply have poor verbal skills (not to be confused with low intelligence). Others are not fluent in spoken English. In such instances, a person's tendency to reticence will be accentuated by anxiety and the inhibitions associated with talking to a physician who may be articulate and of a different class and cultural background. Still other patients are quite capable of talking but are anxious, embarrassed, angry, mistrustful, or evasive and will not speak freely until comfort and trust have developed. For a chronically withdrawn or suspicious person, ease in talking may not develop even after many visits. Still other patients have learned that their physicians want them to be reticent. Silence may also be associated with depression and other serious disorders of mental status.

Many reticent patients will eventually begin talking more freely in response to the open-ended, nondirective interviewing approach, especially after initial long periods of silence. For others, however, the tension resulting from your silence and other efforts to get them to talk only heightens their anxiety and the tendency to be reticent. A number of tactics may then be useful. First, the interviewer should do more of the talking, thus taking the pressure off the patient while also demonstrating the desired interview behavior. Do more explaining and even consider talking a little about yourself. Second, turn the conversation to neutral topics or engage in "small talk" for a while to make it easier for the patient to participate. Third, be respectful and unhurried and respond to the patient's utterances with pleasure and encouragement. Fourth, use very directed inquiry, trying to avoid leading questions, yet only relying on the patient for brief, simple responses, as described for overtalkative patients. Get the patient talking, if only briefly. Finally, for information on the patient's feelings, you may have to express what you think they are (e.g., "My God, you must have felt up against the wall." "You look down." "You look blue.") and then seek confirmation. You also may need to rely heavily on nonverbal cues and "intuition."

Communication Disabilities

Defects in vision, hearing, or speech inhibit or prevent communication. Difficulty in communication is often mistaken for impaired mental capacity; remind yourself that such disabilities do not imply low intelligence. Also, patients who cannot communicate normally tend to be isolated, and they particularly benefit from your patience and eagerness to relate to them as you would with unimpaired persons. Use touch and other nonverbal methods to convey your interest.

Hearing-impaired patients may be able to communicate well with sign language, in which case a translator can be helpful. They also may be able to read lips. If so, make sure the room is well lit, then sit nearby and speak slowly and clearly but normally. If the patient can use a hearing aid, be certain it is in place. Finally, you may need to communicate in writing, presuming the patient is literate. This can be time-consuming, but may be facilitated by using a prepared history form (a printed questionnaire).

Blind patients can communicate with words, but they may need verbal explanations for many matters that are rarely attended to consciously by sighted persons. For instance, interviewers should consider describing themselves and others present and orienting the patient to the surroundings. Explain what you are doing. Other suggestions for working with the blind include using touch and making sure to negotiate with the patient about what kind of help they want, for instance, in moving about the room or office, changing clothes, or getting home. Remember that many handicapped persons are justly proud of their independence and want or need little assistance.

Various disorders of speech may be encountered. Aphasic or dysarthric patients are sometimes better understood by close family members, who can serve as translators. Mute patients who can communicate with sign language will benefit from a translator. Some patients who have had a laryngectomy can talk with esophageal speech, produced in a manner similar to belching, while others use prosthetic devices or rely on lip-reading. At times, written communication may be required, presuming again that the patient is literate and otherwise capable of employing written language. Ask patients to write out their medical history or to fill out a history questionnaire, preferably before the visit.

Language Barriers

When patients cannot speak well in a language you understand, even after your encouragement, a translator is required. Translated interviews are slow and rarely allow for a very intimate doctor-patient relationship and thus can be frustrating for both parties. Acknowledge the difficulty.

We may have some difficulty getting to know each other.

Let's do our best to understand each other.

Make a special effort to maintain eye contact with the patient. Address your questions to the patient, even though the translator will be speaking for you. Liberal use of touching and other nonverbal communication may be helpful. Prepared history forms allow the interviewer time to be used for addressing key issues, solidifying a relationship, rather than gathering standard data. For complicated problems and long-term care, consider helping the patient find a physician who speaks the same language.

Translators need instructions and training. They should be familiar with medical terms in both of the languages that are being used. Their impressions of the patient should be sought, but they should be asked to translate a complete report of what is said, rather than filtering, summarizing, or explicating. They should maintain confidentiality and assure the patient of privacy. In general, family members or friends make poor translators for discussions of personal matters, but can handle many other aspects of the medical history and offer their opinion about "What do you think your mother has?"

THE DOCTOR AND THE SOMATIZING PATIENT

A "functional" illness means that the patient has had a problem which he tried to solve with an illness. The illness enabled him to complain, whereas he was unable to complain about his original problem.

Michael Balint
The Doctor, His Patient and the Illness

When patients come to the doctor with bodily complaints, the customary clinical mandate is to diagnose an underlying medical disorder and, where possible, to provide effective treatment. Frequently, however, somatic distress cannot be fully explained by a physical disease. In such circumstances, the clinician may wonder if a medical diagnosis has been missed, yet a vigorous pursuit of a physical basis—ruling out organic disease—often proves fruitless. Many of these patients are "somatizers" whose distress and communication are best understood primarily as a response to psychosocial conditions.

Many patients somatize transiently and get better quickly, perhaps with some help from a physician. Others have a long-standing pattern of presenting with somatic complaints and require care that is exacting and trying but only ameliorates their distress, rarely curing it. The latter patients often cause havoc for clinicians, themselves, and their families.

By becoming familiar with somatization, you can learn to identify psychological diagnoses early in your clinical evaluations. A failure to recognize somatization promptly—"missing the forest for the trees" by focusing on individual symptoms rather than on the overall picture—may lead to useless and expensive diagnostic efforts, some of which are counterproductive or even harmful to patients, as well as exasperating for the doctor.

Patterns of Somatization

Somatization (which has sometimes been called "functional" illness) generally falls into one of six categories.

Categorizing Somatization

Psychophysiological reactions
Psychological events precipitate physiological states, such as irritable bowel, hyperventilation, or tension headache, which, in turn, cause somatic distress.

Amplification of normal or minor bodily sensations
Normal physical sensations and minor somatic complaints are exaggerated or responded to as serious, often in response to stress.

Hypochondriasis
The patient has recurrent beliefs of having a serious illness or is preoccupied with fears of a grave condition.

Somatization disorder
The patient persistently reports multiple bodily sensations that cannot be fully explained by a physical diagnosis.

Conversion disorder (hysterical neurosis, conversion type)
A loss or alteration of body function develops in response to psychological stress.

Chronic pain states (somatoform pain disorder)
A persistent preoccupation with pain occurs in the absence of a medical condition to explain the pain.

While the term "somatization" is generally used to describe how physical complaints may reflect psychosocial processes, you should be aware that the latter four categories—hypochondriasis, somatization disorder, conversion disorder, and somatoform pain disorder—are formal psychiatric diagnoses and, along with a few other chronic conditions, are subsumed under the title Somatoform Disorders. Patients with these conditions should be distinguished from persons with depression, schizophrenia, anxiety disorders, or other major psychiatric conditions that may lead to bodily complaints, delusions, and preoccupations. Indeed, some persons who eventually are considered to have a psychiatric disorder present initially with physical symptoms. Also, somatizers *unintentionally* develop symptoms that mimic physical disorders and thus are distinguished from patients who consciously try to deceive the physician. As an introduction to somatization, the first four of these six categories are discussed below.

Patients with Psychophysiological Reactions

The interplay of mind and body is important in all illnesses. When psychological factors play a particularly prominent role in the initiation, exacerbation, or perpetuation of physical distress, the condition is often referred to as psychophysiological or psychosomatic. Examples include some cases of eating disorders, asthma, and hypertension.

Psychophysiological reactions are the responses of the body to the mind and may cause physical discomfort as surely as more tangible disease agents. Such reactions should be familiar to anyone who has felt sweaty, shaky, or "sick to the stomach" when anxious. Clinically, we readily recognize how angina may be provoked by emotion or how depression may aggravate pain, just as we know that a variety of physical conditions can incite psychological reactions (e.g., anxiety is provoked by hyperthyroidism).

In the care of patients with *transient* psychophysiological reactions, most clinicians are comfortable.

A 20-year-old college student experienced repeated bouts of chest discomfort, sweating, and palpitations during a stressful examination period. His physical examination was normal. He was concerned about cardiac disease, since his father had died of a heart attack. An electrocardiogram was normal. He was reassured about his heart, while the relationship of his symptoms to stress was discussed. His concerns over his school performance were reviewed. His symptoms remitted after his second visit.

▲

After evaluating such somatic complaints, clinicians can relieve the patient by offering a physiological interpretation and occasionally by prescribing measures for symptom control, such as medication, relaxation exercises, diet, or physical therapy. *Persistent* psychophysiological disorders—such as chronic tension headache, irritable bowel syndrome, and hyperventilation—are discussed in standard medical texts.

Patients Who Amplify Bodily Symptoms

Emotional states modulate everyone's perception of bodily sensations, leading to "psychological overlay." Many persons present to physicians with minor problems or no recognizable disease but can be understood as having developed transient somatic complaints in association with crises in their lives.

Patients undergoing stress may have an intensified awareness of physical sensations that usually would be overlooked or dismissed and thus may come to the doctor with "growling in the stomach" or "red eyes." Such patients may also experience heightened suffering when they develop a minor physical symptom, such as an everyday muscle ache or sore throat. Some patients, particularly when anxious, experience pain diffusely—"It hurts all over"—although they have a relatively localized source of pain. Others apparently report bodily complaints at times of stress because they simply have little ability to describe their disturbing feelings in psychological terms. They may come from personal or cultural backgrounds in which the expression of emotions is discouraged but in which complaining about physical symptoms is customary and sanctioned. Regardless of the mechanism by which physical complaints substitute for psychological ones, these somatizing patients feel ill and seek out a doctor for attention to their body.

Psychosocial distress also affects how symptoms are interpreted, as described under Triggers in Chapter 10. Patients who have recently faced a serious disease, such as a heart attack or cancer, often feel unusually vulnerable to illness and may develop transient somatic complaints or preoccupations that reflect persistent worry about new or recurrent disease. Similarly, when a person is diagnosed with a dreaded ailment (such as a stroke) or dies of such a disorder, bodily complaints and concerns often develop among the patient's friends and family, and, at times, even among health professionals who identify with the patient.

Patients who are preoccupied with their health and who tend to amplify bodily complaints, particularly in response to anxiety or sorrow, are generally managed without difficulty by performing an appropriate medical evaluation and offering reassurance about their concerns. They are able to "wait and see," letting a good medical examination and "the test of time" prove that nothing serious is developing. When able to relate their worries to their emotional state, they may appreciate tactful exploration of personal stresses and carefully worded explanations about the relation of their bodily complaints to these stresses.

Difficulties With Patients Who Amplify

Some patients are reluctant to attribute their symptoms to stress and are unwilling to look further into their psychological lives to understand and modify their reaction to stress. Others accept explanation and reassurance but demand repeated contacts. Effective reassurance may require persistent pursuit of patient attributions and concerns. Consider questions such as:

> What could I do to help you feel reassured about this problem?

or even a confrontation:

> Can you believe me if I tell you that you're alright?

The physician's notion of what is an appropriate response to a bodily complaint may differ significantly from that of his or her patients. Clinicians tend to be annoyed by patients who seem to overreact or be excessively sensitive to pain or discomfort or who seem overly anxious about the meaning of an illness (just as they may be troubled by a patient who minimizes or denies symptoms). Some physicians, particularly those who are moved to "fix bodies" rather than to "relieve suffering," may be unsympathetic to the "worried well" (or "worried sick")—patients who are healthy by strict medical standards but who present with distress.

Similarly, some patients are even more preoccupied with bodily function than physicians (e.g., some dancers, athletes, or health food devotees). In general, you and your patients hold a spectrum of attitudes about bodily appearance, physical fitness and strength, vulnerability to disease agents, and such normal processes as physical aging. Rather than condemning a particular stance, try to appreciate and tolerate the variety of human attitudes and behaviors.

Patients With Hypochondriasis

Patients with hypochondriasis are persistently preoccupied with disease. They present with complaints that often seem vague, odd, or suggestive of a functional disorder, although they may also have symptoms typical of a medical disease. Despite careful evaluation and reassurance, they continue to worry about their symptoms and the possibility of a hidden ailment. They usually interpret minor or normal bodily sensations as ominous; they are obsessed with recurrent fears that they have a serious disease or impairment. Indeed, many are truly worried that they are dying. Rarely, such patients have fixed beliefs that they have an illness and may show evidence of a serious underlying mental disorder, such as schizophrenia or depression.

A long-standing pattern of such behavior is formally called *hypochondriasis.* Such patients seem to make a career of suffering. They experience their bodies as fragile, vulnerable, and under attack from various diseases, and their preoccupations may lead to significant impairment of their work and social life. They visit the doctor frequently and seem desperate for reassurance, yet unable to benefit from it.

Difficulties With Hypochondriacal Patients

Physicians learn to tolerate a degree of uncertainty about a patient's diagnosis and prognosis. Patients, too, are usually satisfied by a clinical evaluation without being convinced of the physician's infallibility. Hypochondriacal patients, however, are not reassured and seem to demand extreme measures to lessen uncertainty. One management tactic is to undertake extensive diagnostic studies and to explain carefully the clinical findings. Yet, the reassurance resulting from such efforts is often transient. Nothing, including an elaborate workup, detailed discussion, and a benign course over time, shakes the hypochondriac's convictions about lurking disease. Indeed, all the attention to bodily symptoms seems to reinforce their suspicions that they are not alright. The mention of the possibility of turning up a hidden problem heightens concern. An alternative tactic, then, is to avoid communicating any uncertainty that might support the patient's worry. The clinician may offer premature reassurance or falsely portray confidence in a diagnosis. Yet these approaches are rarely convincing or effective. A third alternative is to ignore complaints—"You've 'cried wolf' too many times"—and leave bodily concerns unattended.

Patients with severe hypochondriasis may be quite willing to talk about psychosocial stresses in their lives and may accept some emotional support, but they tend to resist psychological explanations for their bodily preoccupations, as well as any attempts to explain these preoccupations as reflections of their emotional state. Therapeutic enthusiasm is easily lost as the patients do not give up their symptoms and thus disappoint the physician about the value of medical attention. Maintaining a relationship and an interest in the patient may enhance the patient's functioning.

Patients With Somatization Disorder

Somatization generally begins before the age of 30 and has a chronic, fluctuating course. Patients have multiple, vague bodily complaints, affecting a number of organ systems. The review of systems is often "positive," and as soon as one symptom is addressed, another one pops up. Several other features suggesting this diagnosis deserve note:

1. The symptoms are often described as disabling, yet, while the patient is clearly worried and upset, he or she appears well and seems to be eating, sleeping, and carrying out activities of daily living.

2. The history often reveals that the complaints are long-standing, yet the patient is overtly demanding and conveys a sense of urgency—"You've got to help me . . . I don't know how I can live with this . . . I can't stand it any longer." The complaints may regularly be described as "worse than ever before," which is worrisome on initial visits, but less so when such a statement has been repeated on many subsequent visits.

3. The history may reveal that the patient perceives himself or herself as sickly for years—"I can't remember when I last felt well"—and that illness has caused long-standing disruptions in his or her life—"I don't know how my family stands it."

4. Many physicians have been consulted and multiple medications have been tried. The patient may have undergone repetitive procedures, including surgery for which the indications may be questionable. A variety of diagnoses have been offered. Nonetheless, the patient (and perhaps the interviewer) has no clear idea of what is wrong.

5. "Nothing helps." The patient has been exasperated, as may have been many physicians and family members. Occasionally, a treatment will work briefly, but relapse occurs soon thereafter. In general, medical care is described as useless. The patients often complain of the side effects of prescribed drugs, and may have been labeled "help-rejecters." Despite therapeutic failures, the patient continues to present with the expectation of finding quick relief.

6. The patient may seem to parade suffering. Nobody has suffered quite as much, had such a complicated, inscrutable problem, seen so many illustrious physicians, or found so little help. These patients tend to reject any observation that they look well or seem to be functioning better.

7. The patient will be quite unwilling or unable to entertain a psychological basis to his or her complaints. While persons with chronic physical conditions often note how their emotional state affects the perception of pain, patients with somatization disorder tend to deny any such relationship. The patient may begin the interview by letting you know that "I'm not just making this up or imagining it," and may report with considerable annoyance how some doctor said, "It's all in your head" or "There's nothing really wrong with you," thus warning you not to try such an interpretation. One patient, when invited to discuss considerable psychosocial problems, aptly said, "How can I talk about my feelings when my feelings are pain?"

Difficulties With Patients Who Have Somatization Disorder

1. *Uncertainty about giving the right amount of attention to bodily complaints.* A natural tendency for the clinician dealing with patients who

have multiple, vague bodily complaints is to "rule out medical disease." The clinician who works with a somatizing patient will constantly be considering the pursuit of further diagnoses, trials of new treatments, or perhaps, repetition of previously negative studies. The inevitable false positive or equivocal tests lead to further procedures. In the process of diagnosis and treatment, these patients may develop adverse drug reactions and long-term complications from procedures.

Even if the patient has been "crying wolf," the physician worries that a "real" problem will emerge and be overlooked amidst the other complaints. Additionally, a number of patients with illnesses that may present with vague problems and may be difficult to diagnose (e.g., multiple sclerosis or systemic lupus erythematosus) have incorrectly been labeled as somatizers. A clinical necessity in dealing with such patients is remaining alert to the possibility of medical disease while not overresponding to bodily complaints.

A focus on specific symptoms runs the risk of failing to recognize and address the overall pattern of somatization. However, despite the futility and occasional harm of continually searching for new diagnoses or attempting to treat unlikely underlying disorders, these patients seek and appreciate any attention given to their bodily complaints. They become impatient when the physician stops searching and tries to reassure them or says, "I cannot find anything wrong. Let's just try to live with this," especially if this shift in approach means less attention. They may be critical of their care, but nonetheless, they often appreciate a physician who, despite repeated failures, does not get angry about their puzzling complaints and their demanding, plaintive manner, and is able to stick with them in the elusive search for comfort.

2. *Discouragement with one's efforts.* As the physician confronts failure in making a clear diagnosis or providing relief, discouragement mounts. Insofar as physicians focus blame on themselves, they may become overwhelmed by the patient's demands. Feeling helpless, they may try increasingly desperate measures—studies with very low likelihood of confirming a diagnosis or treatment methods of questionable indication.

3. *Frustration with patient.* Alternatively, the patient may be blamed for not responding to medical treatment, and the angry physician perceives the somatizer as an annoyance, "poor historian," malingerer, or a moral reprobate who should take responsibility for his or her problem. Derogatory labels, such as "turkeys" and "crocks," may be applied.

Tactics of Communication and Care for Hypochondriasis and Somatization Disorder

1. Provide a sound medical evaluation, but avoid excessive interventions, particularly medications and procedures that may have side effects. Consider citing the patient's experience of the futility or toxicity of previous investigations and treatments to justify your restraint. Rather than immediately pursuing every problem, favor a slow, sequential approach, perhaps addressing one problem at a time or

temporizing before moving ahead with additional studies. Judiciously and tactfully disregard those complaints that are unlikely to reflect a significant underlying medical disorder.

2. Elicit and address the patient's attributions.
3. Provide a clear, simple explanation of your findings and provide appropriate reassurance, but do not expect the patient to feel relieved.
4. Do not dismiss patients or their complaints. These patients suffer from their symptoms and worry as surely as do persons with an underlying physical problem, and they do not have voluntary control over their condition. They are ill. Moreover, they seem to need the attention derived from being sick, and their physicians are often highly important figures in their lives. Indicate your own certainty about the lack of a serious underlying physical problem but also acknowledge and validate the patient's persistent discomfort.

> I have examined you carefully and everything seems fine. I find no serious abnormality in your body. On the other hand, I know that you have been troubled with these symptoms for a long time and that it must be difficult for you not to get relief.

> I see that you have been very worried, but I feel confident that we are not dealing with a serious physical problem here. I think we will need to work together now to keep an eye on these symptoms and see what we can do to help you.

Empathize with the patient's dilemma.

> This must be terrible for you.

> It sounds unbearable.

Applaud perseverance and strength of character.

> You've really put up with a lot.

> This condition has been quite a burden.

5. Do not proclaim your psychological diagnosis with the expectation that the patient will accept it. Do not try to convince patients that they have an emotional problem. You must adopt an unusual therapeutic stance in which you tolerate the patient's requirement that the condition be viewed primarily as a physical one, while believing that psychological factors are of foremost importance.
6. Gently direct the conversation toward psychosocial matters. Perform a careful psychosocial assessment and encourage the patient to explore problematic areas. Attend to emotional distress. The process of providing psychosocial support is generally conducted in parallel with "body talk" and without explicit attempts to relate psychological issues to somatic complaints. You know that the source of the pain is not physical, so you try to address the psychosocial realm, yet you may not share an explicit contract with the patient to discuss emotional issues. You slowly but persistently shift the topic of clinical conversation from the body to the patient's social and psychological life. Some patients eventually learn to relate their bodily symptoms to emotional matters, but usually only after many years of help. Even over the course of a few visits, though, successful psychosocial support may promptly diminish the intensity and severity of the somatoform disorder.
7. Foster a long-term relationship, focused initially on the patient's persistent physical suffering. Somatizing patients benefit from an ongoing relationship in which

the clinician has the delicate tasks of listening carefully to complaints, taking the patient seriously, acknowledging suffering, and being reassuring, and yet being well aware of the psychological basis for the condition and not responding to every symptom as evidence of a serious problem. Initially, this may mean tolerating the patient's bodily preoccupations and showing more attention to physical complaints than they deserve from a strictly medical viewpoint.

Visits typically begin with a litany of physical complaints. The focus of discussion can later turn to psychosocial matters, and patients may eventually accept having most of their office time address such issues. Typically, however, the patient ends the visit by restating physical problems.

8. Establish a primary care provider. These patients generally do better when a single clinician coordinates and helps contain their care. Discourage a pattern of obtaining help from multiple specialists and make sure that everyone involved in the patient's care is familiar with the overall approach described in this section.

9. Schedule regular appointments, perhaps once a month, regardless of whether the patient is feeling better or worse. "Prescribe the doctor," but do not make attention contingent upon the patient having physical complaints.

10. Attend to the family. Such patients often cause serious psychosocial problems among family members, while the response of the family to the patient's condition may serve to reinforce an unfortunate pattern of behavior.

THE DOCTOR AND THE DYING PATIENT

To cure sometimes, to relieve often, to comfort always.

Folk saying

Death destroys a man; the idea of Death saves him.

E. M. Forster

Avoidance of the Dying

Clinicians often avoid the dying, thus hindering their own learning about terminal illness, while also depriving the patient of good care. Avoidance is partly an instinctive response to perceived danger—the prospect of being touched by suffering. Physicians may also view dying patients as their failure; feeling troubled or even ashamed about defeat, they withdraw attention. Furthermore, many clinicians are frustrated that they cannot rescue the terminally ill and they do not appreciate the many satisfying opportunities to provide such patients with comfort and support.

Among common avoidance behaviors are frank neglect (not going into a patient's hospital room on rounds, saying "nothing more can be done"); shunning conversation (not sitting down to talk on rounds, being "too busy"); and various, often unconscious, tactics of steering the discussion away from upsetting matters (for instance, by lecturing, focusing on technical interventions, being excessively optimistic, not attending to affect, or otherwise evading the patient's anxiety and sadness and such difficult topics as the prognosis and the limited options for care).

Being aware of such impediments to the care of dying patients, you may need a bit of courage and resolve to plunge yourself more deeply into their special world. You may want to read about "death and dying," view educational movies or videotapes, observe model interviews, and eventually talk directly with terminally ill patients. Books and demonstrations introduce you to what is known about terminal care and help you make sense of your clinical interactions (as well as initially lowering your apprehension), but cannot substitute for personal encounters with the dying.

Talking With the Terminally Ill

What can one say to a dying person? How does one understand what the patient wants to discuss? More important than what you say is what you let patients tell you. Listen to your patients' agendas, and you will often find them bringing up the very topics that you thought should be explored.

Do not assume that your patient is fragile. Particularly with articulate patients, you can explore many important areas with rather direct questions.

> What is your understanding about what is happening to you?
> > How did this illness begin?
> > How has it been treated?
> > What is happening now?
> > What have you been told?
> > > What do the doctors say?
> > > Your family?
> > > What do you make of it?
>
> What has this illness been like for you?
> > How has it affected you physically?
> > > Emotionally?
> > What has been difficult about this illness?
> > Have you been sad? Frightened?
>
> How have you been helped?
> > What gives you strength?
> > How have you been helped by family and friends?
> > By doctors? Nurses? Other health care people?
> > By your minister [priest, rabbi, other]?
>
> Have there been other tough times you have had to face?
> > Have there been serious losses before?
> > What was it like for you? What helped you?
>
> Have you been thinking about dying?
> > What kinds of thoughts have you had?
> > What worries?
>
> How have your family (or close friends) been affected?
> > What have you discussed with them?

A Few Basic Concepts in Working With the Dying

People tend to die as they live. Much of the day-to-day care of the dying is quite similar to the ordinary care of patients less ill. Nonetheless, a number of issues stand out in the care of the dying. The following concepts apply particularly to chronically ill persons—the cancer patient, the person with a progressive neurologic disease or with end-stage heart or lung disease—rather than persons with an acute, life-threatening condition (see Quick Tips: Additional Themes To Recognize in Working with the Terminally Ill).

QUICK TIPS

Additional Themes To Recognize in Working with the Terminally Ill

- Sadness, loss, grief, depression
- Loss of the future—not seeing children grow up; missing anticipated anniversaries or retirement
- Guilt, self-blame
- Anger, frustration, bitterness, resentment—"Why me?"
- Being a burden—fears of helplessness, loss of self-control and of excess dependency on support systems, either "formal" (professional) or "informal" (family and friends)
- Fears of abandonment
- Loss of self-esteem, identity, dignity, respect—being "only a patient," being pitied
- Fears of death or extinction (uncommon) vs. fears about the moment of death (common) vs. fears about the process of dying (nearly universal—concerns about pain, physical suffering, isolation, loss of control, and other factors)
- Existential and religious concerns—guilt, the significance of suffering, the meaning and value of one's life
- Setting things right—reconciliation and using remaining time for reconciliation
- Practical concerns—unfinished business, wills, custody, arranging for the funeral

---

Alleviating Suffering

Terminally ill patients will die despite our most strenuous ministrations and, in the process, they and their families and close friends will almost inevitably suffer. Nonetheless, clinicians can contribute enormously to the quality of remaining time—not by preventing death, but by comforting the dying and easing their passing. Physicians, in their ability to relieve discomfort, have a unique role in dying patients' lives. While so much medical training focuses on using symptoms as clues to the diagnosis of an underlying illness and on trying to cure that illness, terminal care is often primarily symptomatic care. Concerns about physical suffering and disfigurement are often foremost in the patient's mind. The physician has a special responsibility to relieve pain, nausea, dyspnea, constipation, and so on. In addition to such comfort measures directed at physical suffering, doctors help patients and their families live with a fatal illness and cope with the inevitable psychological crises by explaining the illness, attending to emotional support, and, when a person is being cared for in the home, by providing supportive services there.

Combatting Isolation

Dying is often a lonely process. Patients harbor fears, concerns, and wishes that are often not readily shared. The patient's closest companions may be too overwhelmed by the prospect of loss to discuss openly such personal thoughts and feelings. The patient may censor difficult emotions to protect loved ones from distress. The clinician, in being able to listen to painful feelings—encouraging their expression, tolerating upsetting discussions, and reflecting emotions—can rescue patients from disabling isolation and help them bear their suffering. Of course, you help simply by attending and by sticking with the patient, but availability—not just physically but emotionally—is a key quality and an antidote to the patient's isolation. The doctor should be a person whom the dying patient does not have to protect from upsetting feelings or thoughts.

Facilitating Life Review

Dying, as with any prolonged crises, is a period in which going forward involves looking back on the past. Patients find strength and meaning in reminiscing. They review and rework disappointments, and sometimes develop new strategies for the future. The clinician should encourage their reconstruction of the past and will be rewarded by sharing in reflections on the personal meaning of a unique life. Patients' talk about who they were and what they did is rarely "morbid," depressing, or focused on death. While you facilitate the process of review, you also develop useful insights into a patient's coping style.

Addressing Worries

Terminally ill patients are often anxious, faced by the decay of their bodies. They ride a roller coaster of remission and relapse, despondency and hope, loss and adjustment to loss, while seeking reassurance about an uncertain future. They monitor themselves for signs of progressive disease and they anticipate crises—some realistic, some fanciful. They harbor fears and often interpret the verbal and nonverbal behaviors of the health care personnel without explicitly checking out whether their notions are correct.

Attend to your patient's information needs, being aware of their reluctance to speak openly about some worries. You will find many important misinterpretations. In particular, pay attention to patients' attributions and attendant concerns.

What do you make of how things are going now?

What are your concerns about this new symptom?

What are your thoughts about the test results?

What is your understanding about the treatment?

Needs for information fluctuate with time, and you may be surprised to find how a fact that was discussed openly one day may be lost to awareness on the next day, then rediscovered or relearned later. Denial is a fluctuating defense that may vary enormously from moment to moment, reflecting the patient's emotional state, the setting of the discussion, and the interviewer's relationship with the patient.

For many patients and family members, anticipation of problems and rehearsal of management strategies can be very helpful:

> It is possible, as you suggested, that your shortness of breath may worsen. If you feel that your breathing is worse, you could increase the oxygen to 3 liters per minute, but I would also like you to call me.

> You may find your husband getting drowsier and drowsier now, and he will be less able to take care of himself—cleaning himself, feeding, getting to the bathroom, and so on. As this happens, the nurse and I will visit and make sure everything is taken care of. He won't be able to take his pills. It's likely that he will gradually go to sleep before he dies.

Facing Facts Openly

While physicians always fear harming patients with frank discussions of distressing information, the dying almost invariably can protect themselves from being overwhelmed by "bad news." They have both unconscious defenses as well as conscious methods for momentarily keeping themselves from full awareness of topics they wish to avoid. As a beginner, you may be surprised how patients may dismiss what you said. A much more frequent problem than being unwittingly intrusive or confrontational with patients is to avoid talking to them about painful facts. You should respect denial, but generally not encourage it or engage in it yourself. Remember that talking about painful reality does not create the circumstances or the pain; the patient's dilemma is a fact that is generally best dealt with as openly as the patient will tolerate.

■ CONCLUSION

As you come closer to the dying, you see that they will not harm you, though they touch you with sadness. They may not even make enormous demands on you, except that you listen. Active listening is therapy for the patient, while for you it is a remarkable opportunity to learn how people make sense of their lives and the crisis of approaching death. Professionals with an interest in the care of the dying describe their work not only as challenging, difficult, and sometimes sad, but also as extremely gratifying—a treasured personal lesson on how suffering is borne, how cherished relationships may transcend the pain of loss, and how limited time should be savored.

SUGGESTED READINGS

Introduction to "Difficult Dyads"

In addition to standard textbooks on psychiatry (including the *Diagnostic and Statistical Manual of Mental Disorders—DSM-IV*) and on psychiatric aspects of general medicine, the following may be useful:

Balint M: *The doctor, his patient, and the illness,* New York, 1952, International Universities Press.

Enelow AJ, Swisher SN: Emotional and behavioral responses to illness and to patients. In Enelow AJ, Swisher SN: *Interviewing and patient care,* ed 4, New York, 1996, Oxford University Press.

Groves JE: Taking care of the hateful patient, *N Engl J Med* 298-883, 1978.

Kahana RJ, Bibring GL: Personality types in medical management. In Zinberg NE, editor: *Psychiatry and medical practice in a general hospital,* New York, 1964, International Universities Press.

Lipsitt DR: Medical and psychological characteristics of "crocks," *Int J Psychiatry Med* 1:15, 1970.

Shapiro D: *Neurotic styles,* New York, 1986, Basic Books.

Williams WC: A face of stone. In *The farmer's daughters: the collected stories of William Carlos Williams,* New York, 1961, New Directions.

Zborowski M: Cultural components in response to pain, *J Soc Issues* 8:16, 1952.

Zola IK: Culture and symptoms: an analysis of patients' presenting complaints, *Am Sociol Rev* 31:615, 1966. Reprinted in Zola IK: *Socio-medical inquiries recollections, reflections, and reconsiderations,* Philadelphia, 1983, Temple University Press.

The Sad or Crying Patient

Bowlby J: *Attachment and loss,* vol I, *Attachment* (1969); vol II, *Separation: anxiety and anger* (1973); vol III, *Loss: sadness and depression* (1980), New York, Basic Books.

Lazare A: Unresolved grief. In Lazare A, editor: *Outpatient psychiatry: diagnosis and treatment,* ed 2, Baltimore, 1988, Williams & Wilkins.

Lewis CS: *A grief observed,* New York, 1963, Seabury Press.

Lindemann E: Symptomatology and management of acute grief, *Am J Psychiatry* 101:14, 1944.

Osterweis M, Solomon F, Green M, editors: *Bereavement: reactions, consequences, and care,* Washington, DC, 1984, National Academy Press.

Parkes CM: *Bereavement: studies of grief in adult life,* New York, 1972, International Universities Press.

The Anxious Patient

Freud A: *The ego and the mechanisms of defense,* New York, 1966, International Universities Press.

Kahana RJ, Bibring GL: Personality types in medical management. In Zinberg NE, editor: *Psychiatry and medical practice in a general hospital.* New York, 1964, International Universities Press.

Nemiah JC: *Foundations of psychopathology,* New York, 1961, Oxford University Press.

Weisman A: *On dying and denying: a psychiatric study of terminality,* New York, 1972, Behavioral Publications.

Communication Styles and Communication Barriers

Greene MG, Majerovitz SD, Adelman RD, Rizzo C: The effects of a third person on the physician-older patient medical interview, *J Am Geriat Soc* 42:413, 1994.

Huntly RA, Helfer KS, editors: *Communication in late life,* Boston, 1995, Butterworth-Heinemann.

Seattle, 1994. Pacific Medical Center: Cross-cultural health care project: a report.

Ryan EB, Meridith SD, MacLean MJ, Orange JB: Changing the way we talk with elders: promoting health using communication enhancement model, *Int J Aging Hum Dev* 41:89, 1995.

Silliman RA: Caring for the frail older patient: the doctor-patient-caregiver relationship, *J Gen Intern Med* 4:237, 1989.

Waitzkin H, Britt T, Williams C: Narratives of aging and social problems in medical encounters with older persons, *J Health Soc Behav* 35:322, 1996.

Woloshin S, Bickell NA, Schwartz LM, et al: Language barriers in medicine, *JAMA* 273:724, 1995.

The Somatizing Patient

Adler G: The physician and the hypochondriacal patient, *N Engl J Med* 304:1394, 1981.

Barsky AJ: Patients who amplify bodily sensations, *Ann Intern Med* 91:63, 1979.

Barsky AJ, Klerman GL: Overview: hypochondriasis, bodily complaints, and somatic styles, *Am J Psychiatry* 140:273, 1983.

Drossman DA: The problem patient: evaluation and care of medical patients with psychosocial disturbances, *Ann Intern Med* 88:366, 1978.

Engel GL: "Psychogenic" pain and the pain-prone patient, *Am J Med* 26:899, 1959.

Lipsitt DR: Medical and psychological characteristics of "crocks," *Psychiatry Med* 1:1, 1970.

Mechanic D: Social psychologic factors affecting the presentation of bodily complaints, *N Engl J Med* 286:1132, 1972.

Smith RC: Somatization disorder: defining its role in clinical medicine, *J Gen Intern Med* 6:168, 1991.

The Dying Patient

Cassell EJ: *The healer's art,* Boston, 1985, MIT Press.

Cassel EJ: The nature of suffering and the goals of medicine, *N Engl J Med* 306:639, 1982.

Cassem N: Treating the person confronting death. In Nicholi AM Jr: *The new Harvard guide to psychiatry,* Cambridge, Mass, 1988. Harvard University Press.

Despelder LA, Strickland AL: *The last dance: encountering death and dying,* ed 4, Palo Alto, Calif, 1996. Mayfield Publishing.

Gonds TA, Ruark JE: *Dying dignified: the health professional's guide to care,* Menlo Park, Calif, 1984, Addison-Wesley.

Grollman EA: *Talking about death: a dialogue between parent and child,* ed 3, Boston, 1991, Beacon Press.

Kubler Ross E: *On death and dying,* New York, 1969, Macmillan.

Spiro H: What is empathy and can it be taught? *Am Intern Med* 15:843, 1992.

Tolstoy L: The death of Ivan Ilych. In *Great short works of Leo Tolstoy,* New York, 1967, Harper & Row.

Weisman AD: *Coping with cancer,* New York, 1979, McGraw-Hill.

CHAPTER 14

CARRYING OUT A PLAN

"Patient Satisfaction: A Business Imperative for the 90's" (with complimentary breakfast).

FLYER

CONFLICT: NEGOTIATION AND MANAGEMENT

Conflict is inherent in the clinical encounter. Patients and doctors often have different views about how they should relate to each other, the nature of the illness, and the preferred goals and methods of diagnosis, treatment, and prevention. Remarkably, these divergent perspectives rarely produce overt clashes, since patients and doctors, with little conscious effort, tend to accommodate to each other and maintain a semblance of agreement. However, when significant conflicts are not reconciled, both participants may be dissatisfied: the patient may not cooperate with medical advice, while the physician may become irritated or lose interest in the patient.

This chapter characterizes common forms of clinical conflict. To recognize differing viewpoints and arrive at decisions that support effective and personal care, we suggest that physicians ask a few simple questions, such as:

How do you think we should approach this problem?

How would you like me to help you?

What do you want to do now?

Next, techniques are reviewed for managing conflict. We highlight the concept of "negotiation," a style of conflict resolution that applies egalitarian values to the doctor-patient relationship.

Conflict in Various Phases of the Encounter

Conflict may arise in the earliest moments of the interview, as the patient and physician first establish a relationship, particularly as they decide which problems to discuss and how. Who will do the talking? How much detail will be provided on what matters? Which problems will be addressed during this visit, and in what order? The patient typically has one notion of how to tell the story of the illness; the doctor may want to hear only some of the account and usually desires to direct the flow of information:

A 70-year-old man with foot pain wanted to tell a lengthy story about standing all day at his job and about how tight shoes were contributing to his problem. His physician quickly took control of the interview, gathering information useful for the diagnosis

226

of peripheral vascular disease or gout. Although the physician discussed his findings and opinion thoroughly, the patient later complained that he did not get to describe "what my problem was" and noted that "the doctor didn't explain anything," by which he meant that no advice was given about his prolonged standing or about wearing special shoes.

▲

Commonly, during the initial phases of the interview, the doctor and the patient make accommodations to each other's preferred approach to telling the story of the illness, and settle into a pattern of information exchange that is acceptable to both. In many instances, the physician controls the agenda by asking serial questions, while the patient exerts influence by the manner in which he or she answers questions. Patients may be dissatisfied with a visit if they never get to tell their story fully or if they feel that the physician focused on the wrong problem or was inattentive to important details. In such situations, patients leave feeling disgruntled; rarely, however, do they confront the physician with their disappointment.

Throughout the interview, common sources of conflict arise from doctor-patient differences: (1) in the meaning of terms and language ("This job is giving me hypertension"), (2) in appreciating the emotive significance of the patient's problem ("Your hair may fall out, but it will grow back later"), (3) in views of etiology and pathophysiology ("I'm hardly eating anything but I still gain weight"), and (4) in preferred goals and methods of diagnosis and treatment ("I want an antibiotic"). Fortunately, both the patient's and the physician's perspectives on the problem and its management may be modified by their evolving appreciation of and accommodation to each other's views. For instance, physicians may recommend diagnostic tests and therapeutic interventions in response to the patient's explicit requests and expectations.

Patient: Gee, Doc, I've had this headache for 6 months. Don't you think I need a CAT scan?

Doctor: Seems reasonable, but first let me go over your examination.

Likewise, conflict may be avoided. Thus, when a physician suspects that patients would not want a diagnostic or therapeutic procedure (e.g., because they seem uninterested, lack insurance coverage, might find the procedure too troublesome, or have difficulty coming back to be tested), he or she may not even suggest the procedure.

Moreover, even if the patient's perspective is hidden or not elicited, the physician's handling of the visit may satisfy the patient.

An elderly woman presented to the office with chest discomfort. She was worried about a heart problem but did not openly state her concern. She was appreciative when the physician carefully elicited a description of her symptom and then examined her thoroughly, including attention to her heart. She noticed that the physician did not seem alarmed by her complaint or physical findings. She readily accepted reassurance that her pain was "not serious," interpreting the statement to mean that her heart was fine. Although her attributions were not made explicit and her concerns were not addressed directly, she left the interview feeling sure that she had been properly checked for heart disease.

▲

Conflict frequently emerges in the exposition phase of the interview when an assessment and a plan are offered. Ideally, a treatment plan should be developed that is mutually satisfactory to both patient and physician. The means to this end may require education and negotiation. Consider the elaborate give-and-take occurring around two middle-aged patients, each presenting to their physicians with a painful left shoulder. In both cases, the diagnosis, based on history and physical examination, is tendinitis. Treatment generally consists of resting the shoulder, applying heat, and taking medications to reduce the inflammation and pain. In both situations, the doctor and patient must determine what additional diagnostic steps are needed (including measures to reassure either party about the seriousness of the problem) and what kind of treatment will be used.

A Patient Primarily Concerned About Pain Relief

In the first case, the physician is relatively confident about the diagnosis but is inclined to seek further confirmation. She suggests obtaining a shoulder x-ray. The patient, however, does not want to bother with tests; he has concerns about "unnecessary radiation." He does not believe that the discomfort signifies a serious condition, but he wants relief from his pain. His goals are uninterrupted sleep tonight and an ability to function at work tomorrow. The physician reconsiders the need for an x-ray, suggesting that it could be obtained later if the discomfort persists or worsens. Moreover, since the antiinflammatory regimen may not provide prompt relief, the physician also offers to prescribe medication for pain relief. The patient, however, does not want so many pills; he would like to start with only one medication, but also would like to be sure that the physician is available by phone over the weekend if the first treatment does not provide adequate relief. The physician replies that she is not going to be available and suggests that the patient accept a prescription for the pain medication, but only fill it later if needed. The patient agrees.

A Patient Primarily Concerned About the Meaning of Tendinitis

The second patient is concerned about the possible seriousness of his illness but is suffering little physical discomfort. He initially accepts a prescription for an antiinflammatory drug. When the directions for taking the medication are reviewed, however, the patient reveals that he probably will not take the drug. The physician suggests that the medication might speed recovery but also predicts that the tendinitis will probably resolve in a few weeks with heat and rest. The patient decides to use heat and rest and prefers to wait a while before taking medication. Also, he wants a shoulder x-ray and an electrocardiogram. The physician elicits the patient's specific worries—metastatic cancer and a heart condition—and she states a strong doubt that the pain is a sign of "something serious, such as cancer or heart disease." She proposes that an x-ray be obtained later only if the pain persists or worsens despite treatment. She also states that an electrocardiogram would not be helpful for evaluating this shoulder pain, but since the patient is concerned about heart problems, perhaps he would like to obtain a baseline electrocardiogram and serum cholesterol.

At this point, if the patient accepts the physician's advice and is reassured, a mutually satisfactory plan has been achieved. If the patient still wants an x-ray, the physician might: (1) elect to do the procedure for the patient's reassurance and to maintain an alliance, (2) bargain for the patient to try a brief course of therapy before obtaining the x-ray, or (3) stick firmly to her initial plan, carefully explaining her reasoning, acknowledging the patient's viewpoint, and possibly enduring the patient's displeasure.

▲

Conflict Over the Relationship

Conflicts about the doctor-patient relationship are common but are subtle, rarely discussed in the encounter, and often difficult to recognize. For instance, one patient may dislike a highly authoritarian approach by the physician, another will resent an egalitarian style, while most patients want some of each style at different times. Likewise, a physician may prefer patients whose behaviors are diffident or assertive. Patients may not only bring requests for straightforward medical expertise, but also present with needs and desires for succor, friendship, encouragement, acceptance, sympathy— wishes that may not be fully conscious or readily communicated and which the physician may not appreciate or may simply feel are unacceptable. The very nature of the doctor-patient relationship—who is supposed to do what with whom—can be in dispute.

Differences in how patients and doctors prefer to work together— conflicts in the relationship—are difficult to separate from conflicts about the nature of the problem and the goals and methods of care. In practice, such conflicts are often inseparable. For instance, some patients seek a physician who is extremely kind, understanding, and tolerant; their additional preferences about treatment or information-sharing are often subservient to these interpersonal goals. Likewise, discussions about missed appointments, noncompliance, and contacting the physician when problems arise may seem to be about the goals and methods of care, but also reflect conflicts about the relationship. Many festering clinical dilemmas in which patients are labeled as "hateful," "difficult," or "problem patients" can be at least partly understood as conflicts in negotiating a mutually satisfactory relationship.

Negotiation in the Encounter

The manner in which clinical conflict is handled reflects core values about the doctor-patient relationship. The term "negotiation" is used to describe an approach to conflict management that is based on egalitarian values. In our view, medical care ideally is a collaborative process between partners—the doctor and patient—who are joined in helping the patient. When satisfactory negotiation occurs, these partners, despite their different expertise, maintain mutual respect and a desire for consensus. Negotiation proceeds best when the importance of the personal perspectives of both participants in the relationship is recognized and when the process and outcome of the encounter reflect active attention to such perspectives.

The doctor-patient relationship differs from other encounters in which negotiation is a recognized feature. In a business transaction, for instance, negotiation is motivated primarily by self-interest. In a married couple's negotiation, a gain for one partner may entail some loss for the other. In the clinical encounter, both parties should have the same basic goal of helping the patient. Of course, physicians, too, can negotiate from a perspective that might be considered selfish, for example, not wanting to make a house call at night, resisting the addition of another patient into a busy schedule, or acting on behalf of "third parties"—colleagues, the practice, the hospital, the insurance company, the profession, or government—rather than for the patient (e.g., trying to avoid hospital admissions or to reduce health care costs, wanting not to disturb a colleague on the weekend, limiting access to disability and welfare benefits).

Effective negotiation requires the following four broad conditions.

Conditions for Effective Negotiation

1. **The patient needs authoritative information and medical advice to make informed decisions.** For the patient, the encounter is for learning; the physician must transmit information about diagnosis and treatment, including reasonable options.
2. **Both parties accept the legitimacy of differences, of conflict between each other's views; both attempt to solve problems jointly.** Negotiation should be distinguished from a laissez-faire or passive attitude on the part of the patient or the physician.
3. **The outcome is approached flexibly,** recognizing that one's goals may not be fully met and that complete accord may not be attained.
4. **The patient's autonomy in decision-making is recognized;** the patient is ultimately responsible for his or her well-being.

In the actual clinical encounter, these conditions are not regularly met. The patient's position in the negotiation process may be bolstered by contemporary social pressures for "activated" patients, consumer participation, and self-care, but physician dominance is favored by the enormous disparity in clinical knowledge and experience between the two parties, especially in acute care settings. Many patients, so anxious about their well-being, will readily accept a passive role, trusting a paternalistic physician who offers certainty. Patients even say, "You decide," when options are offered. Moreover, by tradition and habit, physicians tend to exercise their authority, exerting what Balint called the "apostolic function":

> *Every doctor has a vague, but almost unshakably firm, idea of how a patient ought to behave when ill. Although this idea is anything but explicit and concrete, it is immensely powerful and influences ... practically every detail of the doctor's work....*

Regardless, negotiation is a style to which clinicians may aspire, especially in the chronic care setting, which constitutes the bulk of ambulatory medical practice.

A key moment for encouraging negotiations is the beginning of the exposition phase. The physician's manner—particularly how he or she initiates the discussion of the diagnosis, presents management options, invites questions and suggestions from the patient, and involves the patient actively in the decision-making process—has a strong impact on how conflict will be managed. With little conscious effort, the interviewer's behavior may strongly influence whether the relationship will follow an authoritarian-passive interaction or more mutual participation. If the latter is favored, the presentation of a plan can be seen as an initial proposal that might include alternatives for review by the patient as well as opportunities for the patient to introduce further options. Interest in how the patient evaluates various proposals—what meaning and utility the patient attaches to them—is essential. The possibility of disagreement must be recognized and its expression encouraged. A plan is sought that suits the needs of the patient who, ultimately, will carry out treatment. Note the following examples.

Authoritarian Style
The physician begins the exposition phase by saying, "You have a tension headache," and then gives a description of the etiology and pathophysiology of the complaint. Next, such a physician says, "Take this medicine whenever you feel one coming on. I will see you in a month to find out how things are going." The patient is given no encouragement to express his or her ideas. Conflict recognition and resolution are not among this physician's explicit goals for communicating about the diagnosis and treatment.

Egalitarian Style
Another physician says, "You seem to have a tension headache. What are your thoughts about it?" If the patient rejects the diagnosis, the physician explores the basis of the divergent views. If the patient accepts the diagnosis, the physician may next want to explore the patient's understanding about this condition: "What do you know about tension headaches? What are your ideas about why you might have one?" The patient is given a variety of opportunities to learn about the illness.

Later, this physician might introduce a management plan by saying, "There are a number of ways to proceed now, and I would like to review these with you. To confirm the diagnosis, I do not think you need any more tests. To treat your condition, we should consider a few approaches." The patient is encouraged to present his or her viewpoint (e.g., about the need for tests) and to participate, insofar as personally desired, in decisions. A few management options may be offered, and the patient may be asked if he or she has any other suggestions. Does the patient want pain-relieving treatment, or reassurance, or both? If treatment is requested, does the patient prefer medication, counseling, or behavioral intervention? The physician gives his or her opinion on the benefits and disadvantages of each treatment and seeks the patient's personal evaluation of each option. If reassurance is sought, what patient concerns need to be addressed, and how? Finally, how and when should follow-up be arranged?

▲

Recognizing Conflict

A review of audio and video recordings of clinical interviews reveals that negotiation of doctor-patient differences is often missing because conflict is simply not recognized. The physician cannot begin to manage conflict without appreciating the patient's perspectives: (1) the definition of the problem, (2) attributions (ideas about etiology, pathophysiology, and meaning of illness), (3) desired goals and methods for handling the problem—the requests, and (4) reactions to the proposed plan, including both diagnostic and therapeutic aspects. The clinician should listen throughout the interview for the patient's goals—immediate and long term—for the doctor-patient relationship and for managing his or her own health. Most important, how does the patient's "agenda" for the visit differ from the physician's? An effective interview should recognize, respect, and encourage the expression of divergent viewpoints.

Unless coaxed, patients regularly fail to present direct information about their perspective on the illness and its management, particularly their "requests." Nonetheless, they generally give hints during the interview about their attributions, and when questioned carefully, patients uniformly have requests. Ordinary questions will elicit the patient's perspective.

> What do you make of the problem?
> What are your thoughts about what is wrong?
> What are your concerns?
>
> How can I help you?
> What do you hope to achieve in this visit?
>
> What ideas have you had about how to figure out what is wrong?
>
> What are your thoughts about treating this problem?
>
> How should we follow up on this matter?
> When do you want to come back to see me?

(See also in Chapter 10 the section Attributions and the topic Assessing the Meaning of Illness in the section Psychosocial Assessment.) When regularly asked about their perspective, patients soon learn to assert their ideas with less encouragement; eventually, they may spontaneously present their attributions and requests as a routine feature of telling their story.

With encouragement, patients also learn to negotiate over the several elements of the encounter. Common conflicts occur over the following:

Recognizing Conflicts _____

Definition of the problem
- Seriousness:

> Doctor: You need to be admitted.
> Patient: Gee, not now. I've got work to do.

- Urgency:

  Doctor [over the telephone]: It sounds like a virus.
  Patient: I've got to see you right away. I could have pneumonia.

- Relationship of physical complaints to psychological state or behavior:

  Patient: It's not in my head.
  Doctor: I think it's tension.

- Standard medical explanations (diagnoses, etiology, pathophysiology) vs. popular, lay, or culturally derived attributions

Goals of care

- Relieving physical distress with somatic therapy, explanation, or reassurance:

  Doctor: Here, take this prescription.
  Patient: I just want to know what it is.

- Curative vs. symptomatic treatment (e.g., for a diarrheal illness)
- Cosmetic vs. noncosmetic purposes (e.g., balancing disfigurement vs. optimal surgical outcome)
- Accuracy and certainty in diagnosis vs. attention to cost, convenience, and symptomatic relief
- A focus on immediate treatment vs. long-term preventive measures

Methods of care

- Standard medical treatments vs. lay treatments
- Timing—differing perceptions of urgency of diagnosis and management (e.g., beginning immediate treatment for a presumed infection vs. waiting for a culture to confirm the appropriateness of antibiotics)
- Somatic vs. psychosocial treatment (e.g., antidepressants vs. psychotherapy)
- Resource commitment (time, money, energy) to therapeutic and diagnostic activities vs. to other priorities (family, work, recreation)
- Patient desire for greater communication, attention, and education vs. physician's desire for speed and efficiency

Doctor-patient relationship

- Authoritarian vs. mutual participation
- Technical vs. personal relationship
- Time devoted to the relationship (e.g., frequency of contact; communication only through scheduled appointments vs. after regular office hours)

Managing Conflict

At times, doctors and patients may choose to "set agendas," establish a "contract," make agreements, openly bargain or compromise, or employ other explicit strategies for conflict resolution, including calling in third parties, such as family members. Much conflict, however, is unstated and is handled with little explicit discussion or even conscious awareness. Often the patient or doctor simply decides to accommodate, deferring to the other's expertise or request, perhaps assuming that the other party holds a firm viewpoint. Insofar as both parties are skillful at setting forth their own perspectives and recognizing each other's, clinical care can be successfully carried out without much explicit discussion. Unfortunately, well-intentioned efforts based on faulty assumptions (e.g., the doctor thinks the patient wants a test or the patient thinks the doctor will be mad if a suggested treatment is not followed) can lead to frustration of both parties and to mutually unsatisfactory outcomes.

The physician should be familiar with a variety of approaches for conflict management, ranging from the most subtle accommodations to formal contracts. Also, ongoing monitoring of conflict is an important feature of follow-up visits. The following "techniques" may be useful in conflict management.

Techniques for Managing Conflict

- Form a relationship that favors the expression of the patient's perspective

  > How would you like us to help you?
  >
  > I'd like to hear your thoughts about what I propose.
  >
  > I hope you understand the treatment options and my recommendation. I want to find a plan that you approve.

- Clarify the conflict and the patient's perspective. Beware of those requests with important implications for treatment planning (e.g., "What did you hope I could do for you?"). Also, clarify your viewpoint. Seek mutual understanding.

  In general, whenever conflict occurs, go back to basics, namely understanding different perspectives on the definition of the problem and on the goals and methods of care, based on divergent knowledge, attitudes, and beliefs. Avoid simply overlooking disagreements in the hope that a disgruntled patient will follow a suggestion, especially in the presence of signs to the contrary (nonverbal expressions of dissatisfaction, "accidentally" missing an appointment, or forgetting to follow advice).

- Recognize, acknowledge, and respect your patient's stance (e.g., "I can see what you are saying now," or "I see your point"). Rather than focusing on a position or outcome (e.g., whether or not to be admitted to the hospital), the parties in a conflict should try to state their viewpoints in terms of the basic principles, values, or constraints that presumably led to such a position, for example:

  > Patient: I know I have a serious illness, maybe cancer, and that I will not get a quick diagnosis unless I'm admitted to the hospital.
  >
  > Doctor: I agree you need a prompt and thorough evaluation, but I think we can get the necessary tests done readily without hospitalizing you, and that we won't risk any serious delay. What if I can promise you to get all the x-rays, blood tests, and consultations you need in this week? Would you agree?

- Try to take the other side: what is the other person's stake in a particular solution? Restate the other person's position and its premises to show your interest in his or her stance and to determine if you understand it properly. Encourage the patient to do the same, making sure the basis for your viewpoint is well communicated:

> This is how I understand what you are saying. . . .
>
> What would you do if you were in my shoes?

- Preserve and strengthen the relationship, rather than merely attempting to reach a quick solution. Show your continued respect for the patient's values, even if you differ. Emphasize the patient's stake in the problem and your recognition of its importance to the patient. Underscore areas of agreement and aim at further joining of purposes.

> I see why this matters so much to you.
>
> I think we agree on what we are trying to accomplish here, but we still have different notions of how to do it.

- Invite criticism of your viewpoint and plan. Demonstrate how the relationship can tolerate disagreement while reaching for satisfying solutions. Admit error or misunderstanding, and, where appropriate, apologize.
- Educate by transmitting appropriate information. What do you see differently than the patient about the likely outcome of various options? How do various methods meet agreed-upon goals?
- Persuade and argue. Make appeals to professional expertise.
- Manipulate contingencies, using exchange, bargaining, and counterproposals, for example:

> Well, would you do it after Christmas?
>
> How about if I were the one to draw the blood sample?
>
> Let's say we get the x-rays you want, but you also agree to try this medication for a few weeks.

- Compromise or give in. Show your flexibility and willingness to make concessions, giving the patient a sense of control. Avoid ultimatums. Generate options, devise solutions, and present alternatives that satisfy the patient or meet both parties' wishes.
- Tolerate the other's viewpoint. You may "bite the bullet," agree to disagree (perhaps with attempts to find common ground), or hope that the other person will change later. Even when significant differences in viewpoint are not settled, a relationship can still be maintained in which conflict is recognized and respected. Also, negotiation can often be carried out over time, so both doctor and patient may choose to delay settlement on important issues, hoping that time will lead to a favorable outcome. A good general rule in negotiating serious conflict is not to insist on immediate total agreement.
- Enlist third parties for mediation, arbitration, or adjudication, for example:

> Since we disagree about this matter, I wonder if it would help to have you see a specialist to get another opinion?
>
> Can we get your wife to help us with this matter?

- State your limits. Consider setting terms for continuation of the overall relationship or specific features of the relationship:

> I can only prescribe this treatment after checking you properly.
>
> I am willing to be your doctor and help you with this pain problem if you agree to be seen monthly and to obtain all your prescriptions through me.

• Renegotiate

> We did not get very far with this plan. Let's make a new one.

■ CONCLUSION: WHY NEGOTIATE?

Most encounters between patients and doctors have satisfactory outcomes. Most patients are ready to defer to the physician's expertise. Why focus on conflict and its resolution?

On the one hand, conflict recognition and management can be viewed as techniques that need to be employed only when problems arise in the doctor-patient relationship. Under ordinary circumstances, usual practices are satisfactory; attention should be directed to settling differences only when conflict is obviously present (e.g., the patient and doctor are overtly dissatisfied, the patient is noncompliant).

On the other hand, a host of studies on doctor-patient communication suggest that conflict is common and has significant sequelae. Surveys report that patients are dissatisfied with the limited explanations they receive. Noncompliance is ubiquitous and often has serious consequences. Malpractice suits are burgeoning. Many patients find that conventional medicine fails to address their special needs. Meanwhile, with consumerism and an increased supply of doctors, patients are more likely to seek personalized care that promises them a greater role in decision-making, while physicians may feel that they cannot afford to dismiss such demands.

From a more personal point of view, we find that attention to conflict helps make clinical care more effective, efficient, and gratifying. Many of the vaguely perceived problems of daily medical work with patients become explicit and more manageable when conflict is elicited and an atmosphere of negotiation is established. Greater attention to the patient's perspectives opens the physician to an appreciation of the varied ways illness is experienced and of the complexity and delicacy of the task of providing personal care.

EDUCATION AND PERSUASION FOR COMPLIANCE

> *Life is short, and the Art long; the occasion fleeting; experience fallacious, and judgment difficult. The physician must not only be prepared to do what is right himself, but also to make the patient, the attendants, and the externals cooperate.*
>
> *First Aphorism of Hippocrates*
>
> *Compliance is that state of grace when the patient does what the physician reasonably wanted . . .*
>
> *Richard N. Podell*

Patient compliance—following medication regimens, keeping appointments (for visits, tests, and other treatment), changing behaviors (e.g., eating, exercising, smoking, and drinking), and otherwise performing self-monitoring and self-treatment—is critical to the effective management and prevention of medical disorders.

Studies indicate that 20% to 80% of patients do not comply with medical advice. However, these dismal statistics are based on a rigid definition of compliance as all-or-nothing adherence to the physician's instructions. In fact, patients generally neither attend perfectly and obsessively to a physician's preferred plan nor totally neglect it. Their intentions to comply reflect a variety of personal understandings and attitudes about treatment, while their actual behaviors may depart markedly from what they intend to do and even from what they perceive they have done.

Nor should the blame for noncompliance necessarily rest on the patient. A number of physician-generated problems are common, including errors in writing prescriptions, failure to explain clearly the purpose of a medication or how to take it, not indicating why the patient should return for an office visit, or not negotiating a suitable appointment time, failure to properly relabel pill containers when the directions are changed, and many instances of unclear instructions about diet, exercise, and other treatments. Moreover, prescribed regimens may be unrealistically demanding on time, energy, or financial resources.

The terms "compliance" and "adherence" may carry the unfortunate connotation that the patient is subservient to the physician. Moreover, clinicians too often simply resort to scolding, lecturing, or making authoritarian demands on noncompliant patients. Rather than presuming to reprimand your patients, try to understand what went wrong and how you can help them (see Quick Tips: Techniques for Promoting Compliance).

QUICK TIPS

Techniques for Promoting Compliance

- Education—Inform your patient about the rationale of your proposed plan.
- Motivation—Explore attitudes and help foster favorable ones.
- Behavior—Offer simple suggestions that help your patient follow treatment.
- Technical solutions—Simplify and customize your regimen to best suit your patient.
- Monitoring—Monitor adherence in a nonthreatening and nonjudgmental way.

Patient Education

Is noncompliance a reflection of inadequate knowledge? Does the patient understand the rationale for treatment? Does the patient understand the regimen?

A first step in promoting compliance is to assure that the patient understands the management plan and has the knowledge to carry it out. Does the patient know about the diagnosis and therapy? Have the immediate and long-term health risks and treatment benefits been communicated and appreciated? In particular, what are the expected outcomes and potential side effects of the proposed treatment?

In providing patient education, instructions should be adapted to the patient's language and knowledge level. Directions should be explicit and as simple as possible. Use multiple modes of communication—speech, writing, and audiovisual materials—to reinforce knowledge. Printed medication instruction sheets are commercially available. Similarly, enlist other members of the clinical team—nurses, physician assistants, nutritionists, physical therapists, pharmacists—and family members in the education of the patient.

Consider the following:

- Emphasize and repeat important messages.
- Write out the medication schedule. Make a daily or weekly calendar that indicates when pills should be taken.
- Be very clear with directions. Beware of terms such as "four times a day" or "with meals," which may have a different meaning to the patient than to the clinician.
- Clarify how the patient should respond (e.g., continue the medicine or stop it) if he or she begins to feel well or has some side effects. Elicit and address common fears of toxicity or of becoming dependent on medication.
- Explain what you mean when instructing a patient to take a medication as needed (*prn*).
- Be clear about when the medication can be stopped. If the current prescription expires, should the patient discontinue the medication or renew the prescription?
- Finally, to assess patient understanding, get feedback. Have the patient repeat key elements of the plan and its rationale.

Motivational Strategies

Now that the patient is well-informed, what is his or her attitude toward this management plan—its costs and benefits—and how can favorable attitudes be fostered?

Discrepancies between the patient's behavior and the doctor's expectations often arise because the two have failed to develop a mutually agreeable plan and sense of partnership. Instead of scolding a patient for behavior you do not favor, explore the patient's perspective, particularly as it differs from your own. Does the patient recognize the problem as serious? What aspects hold particular concern (and hence are most likely to motivate behavior)? How does the patient feel about undergoing diagnostic procedures or treatments? What seem to be the personal benefits as well as the barriers, such as cost, inconvenience, and undesired effects on physical and psychological well-being? Anticipate problems.

What could go wrong in trying to carry out this plan?

When the patient's perspective is recognized, a mutually acceptable plan can be negotiated. If necessary, address conflict and consider adjusting treatment plans to suit the patient. When you and the patient share a common view of the illness and its management, you can seek and expect clear commitment to the plan and may clearly assert this expectation.

Use your understanding of what motivates the patient to be persuasive and help strengthen resolve. For instance, in discussing smoking cessation, you might appeal to a particular patient's concerns about appearance (wrinkles), well-being of the family (avoiding the effects of passive smoking on others; being healthy enough in 15 years to support a growing child), short-term comfort (diminished cough), finances (the expense of cigarettes), or various illnesses (lung cancer, throat cancer, emphysema, heart disease). Personalized messages are more likely to be motivating than generic stern advice or fear-laden warnings.

A positive, affiliative, doctor-patient relationship is important for making the patient ready to receive patient education and to negotiate about treatment. Beware of the downward spiral in which noncompliance alienates doctor and patient, leading to worsening compliance and increasing frustration. When compliance is a problem that has undermined the relationship, work on building rapport. Consider focusing less attention on noncompliance until further intervention is likely to be successful. Spend more time on patient education to build a relationship that can foster compliance. Sometimes, increased contact between patient and doctor—more frequent or longer visits, or simply allowing more time for the relationship to evolve—is necessary to promote compliance. When the doctor and patient are allies, they can jointly plan for return visits, referrals, and various methods of reviewing and promoting compliance.

Support the patient's capacity to carry out the plan by providing rewards or reinforcement. Recognize success and offer praise for successful adherence. Be encouraging; acclaim even the smallest accomplishment.

Additional sources of reinforcement include the spouse, family, and, when present, home care staff (visiting nurses, home health aides, homemakers) who may encourage, remind, and monitor the patient.

Behavioral Techniques

How can this regimen best be enacted?

Make personalized plans that are organized around the routine of the patient's life, using everyday events as cues for pill-taking. Suggest that the patient keep medication containers in a conspicuous place. Instead of prescribing by the clock, prescribe by the patient's usual activity. For instance, pills are more likely to be taken at a daily event (getting up in the morning, a meal, brushing teeth, coffee break, going to bed) than in the middle of an activity. Rather than saying, "take these four times a day," ask:

> When would be a good time during the day for you to remember to take the medicine? When do you get up? What do you do when you get up? How about bedtime? How many meals do you usually eat a day? When? Where? Could you take a pill during those two meals you eat at home? What kind of reminders would be helpful?

A second behavioral strategy, particularly when seeking major changes in a patient's life, is to start with a few simple suggestions. Prioritize your plan and select some critical aspects of the regimen, preferably ones that can be realistically accomplished. As the patient masters these behaviors, you can gradually add on further measures. Success with earlier steps will be a source of encouragement and will provide a sense of mastery and confidence.

Help patients recognize and enjoy success. Identify how patients feel personally rewarded by healthful outcomes and use your understanding to reinforce a sense of accomplishment.

> You've achieved your goal of controlling your blood sugar without having to take injections.

> Your stamina and breathing capacity have really improved, and it looks like you are going to be able to do a lot more exercising without getting winded.

The physician's encouragement and praise are also an important source of reinforcement. Some patients benefit from constructing rather simple systems of reward, as, for instance, when a patient who is cutting down on smoking finances a special treat from the money that has been saved from not buying cigarettes.

Technical Solutions

What adjustments in the treatment regimen can promote compliance?

Simplify the regimen. Many inpatient pill-taking schedules are transferred to the outpatient setting where patients find them disruptive, complicated, and confusing. Favor medications that are easy to take. Pills should be administered on as few occasions a day as possible. Choose once-a-day and long-acting preparations. Regimens requiring more than four administrations a day are rarely justified, and even twice-a-day administration is difficult. A properly followed three-times-a-day regimen is often preferable to an erratically followed four-times-a-day schedule. If possible, patients should not be asked to take medication during their usual hours of sleep. Stop nonessential treatments.

Compromise for the sake of compliance. For instance, liquid antacids may work better than pills, but the pills may be easier to carry around and thus may be taken more regularly.

In the course of a day, patients may forget whether they have actually taken their pills. Calendar packs, used routinely for birth control pills, obviate this problem. Consider a pill administration regimen in which all the pills that should be taken during a day or week are poured into marked envelopes, cups, or commercially available medication containers that allow assessment, at a glance, of what has been taken or forgotten. Similarly, medication calendars serve as reminders about when to take medication, and the patient can cross out the times when pills were administered. Timers (including some that serve as tops for pill containers) can be used to remind the patient when a medication is due.

Assess problems in obtaining prescriptions, filling them, paying for them, having medication delivered to the home, opening pill containers, and monitoring when the medication is running out and needs to be refilled. Cost is an often overlooked barrier to compliance. Beware of childproof containers that also foil slightly disabled adults. Enlist the spouse or family members to remind, encourage, or supervise the patient.

Compliance with appointments can be promoted in several ways. Patients will benefit from reminders that can be provided either in writing or through telephone calls. When a patient "no-shows," seek information on why the appointment was missed; do not just reprimand the patient or overlook the problem. Assist the patient with scheduling and transportation for office visits or tests, and avoid long waiting times.

Monitoring

How can adherence be assessed?

The assessment and reinforcement of compliance are regular parts of follow-up care. Heightened attention to adherence is particularly important when regimens are complicated, long-term, aimed at prevention rather than immediate relief of distress, or involve significant behavioral change.

Studies indicate that physicians are generally poor predictors of which patients are noncompliant. Assume that adherence is imperfect and monitor it in a nonthreatening, nonjudgmental fashion. Begin with questions that directly assess patient behaviors.

How did it go with taking these new medicines?

Did you have any difficulties remembering to take them?

Many people have difficulty taking this sort of medication.

> About how often would you say you remembered to take it?
>
> What are the circumstances in which you tend to forget them?
>
> What do you do when you miss taking your medicine?
>
> Did you notice any side effects? Any other concerns about continuing the medication?

In reviewing the medication regimen, beware of yes-no questions (e.g., "Are you taking the medication?"); this form of interrogation will "lead the witness" and not require any demonstration of knowledge by the patient. Have the patient generate a full description of the regimen—the name, purpose, dosage, and schedule.

> What are you taking?
>
> What do you call the pills?
>
> What are they for?
>
> Do you know the size or strength?
>
> How many [or how much] do you take at a time?
>
> When do you take them?

Many patients can become allies in monitoring compliance and may even keep records on their behavior, (e.g., a meal diary or a pill count).

Alternatively, rather than obtaining compliance information from the patient, seek "objective" measures. A key tactic is to ask patients to bring all their pill bottles to the office, allowing you to deal with the medicines themselves. For some patients, you may want to review pill containers at every visit. Count pills or estimate how many were taken. Note whether refills were obtained.

Additionally, for some medications, serum drug levels may provide an indirect measure of compliance. Similarly, the outcome of treatment (e.g., the blood pressure, weight, or cholesterol level) may give some indication of compliance.

When there are significant discrepancies between patients' medication reports and other measures of compliance, the physician faces a difficult communication task. Try to present the information in a nonjudgmental fashion. Consider asking the patient to respond to your observations. Alternatively, simply advise the patient that you have indications that compliance is a problem.

■ CONCLUSION

Noncompliance is a constant challenge in clinical work and a commonly underestimated hindrance to optimal care. In promoting compliance, review the following issues: Does the patient really understand the regimen? Do the patient and doctor have a mutually recognized assessment of the benefits and costs of the management plan? If the problem is not merely a matter of understanding and attitudes, look for motivational strategies that reinforce and reward compliance. Redesign the treatment to make it easier and more acceptable. Find technical and family supports that enable the patient to carry out the regimen. And always monitor compliance. The physician needs to acknowledge and accept nonadherence, while at the same time seeking ways to promote compliance. Rather than being personally offended by limited adherence to a regimen, work together with the patient to identify and overcome barriers.

SHARING BAD NEWS

The communication of "bad news" may be difficult for both the patient and the doctor. Although clinicians frequently convey unsettling information, students rarely receive guidance in this task. Many kinds of information may be distressing to patients. See the following for some common examples.

Types of "Bad News"

The diagnosis of an everyday illness

> You've got bronchitis.
>
> You're coming down with mono.

An abnormal examination finding or test result

> You have a heart murmur.
>
> Your blood level is low.

The need to use medications or undergo procedures

> You should take this diuretic daily.
>
> Your condition requires an operation.

The identification of a chronic illness or disability

> We can't cure this arthritis, but we can provide some relief.

The onset of a fatal illness or its progression

> The biopsy shows lymphoma.
>
> It looks like the cancer has gotten into your bones.

The long-anticipated demise of a chronically ill octogenarian or the sudden death of a loved one

> It's over.
>
> We tried everything.

In sharing these many kinds of bad news, patients and doctors bring their own values, emotions, personality, and knowledge to the discourse. No simple formula can be found to manage such matters. This chapter focuses on the example of "telling the truth" to cancer patients in order to identify and illustrate common issues in conveying "bad news."

Truth-Telling About Cancer

Interviewers who are tactful and comfortable about discussing painful facts can regularly elicit from patients a frank acknowledgement of cancer; less confident interviewers may report that the patient "denies cancer." Although many patients shun distressing facts, total avoidance of the truth about the diagnosis, treatment, and prognosis of cancer is uncommon and nearly impossible to achieve.

Clinicians have recognized that most patients desire and benefit from information that reduces uncertainty, allows for realistic actions, and promotes reassurance. Patients generally sense when the truth is not being told; concealment may lead to suspiciousness and heightened anxiety. Withholding information prevents patients from participating fully in their care and making proper plans and often isolates them from those persons, usually family and physicians, who should be important sources of support. While bad news may inevitably cause anxiety, sadness, and other disagreeable feelings, these dysphoric affects generally pass quickly. Hopelessness or giving up is commonly thought to be the worst consequence of hearing the truth, but dying patients who continue to be able to enjoy some of life's rewards rarely give up after "hearing the worst."

These generalizations, of course, may reflect little about what a particular patient wants when actually faced with bad news (nor about how a physician actually behaves). While "full disclosure" may be a worthwhile clinical goal, a decision on truth-telling should not rely on *a priori* notions that "all the facts" should be announced at one visit, but rather on sensitivity to the needs of the patient in a particular situation.

Moreover, information-sharing is a complex process, and the patient and doctor often must engage in repeated discussions to clarify understanding. Truth is not conveyed in a one-word diagnosis or even a few sentences. The patient's information-seeking and comprehension begin well before the illness and may reflect long-standing attitudes about the world and whether to deal with uncertainty by either obtaining or ignoring information. The patient has already heard about cancer, surgery, radiation, chemotherapy, and dying and has ideas about them that may have little resemblance to what the physician wants to convey. The effect of learning distressing news (including the arousal of hope or despair) is best understood not simply as a reflection of interviewing technique but from an awareness of how the patient and doctor experience the facts, of how their unique personal backgrounds influence their interpretations.

Finally, while truth-telling may be viewed as an absolute ethical goal, an end-in-itself, it also is valued as a means for accomplishing other ends—biomedical, psychosocial, legal—and may conflict with other important values. For instance, patients regularly desire truthfulness, but for some cultures, honesty may seem less important than being gentle and protective. The frank truth may sometimes be perceived as cruelty. Patients may say they want information, yet clearly only want reassurance. Informed consent that includes the "full disclosure" of uncertainty and of treatment alternatives may cause "information overload" and create confusion and distress. In many clinical situations, the physician needs to balance conflicting goals: being honest and informative, responding to the patient's personality and preferences, preserving a relationship of confidence and trust, being kind and providing hope, respecting the family's viewpoint, and maintaining professional codes and the law.

A Clinical Guide to the Communication of Bad News (see Quick Tips: Communicating Bad News)

Setting

Choose a private, comfortable place with freedom from interruption. Seek the patient's consent to involve the family. Everyone should be seated. Ensure ample time for discussion.

For serious bad news, telephoning is rarely an acceptable alternative to face-to-face communication. Rather than giving bad news over the phone ("Your biopsy shows cancer"), ask the patient or family to meet you in the hospital, office, or home.

QUICK TIPS

Communicating Bad News

- Choose a private, comfortable place free from interruption.
- Remain calm and composed.
- Listen to the patient.
- Answer questions honestly, clearly, and accurately.
- Communicate information simply and clearly.
- Pay attention to the patient's feelings and support him or her empathetically.
- Ask the patient how to involve the family.

Preparation

A special effort should be made to be calm and composed before presenting distressing information. You may rehearse in your mind a long discussion, but try to identify a few simple goals for the discussion: What does the patient absolutely need to know now?

Listening

Listening and questioning, not just explaining, are key skills in conveying distressing news. The best intentions to divulge fully can lead the physician astray if he or she is not guided by an appreciation of the patient's perspective: what the patient understands, is concerned about, and is able to absorb at the time. The patient's questions and concerns should direct the physician to presenting information that can best be appreciated and retained.

The clinician who knows the patient and who has previously attended to the patient's perspective may begin sharing bad news with a clear sense of what information needs to be transmitted. However, if the patient's personal background is unfamiliar, review the basic facts of the case, allowing for clarification.

> Let's go back over some of the things that have happened during the past few weeks. First, we found that your blood level is low. The tests suggested that your bone marrow was not functioning properly, so we took a biopsy from your marrow. . . .
>
> As you know, you have a spot on the lung. What is your understanding of the significance of this spot?

Patients usually do want to know the broad facts of their condition and its management, but they may want to hear only a little at a time. Information about a disease is often more painful than the disorder itself. Patients often inquire obliquely, since they fear hearing a blunt, frightening fact. They also may want to avoid appearing stupid or being a nuisance with their questioning. The clinician who responds only to bold inquiries will miss the intimations and implicit questions with which most patients signal their concerns.

Educational Strategies

Simplicity and Clarity. Patients, regardless of their intelligence, regularly have difficulty grasping new information presented in the clinical encounter. Anxiety, which is particularly common when facing bad news, impairs learning. Illness itself makes patients regress and lose some of their ability to think rationally and logically. Many brilliant bedside and office lectures have been wasted on patients who are overwhelmed by bad news and unable to concentrate on what is being said. Avoid expositions on topics that reflect your professional interests but are peripheral to the patient's concerns.

In giving information, start with a few plain statements. Be succinct, clear, and simple. Paint a picture with two or three broad strokes. Then, encourage the patient to review what has been said. Let the patient guide you to further elaboration.

Processing Information. Information-sharing takes time and often is a gradual process that should be carried out over weeks, not minutes. Let the patient digest the information for a while. Repeat and review. Set up later discussions to ascertain what was communicated and to address further concerns. Patients should expect that you will tell them as much as they desire to know and that you will help them with any of their difficulties in comprehension.

It's my job to explain these matters to you so that you understand them as well as you want. Tell me if I haven't made myself clear, and don't hesitate to ask questions.

Graded Exposure. Encourage full disclosure and full understanding, but beware of an unswerving determination to convey the "whole truth" without regard to the patient. You may leave the patient overwhelmed and wary. Treat patients as reasonable and courageous, but appreciate their reasons for not wanting to know everything. If the patient veers away from distressing facts, you may use a discussion of somewhat superficial matters to let the patient relax, but then gently steer the conversation toward more troubling concerns. Do not be surprised if you find yourself weaving back and forth between inconsequential and critical topics, or if some difficult subjects are put off for a while.

Graded exposure to disagreeable information can help ease the discussion toward full disclosure. Say, "We've found some evidence of cancer" before saying, "You have cancer in your liver." Say, "The cancer is affecting your bowels" before saying, "The cancer has blocked your bowels completely."

When important information must be conveyed to a reluctant patient, firmness may be required:

It seems that you have some very important decisions to make with your family. I wonder if it wouldn't be helpful to make sure you and I both understand what your medical condition is like now? How do you see things going?

Let's take a few moments to consider how you're set up if your condition should worsen. What kind of decisions and plans should you try to make now in case you're not feeling well enough to handle them in the future?

When speaking to a patient who is avoiding important truths, the physician may want to address the patient as someone with "two minds," speaking to the more receptive "mind" without disturbing the dominant one:

I wonder if there isn't a part of you that is thinking about some of the worst possibilities?

I can see that you want to look on the bright side of things, but I wonder if you don't also have times when you realize that problems might arise.

Fully informed patients often forget or distort what was said. Also, their awareness of distressing truths and their desire for better understanding will fluctuate. They want (and can use) some information now, some later.

Honesty and Accuracy

Answer direct questions honestly and clearly. Avoid the temptation to be overly optimistic. Shun false reassurance. On the other hand, avoid severe bluntness.

Patients and their families are entitled to the physician's best guesses about the likely course of an illness—the prognosis. They may need this information to plan their lives. However, physicians cannot foresee the future and should not pose as crystal-ball readers. Prognostic statements are often taken literally, so avoid false certainty or an overly precise prognosis.

If I could tell you for sure, I would, but I just have to wait and see like you. Some people can be well months and months with a problem like this, while for others it quickly leads to more serious problems. If something develops that suggests to me that the illness is moving quickly or slowly, would you want to stay abreast of the facts?

Support

Attend to feelings provoked by information. Empathy is part of the explanatory process. In the face of suffering and tragedy, the overt meaning of your speech may be far less important than your manner. Your communication of concern will do more to alleviate distress than your choice of words. You comfort the patient by your gentle, caring attitude and your assurances of ongoing support. Let the patient and family know you are available for further discussion and that you will continue to be involved in care.

Observe how patients respond to the bad news, and anticipate their reactions. You can help patients by providing a roadmap of common feelings.

You may feel shocked or confused initially—like you don't know what is happening.

This can be very upsetting, and you may feel somewhat overwhelmed for a little while now—like your life is out of control.

Patients who respond with numbness and shock can be assured (or warned) that they will have more feelings later on.

You may feel like this isn't real—like it really isn't happening to you—but I know it will sink in soon. You may even be surprised when some strong feelings well up.

Patients who react in a highly intellectualized fashion, perhaps becoming preoccupied with technical questions and marginally relevant data, will benefit from help in addressing their feelings.

I wonder how all this is making you feel?

For patients who respond very emotionally and seem overwhelmed or panicked, offer structure.

I know you are feeling like you can barely stand this, but we are going to help you through it all. There is nothing you need to do right away, except tell your family, and I would like to be with you when you do it so that I can answer their questions. I am also going to arrange for you to see a specialist, who can advise us on the best treatment for your condition.

Involving the Family

Ask the patient how to involve the family. A competent patient is entitled to choose how to disseminate information or include others in decision-making. Should the family be present for important discussions between you and the patient? If not, who will transmit information and answer their questions? May you freely discuss the case with a relative or friend who calls? Does the patient wish to delegate some responsibility for decision making to the family?

In encounters with family members, some may want information to be concealed from the patient. Their attitudes and feelings should be explored.

> Tell me more about why you feel this way? How do you think he will react to this information?
>
> What do you think he knows now? What does he think is going on? Why do you think he doesn't know?
>
> How does he feel about truth-telling? Has he expressed a preference to be told or not to be told? Does he want you to protect him from the pain of bad news? Could we ask him more about it? Could I help you ask him?
>
> How has the patient taken bad news in the past? How have others in the family responded?
>
> What do you think he should not be told? How would he react? What would you want him to know?

Among families who insist on withholding major (and often obvious) facts, two patterns commonly emerge. First, bad news has always been handled with concealment in this family. Such a long-standing pattern can be modified, but will not easily admit to substantial change. Second, the family members are deeply troubled by the prospect of the patient being overwhelmed by despair, and they fear that the patient may give up or lose control. This second pattern can be seen in families that ordinarily manage bad news with some frankness. Concealing the truth can be partly understood as a symptom of the family's anguish—a projection of their own sense of being overwhelmed and an expression of both their desire to avoid painful feelings and their difficulty witnessing the patient in distress. Such a response is rarely managed well by confrontation or reasoning. Caretakers who focus discussion on the decision to withhold facts may end up in useless arguments about the value of truth or about how information-sharing should be handled. Such arguments may alienate the family, deflect attention from the underlying anguish, and further aggravate the family's distress. The family's avoidance should be recognized as arising from their vulnerability and insecurity, as a desperate attempt to avoid pain. Address the family's reluctance through counseling and support, a process which often begins with an elicitation of underlying feelings, an appreciation of personal strengths, and a recognition of hopefulness amidst despair. As family coping improves over time, the symptom—avoidance of frank discussion—lessens and often resolves.

Respect for the family's feelings does not preclude a firm insistence on honesty, especially in responding to the patient's questions and concerns.

> I appreciate your explaining these things to me about your father. I certainly will not force anything upon him or try to tell him something he doesn't want to hear. On the other hand, I would not lie to him, and I must answer all his questions honestly.

Realistic Goals in Sharing Bad News

Doctors like to alleviate discomfort, but clinical responsibilities make them the vehicle for delivering painful news. Primitive or magical thinking is common when reality is difficult to face. The physician needs to remember that talking about a distressing condition does not create the problem, nor does ignoring it make it less of a problem.

PATIENT VALUES AND CLINICAL DECISIONS: THE EXAMPLE OF LIFE-SUSTAINING CARE*

The purpose of the interview today is not only to elicit information for diagnosis and treatment and to educate patients about their illness and its management, but also to learn about patients' preferences and values: what do they want for themselves and why? An appreciation of the patient's viewpoint helps the physician negotiate mutually satisfactory clinical decisions—informed choices that are consonant with the patient's wishes and the doctor's medical advice.

Values and preferences are most often addressed deliberately and openly when patients face grave issues: the initiation of treatments with significant morbidity (transplantation), high mortality (resection of ruptured aneurysms), or uncertain risks (new drug trials). In this chapter we focus on situations in which difficult choices must be made about providing life-sustaining care—the decision whether to use cardiopulmonary resuscitation or other measures that may directly affect whether a patient lives or dies. However, as discussed throughout this text, patient values and preferences play an important (though perhaps a less dramatic and troubling) role in everyday clinical decision-making. A tension headache, for example, may be managed in a variety of ways (explanation and reassurance, medication for pain relief, physical therapy, behavioral interventions, and other measures to address the underlying disorder), and the final decision about treatment should reflect the patient's wishes as well as the physician's advice.

Eliciting Values and Preferences

How do patients express their attitudes about treatment options? Without specific inquiry by the clinician, patients often provide a wealth of clues.

> Don't put me in the hospital.

> I just want to get better, no matter what it takes.

Patients tell stories about their past medical experiences or those of friends and relatives.

> I wouldn't want something like that done to me.

*This section was prepared in collaboration with Dr. Linda Emmanuel.

They may complain or express gratitude about how they have been treated before.

> I can't face another nasogastric tube.
>
> They didn't give up on me.

Thus a doctor who has gotten to know his or her patient well may often have a clear notion of how that patient feels about treatment options and may require little explicit discussion to recommend treatment that reflects this particular person's values and preferences. On the other hand, there are obvious dangers in trying to act on the behalf of patients without explicitly checking out their perspectives. Underlying values about such matters as suffering, prolonging life, dying, undergoing procedures, learning about potential risks, and sharing in decision making often need to be elicited and addressed explicitly.

> Doctor [to patient with advanced cancer and partial bowel obstruction who is requesting relief of vomiting]: Would you consider an operation to try to correct the bowel obstruction?
>
> Patient 1: No. Absolutely no more surgery. I want to be let alone. I would rather die this way.
>
> Patient 2: Yes. I am willing to try anything if it will give me a few more months of comfort.
>
> Patient 3: Yes. I want to be rid of this problem once and for all.
>
> Patient 4: What are the chances of it helping me? What would the operation be like? Are there any other things you can do to help me?
>
> Patient 5: You tell me what to do, Doc.

Asking patients about their preferences and values should not be confused with foisting off decisions on the patient: "Here, you decide." Patients, however, can regularly indicate what they want for themselves and do not feel burdened by the inquiry about their values and preferences, though they may, at times, say that they do not want to take an active role in decision-making.

> Would you talk it over with my daughter?
>
> I appreciate learning about what treatments can be done, but you decide, Doctor.

The Process

Today the clinical process for making both critical and ordinary, everyday treatment decisions is often subsumed under the legalistic notion of "informed consent." In practical terms, the process of joint decision-making has four components: (1) the patient is informed about the nature of his or her condition and about reasonable options for diagnosis and treatment, including risks and benefits of various alternatives; (2) the physician's particular advice for the patient is explained; (3) the patient's preferences are elicited; and (4) the physician seeks the patient's approval for a negotiated plan. It is worthwhile noting that only reasonable options need be presented to patients; cardiopulmonary resuscitation or open-heart surgery would not be mentioned when, in the clinician's judgment, such procedures would offer no hope of benefiting the patient.

Informed consent has recently become a medical-legal requirement for some communications with patients, particularly in hospitals. Patients must sign their consent for procedures, such as operations and anesthesia. Moreover, the discussion of risks and benefits for many treatments is no longer a discretionary practice of physicians; it is mandated. Hospitals may require discussion about cardiopulmonary resuscitation (CPR) and Do-Not-Resuscitate (DNR) orders for some or even all patients.

> We know and you do, too, that you're back in heart failure. As we've discussed in the past, things can get worse with your heart and lungs. We need to get your views about what to do if your heart stops beating or your lungs fail to breathe. First, if your heart suddenly stops, what would you want us to do? Let me explain. Have you heard of electrical stimulation of the heart and mechanical respiration for the lungs? Would you want to have us try electrical stimulation to keep it going? What are your wishes? Second, if your breathing fails, would you want us to try to assist your lungs with mechanical respiration?

Unfortunately, informed consent is often obtained in a perfunctory manner. Rather than occurring in the context of an ongoing doctor-patient relationship in which patients learn to care for themselves and participate in treatment decisions, patients are often informed hastily and with little attention to what they understand, want to know, and hope to discuss. When physicians discuss CPR, their interpretation of the patient's understanding and wishes seems to diverge significantly from what the patient later reports to others. Nor are families very accurate in perceiving a patient's wishes. The patient's response to the communication of risk-benefit information may be markedly biased by the manner in which the clinician presents data. For many patients, though, some straightforward statistical information about the likelihood of successful resuscitation and of functional recovery after CPR, as well as of the morbidity of the procedure—data that clinicians often lack—can be very helpful in decision-making. However, such information may have little meaning to other patients, who, perhaps regressed with severe illness, think and respond in more concrete, intuitive terms, for example, "I trust you doctor. Go ahead." Furthermore, discussions of many important treatment decisions may unfortunately be put off until a medical crisis—a poor time to review values—or somehow only seem to be required when the patient has become incompetent or otherwise unable to express his or her wishes.

An Example: Decisions About Life-Sustaining Care

The broad range of treatment issues on life-sustaining care can usually be directly approached in a surprisingly compact fashion. Because communication at the bedside is so often difficult or even impossible (e.g., the patient is confused, comatose, demented, or aphasic), decisions about life-sustaining and terminal care are now discussed at office visits in advance of anticipated hospitalization. The information can be recorded in the medical record. Indeed, if patients are firm in their responses to questions about life-sustaining care and if they wish to provide "future directives," their choices can be fashioned into a living will that guides (and, in some states, legally directs) later care. Discussion can be repeated during an eventual hospital confinement or whenever circumstances change substantially.

While there are no cookbook formulas for handling discussions about life-sustaining care, some suggestions are offered here on how to introduce this theme and how to sketch out for the patient's consideration some common scenarios and associated treatment options.

Discussing Life-Sustaining Care

Step 1. Get permission to discuss the topic

> Would you be interested in discussing your future care? We want to understand in advance of serious illness what care you would want if you were severely or terminally ill.

Be ready to explore the "not interested" decision of some patients who are reluctant to face any questioning on this theme or the response of others who "want everything done."

Step 2. Review the relationship

If you bring up the subject of options for life-sustaining treatment, patients may mistake this discussion as a sign of your giving up on them. Thus, at the very start, your relationship with the patient needs to be reviewed and your therapeutic attachment reasserted.

> We've been together a long time. Looking ahead, I want to be sure what you want for your future treatment should you become severely ill or even terminally ill. In advance of any hospitalization, I want to understand your preferences and values and to get your directions about your care. In particular, if you were in a coma or otherwise unable to express yourself, you would not be able to discuss your choice and preferences. Now, however, you can give directions about your treatment.

Step 3. Assess the patient's medical status

Raising the topic of life-sustaining care may also arouse some patients' suspicions that they are getting worse. Patients may need to be told if they are stable.

> Let me remind you that right now you're doing fine with your heart and lung condition. You understand that? Even so, we want to look ahead, to discuss your future care should you be in a condition in which you are unable to express your wishes.

Step 4. Outline clinical situations requiring decisions about life-support

I want to discuss some situations—severe illnesses for which you may now want to give us your treatment directions. Specifically, I would like you to tell me how you would feel about some treatments that could be used in these situations.

Situation 1: First, consider a situation where you were in a coma and there was a small but uncertain chance of regaining your awareness and mental function. How would you view the following treatments?

1. Cardiopulmonary resuscitation?
2. Mechanical respiration to keep you breathing?
3. Feedings or fluids given through your veins?
4. Feedings given by tube through your nose or mouth into your stomach?
5. Antibiotics to fight infection?
6. Kidney dialysis to purify your blood?

To make decisions, patients need authoritative, accurate information. You must explain each option and its rationale: what are the various techniques used in life support and what can they do. Thus each question may be followed by: "Do you understand this?" Explanation is then given, if needed.

Encourage patients to respond to each item by asking: "Do you want this? . . ." "Not want it? . . . Or should we try but stop if there is no improvement?"

Afterward, other situations may be posed and the same options considered, for example:

Situation 2: If you were in a persistent coma and might live for a long time but, in the opinion of your physician, had no hope of regaining awareness no matter what was done, then how would you feel about the following treatments?

(See previous list of options.)

Situation 3: If you had brain damage or disease that left you unable to recognize people, to speak meaningfully, or to live independently, but you had no terminal illness (and thus might live for many years), how would you feel about the following treatments that could prolong your life?

(See previous list of options.)

Situation 4: If you had brain damage or disease that left you unable to recognize people, to speak meaningfully, or to live independently, and you also had a terminal illness (and thus would live no longer than 6 months), how would you feel about the following treatments that could prolong your life but not improve your brain damage?

(See previous list of options.)

Step 5. Explore and respond to the patient's choices

Try to come to an understanding of this individual's decisions. What are the patient's notions about the illness and its management and what values or goals underlie stated preferences? For instance, a patient with end-stage pulmonary disease (such as advanced emphysema or lung cancer) might favor "doing everything" in the hope of avoiding severe breathlessness, yet would be better able to achieve the personal goal of avoiding suffering by choosing less-invasive procedures. Patients should appreciate that the decision to forego life-sustaining treatment does not mean that comfort measures or hospitalization will be withheld. Also make sure your own judgment on the problem is well communicated.

Step 6. Assure the patient of the opportunity to reconsider choices
At the beginning and completion of the discussion, the patient needs to be reminded that the specific circumstances of illness cannot be precisely determined in advance. Decisions need to be reviewed periodically and can always be changed.

SUGGESTED READINGS

Conflict: Negotiation and Management

Balint M: *The doctor, his patient, and the illness*, New York, 1972, International Universities Press.

Fisher R, Ury W: *Getting to yes: negotiating agreement without giving in*, ed 2, New York, 1991, Penguin Books.

Friedson E: Client control and medical practice, *Am J Sociol* 65:374, 1960.

Kaplan SH, Greenfield S, Gandek B, et al: Characteristics of physicians with participatory decision-making styles, *Ann Intern Med* 124:497, 1996.

Katon W, Kleinman A: Doctor-patient negotiation and other social science strategies in patient care. In Eisenberg L, Kleinman A, editors: *The relevance of social science for medicine*, Dordrecht, The Netherlands, 1981, D Reidel.

Lazare A, Eisenthal S: A negotiated approach to the clinical encounter. I. Attending to the patient's perspective. II. Conflicts and negotiation. In Lazare A, editor: *Outpatient psychiatry: diagnosis and management*, ed 2, Baltimore, 1988, Williams & Wilkins.

Lazare A, Eisenthal S, Frank A, et al: Studies on a negotiated approach to patienthood. In Gallagher EB, editor: *The doctor-patient relationship in the changing health scene*, (NIH) 78-183, Washington, DC, 1978, US Dept of Health, Education and Welfare.

Ryan EB, Meredith SD, MacLean MJ, Orange JB: Changing the way we talk with elders: promoting health using the communication enhancement model, *Int J Aging Hum Dev* 41:89, 1995.

Szasz TS, Hollender MH: A contribution to the philosophy of medicine: the basic models of the doctor-patient relationship, *Arch Intern Med* 97:585, 1956.

Education and Persuasion for Compliance

Barsky AJ: Nonpharmacologic aspects of medication, *Arch Intern Med* 143:1544, 1983.

DiMatteo MR, Nicola DD: *Achieving patient compliance: the psychology of the medical practitioner's role*, New York, 1982, Pergamon Press.

Haynes RB, McKibbon KA, Kanani R: Systematic review of randomized trials of interventions to assist patients to follow prescriptions for medications, *Lancet* 348:383, 1996.

Miller WR, Rolnick S: *Motivational interviewing: preparing people to change addictive behavior*, New York, 1991, Guilford Press.

Svarstad BL: Patient-practitioner relationships and compliance with prescribed medical regimens. In Aiken LH, Mechanic D, editors: *Applications of social science to clinical medicine and health policy*, New Brunswick, NJ, 1986, Rutgers University Press.

Weiss BD, Coyne C: Communicating with patients who cannot read, *N Engl J Med* 337:272, 1997.

Zola IK: Structural constraints in the doctor-patient relationship: the case of noncompliance. In Eisenberg L, Kleinman A: *The relevance of social science for medicine*, Dordrecht, The Netherlands, 1981, D Reidel.

Sharing Bad News

Billings JA: Sharing bad news. In Billings JA, editor: *Outpatient management of advanced cancer: symptom control, support and hospice-in-the-home*, Philadelphia, 1985, JB Lippincott.

Glaser BG: Disclosure of terminal illness, *J Health Hum Behav* 7:83, 1966.

Pratt L, Seligman A, Reader R: Physicians' views on the level of medical information among patients, *Am J Public Health* 47:1277, 1957.

President's Commission for the Study of Ethical Problems in Medicine and Biomedical and Behavioral Research: *Making health care decisions: the ethical and legal implications of informed consent in the patient-practitioner relationship*, vol 1, Report; vol 2, *Appendices—empirical studies of informed consent;* vol 3, *Appendices—studies on the foundations of informed consent.* Washington, DC, 1982, US Government Printing Office.

Ptacek JT, Eberhardt TL: Breaking bad news, a review of the literature, *JAMA* 276:496, 1996.

Patient Values and Clinical Decisions: The Example of Life-Sustaining Care

Bedell SE, Delbanco TL: Choices about cardiopulmonary resuscitation in the hospital: when do physicians talk with patients? *N Engl J Med* 309:1089, 1984.

Emmanuel LL, Davis M, Pearlman RA, et al: Advanced care planning as a process: structuring the discussion in practice, *J Am Geriatr Soc* 43:1, 1995.

Kasper JF, Mulley AG Jr, Wennberg JE: Developing shared decision-making programs to improve the quality of health care, *Quad Rev Bull* 18:183, 1992.

McKinlay JB, Potter D, Feldman HA: Nonmedical influences on medical decision-making, *Soc Sci Med* 42:769, 1996.

McNeil BJ, Pauker SG, Sox HC: On the elicitation of preferences for alternative therapies, *N Engl J Med* 306:1259, 1982.

Nease RF, Brooks WB: Patient desire for information and decision-making in health care: the autonomy preference index and the health opinion survey, *J Gen Intern Med* 10:593, 1995.

President's Commission for the Study of Ethical Problems in Medicine and Biomedical and Behavioral Research: *Deciding to forego life-sustaining treatment: ethical, medical, and legal issues in treatment decisions,* Washington, DC, 1983, US Government Printing Office.

Stoeckle JD: Do patients want to be informed? Do they want to decide? *J Gen Intern Med* 10:643, 1995.

CHAPTER 15

THE RETURN VISIT

While the initial visit is the usual focus of teaching and studies on the interview, 80% of ambulatory encounters are return visits—"follow-ups." For such encounters, data are sparse on what practitioners actually do and on what communication strategies might lead to better patient satisfaction or understanding or to improved patient care outcomes. The goal of return visits is an assessment of the shared management of the patient's illness, typically focusing on:

- The status of patient's prior complaints, the current physical examination, and a review of tests obtained since the last visit
- The development of new complaints
- Compliance with treatment
- Functional status
- Preventive interventions to reduce the risk of disease and disability
- Psychosocial adjustment

REVIEW THE RECORD AHEAD OF TIME

On return visits, patients should have a sense that the doctor knows them. Before you start the encounter, refresh your memory of the patient's major problems and background. Patients may be disconcerted if you rummage through the record in front of them.

USE A PROBLEM-ORIENTED APPROACH

Review your problem list. When so many patients have multiple health problems, your only hope of efficiently keeping matters straight over months and years is either to have a fabulous memory or to maintain up-to-date problem lists and medication lists. Any new complaint or finding that may have significance for future care or that deserves follow-up should be entered in the problem list. When your patient returns for a visit, a brief review of a carefully constructed problem list saves you the time required to examine the

---

> **QUICK TIPS**
>
> **The Return Visit**
>
> - Review the record ahead of time
> - Use a problem-oriented approach
> - Make a personal connection
> - Let the patient tell his or her story
> - Clarify the reasons for the visit
> - Set an agenda
> - Periodically review the chronic treatment regimen
> - Monitor health promotion and disease prevention
> - Periodically update the review of systems
> - Use your last minutes for explanation
> - If you do not speak directly to the patient about results of tests, send a letter after the visit

---

entire medical record. As noted in Chapter 17, The Medical Record, problem lists and flow sheets can also help you practice medicine more rigorously, and they make information more readily available to other clinicians who use the record.

MAKE A PERSONAL CONNECTION

Early in the visit, if you make a brief personal comment that refers to previous conversations, the patient will feel recognized and remembered, thus quickly restoring a connection with you. Consider placing a few words at the end of your progress notes to remind yourself of important personal topics—"husband's job loss," "upcoming trip," or "sixtieth birthday,"—that were discussed and that might be reintroduced at the next visit.

A personal connection with your patient can be accomplished through "small talk" and the kind of personal comments noted above or by reviewing the major psychosocial events in the patient's life. Update the social history. You may want to use questions that screen for changes in the patient's well-being.

What else has been going on in your life?

Or you may ask about specific issues that you know are important to this person.

How is your wife's health now?

How's the new house?

Anything new between you and that daughter you weren't getting along with?

How are things going at work?

LET THE PATIENT TELL HIS OR HER STORY

Ask the patient, "How have you been?" or "What's happened since your last visit?" In general, use open-ended questions at the beginning of the follow-up interview, just as you would in an initial interview, to survey the patient's problems and appreciate the patient's perspective. Later provide more direction.

CLARIFY THE REASONS FOR THE VISIT

Make sure that both you and the patient develop a common understanding of the overall goals of the visit. Are there new or urgent problems or topics that were not fully addressed in previous encounters or is this truly a "routine follow-up?"

You might begin by asking the patient:

What's happened since we saw you last?

What's on your mind for this appointment?

What should we take care of today?

What do you want to check on?

Next, indicate your own agenda, especially if it differs from the patient's. State your reasons for the return visit, for example, annual checkup, evaluation of medical treatment (blood pressure, edema, depression, pain), review and reinforcement of healthful behaviors (taking medications, exercise, diet, avoidance of alcohol and tobacco), assessment of emotional reactions and coping, or testing to monitor medical treatment (blood sugar, electrolytes, digoxin level).

Okay, but I also want to check your weight and blood pressure and hear about how your diet has been going.

I would like to use this visit to give you a thorough checkup.

Your agenda sounds fine with me.

Seek other requests and concerns:

Any other problems you hoped we could deal with today?

Anything else you want to mention?

SET AN AGENDA

Address urgent problems first. Try to review immediately those problems that are a foremost concern for the patient, even if you view them as minor. If you do not have time to cover both the patient's and your own agenda, prioritize problems and negotiate a mutually satisfactory plan. Beware of trying to do too much at one encounter; consider arranging for later visits to accomplish less-pressing tasks. The workup can be incremental. Save routine, long-term matters for last, but do not postpone them indefinitely.

> You're due for a pelvic, I agree. Could we put that off until your next visit and focus today on these chest pains?

> Let's go over how the diabetes is coming along and let me also check the mole that is worrying you. If time allows, I want to talk with you about breast x-rays and breast self-examination.

> Let's examine your chest and get started on a checkup. We'll finish up at your next visit.

PERIODICALLY REVIEW THE CHRONIC TREATMENT REGIMEN

Either use a medication sheet or include in your notes a list of all the patient's current medications. The questions you should periodically ask about each medication include the following:
- Is the patient taking the medicine as previously directed? Does compliance need to be evaluated or addressed?
- Is this treatment still needed?
- Is this the proper dose and schedule?
- Are there side effects, toxicities, or drug-drug interactions that require attention (e.g., checking for gastrointestinal bleeding with nonsteroidal antiinflammatory agents)?

Similarly, other nonpharmacological treatments (e.g., diet and exercise) need periodic review.

MONITOR HEALTH PROMOTION AND DISEASE PREVENTION

The problem list should identify health promotion as a problem for everyone, as well as indicating important risk factors, such as obesity, smoking, alcoholism, domestic violence, and recent major losses. A computer-based record system or flow sheet may be used to keep track of immunizations, mammograms, serum cholesterol, stool guiaic, pelvic examinations, Papanicolaou smears, and rectal examinations. Counsel patients on health risks and the modifications of hazardous behavior, while also complimenting and supporting them on constructive actions they have taken to improve their health.

PERIODICALLY UPDATE THE REVIEW OF SYSTEMS

A complete review of systems is impractical and unnecessary on most follow-up visits. But selective searching can be employed, guided by the patient's age, sex, and medical condition. For instance, a woman of childbearing age might be asked annually about family planning, while an elderly man might be questioned every few years about vision, hearing, falls, symptoms of prostatism, and social supports.

USE YOUR LAST MINUTES FOR EXPLANATION

Reinforcement—repetition or restatement—is a regular task in follow-up visits. As with initial visits, you need to assess what the patient understands and what the patient wants and needs to know. Ask patients for feedback on essential points: "Now, may I hear what advice you got about your pills and exercise?"

LETTERS TO PATIENTS AFTER THE VISIT

Many return visits today are followed by blood, urine, or other laboratory tests. A statement, such as "I'll let you know if your tests are *not* okay," often provides insufficient reassurance. The patient may still wonder if the clinician got the test results and whether they were normal. Moreover, such a statement tends to discourage later inquiries about test results and to foster a passive role for patients in their health care.

Patients deserve to receive basic information about their health care, including the results of tests performed on their bodies. If you do not speak directly to the patient about the results (e.g., by a telephone call or appointment soon after the tests), write a letter. A form letter may be satisfactory for many tests (e.g., "Your electrocardiogram was normal"), but consider dictating a letter that can serve as part of the patient record and reinforce the messages you communicated in person during the visit, for example:

Dear Mrs. Jones:

This is a report of your visit on 12/13 when your blood pressure was 130/80 and your weight 165. Your special studies showed your EKG to be within normal limits. Your Pap smear was negative. Looking at your blood counts, they showed a white blood cell count of 4800, a red cell count of 4.5 million, and a hemoglobin of 14.5 grams, all normal. Your urine was clear, without sugar, albumin, or any sign of infection. In the chemistries on your blood, you had a blood sugar of 100, a normal value indicating no diabetes. Your cholesterol was 220, a bit higher than optimal, but improved from your previous level of 240, for which I encourage you to keep fats restricted in your diet and to lose weight, as I know you are trying to do. You remember that cholesterol is a long-term risk factor for heart disease. Your stool test for blood was negative.

In sum, I think you are doing well and have your blood pressure under good control. Please keep up with your medications and work on your diet.

Our best wishes,
Dr. Atkins

CHAPTER 16

HOME VISITS AND FUNCTIONAL ASSESSMENT*

While examining an elderly patient during a routine office visit, the primary care physician will probably not discover that:
(1) The patient is eating irregularly, and her kitchen is infested with roaches
(2) Her son yells at her when she forgets little things
(3) The walker she was using in the hospital gathers dust while she lies in bed most of the day
On the other hand, these health and social problems would be evident to a physician who occasionally visits the elderly patient at home. The 3 minutes it takes you to walk in the door, look around, and sit down with the patient—before the examination begins—may teach you more than all your previous encounters with the patient in the hospital or office setting

J.W. ZEBLEY

1.5 million patients use home care services daily.
Over 8000 agencies and 650,000 professionals or paraprofessionals provide the care.
Home care is the fastest growing health service in the United States.

D.M. FOX, C. RAPHAEL

HOME VISITS

Although the home was once the site of most clinical encounters, since the 1940s the location of care has shifted almost exclusively to the physician's office and the hospital. In the 1990s less than 1% of physician visits occurred at home. However, the situation is changing. Increasing numbers of frail elderly, chronically ill, and handicapped patients are making home care a modern necessity and an essential feature of comprehensive health services. Certified hospice programs are mandated to provide terminal care primarily in the home. Moreover, the high cost of hospital care and the availability in the community of technical treatment—intravenous therapy, renal dialysis, chemotherapy—favors more home care.

This chapter reviews the indications for going to a patient's home and then describes the mechanics of the house call. Later sections discuss the functional assessment of the patient, the evaluation of the family's burden of care, and the support of patients and families at home.

---

*Written with Fred H. Rubin, MD, Director, Geriatric Program, Shadyside Hospital, Pittsburgh.

Why Make House Calls?

The great majority of American physicians, even those in primary care fields, do not make house calls. Reasons often cited are inefficient or inappropriate use of physician time, poor reimbursement, and inaccessibility of diagnostic studies. Additionally, many physicians have little or no experience working in this unfamiliar setting. But those who do perform house calls, even if infrequently, generally find them a source of personal satisfaction as well as benefit to patients.

Patients should be seen at home when visits to the office entail serious physical, psychological, or economic hardship. House calls are also useful for some patients who present complex management problems because of psychosocial factors, as when cooperation of the patient and family is a persistent problem or when chronic institutionalization is contemplated. The house call allows the physician to assess functional status, the home environment, the social support structure, and the patient's daily life. One quickly appreciates the interaction of disease, the individual, and the environment— data that otherwise might be elusive. The physician who has made a house call gains first-hand knowledge that allows better communication with the visiting nurse, hospice staff, and other professionals who help maintain the patient safely at home. Moreover, by demonstrating that he or she cares enough to come, the physician strengthens the doctor-patient relationship. The patient maintains a heightened sense of autonomy, assured of ongoing medical supervision while remaining in familiar surroundings instead of going to a bustling, alien office or hospital.

The pronouncement of death is the most common emergency and late-night indication for a home visit. Tasks of the visit include confirming that the patient is dead, preparing the death certificate, helping with decisions about an autopsy and funeral, advising on the disposal of medications, equipment, and supplies, answering the family's questions about the illness and death, communicating sympathy, and assuring ongoing support of the bereaved.

How To Make a House Call (see Quick Tips: Reminders for House Calls)
Getting There and Getting In

Telephone ahead to be sure that the patient and family are ready for your visit. Obtain clear directions for getting to the home and for gaining entrance.

Review the medical chart in advance. Carry your examination tools, paper for recording notes, prescription blanks, and whatever special supplies may be required, such as dressings, urethral catheterization trays, or equipment for obtaining blood or urine specimens.

Notice the condition of the house or apartment and its neighborhood. If nobody answers the door when you knock, it may be because the occupant is bedbound or chairbound, so try to let yourself in.

Your reception in the home will usually be welcome, but also rather unpredictable compared to office visits. The patient and the family control this

> **QUICK TIPS**
>
> **Reminders for House Calls**
>
> - Telephone ahead to be sure that the patient and family are ready
> - Obtain clear directions for getting to the home
> - Review the medical chart in advance
> - Note the condition of the patient's neighborhood and home
> - Find out what the patient does all day and try to view the various sites where he or she spends this time
> - Assess function status and supports and also pay attention to affect and cognition
> - Review medications and diet, including how and where they are managed
> - Examine the house for hazards and note barriers to care or mobility
> - Assure some private time to talk with the patient, as well as privacy in the physical examination, but also try to include the family in the presentation of findings and in decisions about management
> - Allow time for discussion and arrange for follow-up calls

territory. You may be offered food or drink, and may even find a full meal prepared. You may be introduced to a number of relatives and neighbors, be directed to a specific seat or room, or encounter polite silence as the family waits for you to issue instructions.

The Home Interview

In beginning the interview, you may choose first to talk with the patient alone or you may include some or all of the family and friends. A portion of the interview often should be carried out with the family absent, allowing for a confidential exchange in which the patient may be able to speak more freely.

Even though the initial topic of the interview is usually the identification of acute problems, at some point you will want to discuss the living situation. What is the quality of the patient's life? What does the patient do all day? Who are the important people in his or her life? What most impedes the patient from doing what he or she would like to be able to do? Are there sensory or language impairments—problems with sight, hearing, or speech? Does the patient require assistance with any of the activities of daily living: feeding, bathing, dressing, ambulating, or toileting? Are family members or neighbors helpful? Who takes primary responsibility for supervising care at home? How does the patient obtain help in an emergency?

Assessing Medications

Determine what medications are present. Ask to see the medicine cabinet and all medicine containers. Review the medication schedule. Who supervises and administers the schedule?

Physical Examination

Examining the elderly is usually more difficult than with younger patients. Visual impairments may require that you provide brighter light. Hearing loss may require that you speak louder and more slowly. Slower patient responses, even in the absence of cognitive impairment, mean more time is required to accomplish each procedure. The elderly are also likely to have more physical abnormalities than younger patients, though they may be less likely to report every symptom.

Examining the House

A tour of the house can be requested, or you may gain a glimpse of other rooms by asking to use the kitchen or bathroom for hand washing. Where does the patient stay during the day? Where is the television? What cooking facilities are available? Where does the patient sleep? For a disabled person, the family may have already created a "sick room," often a space previously used as a living room, but which now includes the patient's bed, and, hopefully, is convenient to a bathroom.

Are any hazards present that might lead to a fall? Frequent dangers are throw rugs, shag rugs, electrical cords, and thresholds. Is the home secure from outsiders? Is there adequate heat? What physical barriers limit the patient's function? Are stairs necessary to reach the bathroom, bedroom, or street? The bathroom is frequently the site for falls and fractures. Is it safe and accessible? Are grab-bars or a raised toilet seat indicated? How does the patient bathe?

Family Conference

Finally, the entire family can be involved in the presentation of findings and in decisions about management. Allow time for discussion so that everyone is heard. Before leaving, you should be sure that the family knows how to reach you or your preceptor at all hours.

FUNCTIONAL ASSESSMENT

In evaluating patients with chronic disabilities, the precise diagnosis of their medical disorders may be less important than the delineation of their functional abilities. Chronic diseases can rarely be cured, but the function of patients with such disorders can often be improved.

The functional assessment and care of the frail elderly and other homebound patients is generally best provided by a team of health professionals, rather than by the physician acting alone. The visiting nurse might visit frequently, devise medication schedules, provide catheter care, monitor for alterations in chronic conditions, and change dressings. The physical therapist might work with the patient to increase range of motion of joints, promote ambulation with or without assistance, foster more effective breathing and coughing, and improve cardiac fitness. For a patient with arthritis or neurological deficits, the occupational therapist can help with use of household items, such as eating utensils, and may suggest special equipment to perform tasks that would otherwise seem impossible. The social worker can explore the family dynamics, engage in casework with the patient and family members, and help with concrete services, such as applying for day care facilities or assessing eligibility for Medicaid. Case managers allocate resources such as homemakers, home health aides, chore services (for heavy cleaning), and transportation by wheelchair van.

All of these collaborative workers speak a common language of functional status (described more fully later); their services, in turn, are geared toward improving that status. To communicate effectively as a co-worker and leader of the team, the physician must be knowledgeable about functional assessment and ways to improve function. Such assessments allow rational prescription of home supports and decisions about the appropriate site for long-term care. Additionally, a decline in functional ability in an elderly patient indicates the need to search judiciously for an illness that may be presenting as a nonspecific loss of function. In the very elderly, it is common for pneumonia to present as confusion, a myocardial infarction as weakness, and thyrotoxicosis as apathy.

Activities of Daily Living (ADLs)

Assessing Activities of Daily Living

Assessment of activities of daily living and of instrumental activities of daily living helps the clinician evaluate a patient's ability to manage independently at home and avoid preventable illness and injury and assess the need for supportive services. At times, an accurate picture of the patient's functional status needs to be gleaned from the family, home health professionals, or the clinician's own house call.

Activities of daily living (ADL)
- Dressing
- Eating
- Ambulating
- Toileting—getting to the bathroom and cleaning oneself
- Continence of bowels and bladder

Instrumental activities of daily living (IADL)
- Shopping
- Housekeeping
- Ability to handle money
- Food preparation
- Mobility outside the home

Social supports
- Who would assist you if you were ill and needed help?
- Who helps you right now?
- Do you feel you are getting enough help?

Basic performance functions are called activities of daily living, or ADLs. These include eating (need for assistance feeding), bathing (ability to use tub, shower, sponge), dressing (especially managing fasteners and tying shoes), ambulating (transferring in and out of bed or chair, walking on the level with or without assistance, and climbing stairs), and toileting (getting on and off the toilet, cleansing) and continence (bowel and bladder control, use of catheter). For such ADLs, a patient may be able to function independently or may require various degrees of mechanical assistance or the help of one or more persons.

A more complex set of functions are called instrumental activities of daily living, or IADLs. These include preparation of food, light housework, use of the telephone, shopping, ability to handle money, and mobility outside the home.

Numerous rating instruments have been published that assign scores of performance in ADLs and provide a yardstick to measure changes over time.

Two other patient characteristics should regularly be assessed at a home visit: affect and cognition. Disorders of both are prevalent in the elderly. Especially worthy of attention are depression and dementia, which may coexist in the same patient. Untreated depression causes a great deal of unnecessary suffering. Similarly, the physician must be able to recognize early dementia, diagnose reversible causes, and help the patient and family manage irreversible cases. The assessment of affect and cognition is further discussed in Chapter 12, The Mental Status Examination.

Managing the Burden of Care

A homebound patient may need regular assistance with ADLs or medical therapies. Some patients are not easy for families to manage at home: they are incontinent, demanding, or noisy; they may not sleep when the rest of the family does; they may wander into danger or be physically abusive. Sometimes a tremendous amount of help is required to remain at home safely, comfortably, and with proper medical care. Nonetheless, many persons or families willingly accept the challenge of providing safe, effective, and compassionate care for a frail parent or grandparent or other disabled friend or relative. However, outside help is often needed. Homemakers can help with IADL tasks, such as housecleaning, laundry, and shopping. Home health aides can provide personal care, such as bathing and dressing. Numerous other home services are available (see the list in the article by Billings et al. in the Suggested Readings).

Professionals familiar with home care can often foresee difficulties in managing the burden of care long before the family recognizes a serious problem or begins to feel overwhelmed. The physician who anticipates and repeatedly asks the patient and family about the stresses of caretaking will be in a position to recognize problems before they become critical, thus shielding the family from an excessive burden. Services should be provided to prevent or rapidly treat a breakdown in coping with the burden of care. Meticulous planning includes an awareness of and preparation for potential losses of support and for the fatigue and turnover in personnel that commonly occur during a long, taxing illness. Sensible and dependable arrangements to delegate duties should be established so that no person is left with excessive chores and responsibilities. Undependable help may be more troublesome than no help at all.

Even with maximal available and affordable help, families may become overwhelmed. Emergency ward staff often see frail patients brought in and left by the family for a relatively minor problem. Such patients may also appear to be neglected, as evidenced by poor nutrition and hygiene and by untreated medical problems. Contrary to the common myth that families eagerly "dump" their burden on institutions, the family has most likely been providing total care for a prolonged period but is now exhausted of personal and financial resources. Both "dumping" and neglect reflect a failure of the home support system. Many such crises should be preventable when adequate home care supervision and services are available.

Some chronically ill patients eventually require such extensive home supports that placement in an institution becomes a reasonable alternative. A major consideration in making this decision is the extent of family support—many residents of nursing homes could live at home if only they had somebody to take care of them. Conversely, there is probably no one who cannot be managed in a home environment if enough formal resources (nurses, homemakers, home health aides, round-the-clock aides, durable medical equipment) are expended. A physician familiar with the home setting can play a key role in rational decision-making.

COMMUNICATION TASKS IN THE HOME ENCOUNTER

Five important communication tasks in the house call help patients and families manage the burdens of caring for a chronically ill person at home (see Quick Tips: Tasks in the Home Encounter). First is the transmittal of basic information about diagnosis and management. Information-sharing is important not simply because it allows for appropriate technical care, but also because it imparts a sense of control for the lay caretakers, making the future more predictable and manageable for persons who are not used to being re-

---

QUICK TIPS

Tasks in the Home Encounter

- Transmit basic information about diagnosis and management
- Anticipate problems and rehearse responses
- Communicate reassurance
- Understand and address attributions
- Provide encouragement, hopefulness, and appreciation

sponsible for sick patients. The act of explanation should convey the physician's appreciation of lay concerns.

Second is the anticipation of problems likely to arise in the future and the rehearsal of the family in plans for appropriate action. Particularly in terminally ill patients with advanced cancer, some problems are predictable, such as the development of confusion, increased pain, or medication side effects. A review and rehearsal of how to manage the problem will help the family act appropriately when the difficulty arises, inoculating them against panic.

The urine will turn orange with this medication.

He is likely to get more of these black and blue marks, even if he doesn't hit himself. They look terrible but they don't hurt. You don't need to worry about them. Is that okay?

Third is the communication of reassurance. Physicians often reassure without conscious effort. For instance, the physician's demeanor can have a profound effect on the patient and family's feeling of security. Ideally, a sense of "aequanimitas" is conveyed—the physician appears dependable, purposeful, confident, able to bear uncertainty, tolerant, unruffled, yet sympathetic. The physician's manner can communicate a feeling of order and control in a world that otherwise threatens to become chaotic and unmanageable. A thorough, competent evaluation of the patient's condition and a thoughtful explanation may constitute adequate reassurance to many patients.

There's been a setback, but we have some treatment to make the best of it.

The infection is under control.

Specific reassurance, however, requires an understanding of the concerns of the patient and family. The fourth task, therefore, is understanding and addressing attributions. Symptoms, signs, diagnostic actions, therapies, and the behavior of health workers are always interpreted by lay people as having a certain meaning, which may or may not be congruent with a professional viewpoint. Every clinical act—attention to symptoms and signs, tone of voice, facial expression, gestures, and new prescriptions and instructions—can be interpreted by the lay person in such a way as to confirm or deny an attribution, to suggest seriousness or triviality, to create new concerns, as well as to modify old ones. In providing reassurance and relieving anxiety, begin by asking the patient and family members how they perceive things; then deal with their notions.

What do you think could be causing this?

Is there anything special you're worried about?

In addition to the regular tests, is there anything else you'd like me to include now?

Finally, the provision of encouragement and hopefulness to the family is always appreciated. Caregivers commonly believe they are doing an inadequate job; a few supportive words from the physician can be tremendously helpful.

You're doing a great job.

You've made a big sacrifice, and you should feel good about what you've been able to do here.

■ CONCLUSION

In their training, physicians need the vital and humanizing effect of visiting the real-life circumstances of disabled people.

L. R. Lawson

Homebound patients often are chronically ill and suffering from multiple functional limitations; proper clinical management necessitates assessment of the home environment, the social support system, and the family. A house call, particularly the first visit to a patient's home, is a challenging and rewarding experience, requiring skills not readily learned in the office or hospital. The patient must be evaluated in terms of functional status, cognition, and affect, and the physician should attend to the patient's and family's attributes of the clinical situation. If the burden of care is not being adequately managed, the practitioner must either prescribe additional home supports or help the patient be institutionalized.

SUGGESTED READINGS

Billings JA, Rubin F, Stoeckle JD: Home care. In Calkins E, Davis PJ, Ford AB, editors: *The practice of geriatrics*, Philadelphia, 1986, WB Saunders.

Brown LJ, Potter JF, Foster BG: Caregiver burden should be evaluated during geriatric assessment, *J Am Geriatr Soc* 38:455, 1990.

Callahan JJ: Care in the home and other community settings: present and future. In Binstock RH, Cluff LE, Von Mering O, editors: *The future of long-term care: social and policy issues*. Baltimore, 1996, Johns Hopkins Press.

Fox DM, Raphael C, editors: *Home-based care for a new century*, Maiden, Mass, 1997, Blackwell Publications.

Greene MG, Majerovitz SD, Adelman RD, Rizzo C: The effects of the presence of a third person on the physician–older patient medical interview, *J Am Geriatr Soc* 42:413, 1994.

Kane RL, Ouslander JG, Abrass IB: *Essentials of clinical geriatrics*, ed 3, New York, 1994, McGraw-Hill.

Sanford JRA: Tolerance of disability in elderly dependents by supporters at home: its significance for hospital practice, *Br Med J* 3:471, 1975.

Silliman RA: Caring for the frail older patient: the doctor-patient-caregiver relationship, *J Gen Intern Med* 4:237, 1989.

Stoeckle JD, Lorch S: Why go see the doctor? Care goes from office to home as technology divorces function from geography, *Int J Technol Assess Health Care* 13:537, 1997.

CHAPTER 17

THE MEDICAL RECORD

The spirit of the hospital has been ... to have its data so accurately recorded that it furnishes the maximum aid to the advancement of medical and surgical science.

MASSACHUSETTS GENERAL HOSPITAL TRUSTEES (1904)

AN INTRODUCTION TO RECORDS

Medical records are a repository of the information collected about patients, of how the data were interpreted, and of what medical acts were carried out. The record serves the needs of at least six distinct audiences:

1. The clinician who writes the record. Preparing a medical record aids in organizing and remembering information about patients, developing clinical skills, reflecting on the diagnosis and management, and planning continuing care.

2. All the health professionals—physicians, nurses, physician assistants, dieticians, physical therapists, students, and others—who collaborate in the patient's care. These colleagues might use your notes, for instance, when they cover your patient calls on a weekend or when they assume the care of your patient years later. Moreover, with the increasing use of e-mail, fax machines, and computerized medical records, your recent notes may be readily available to other clinicians who are collaborating in the patient's care.

3. Patients. Helping them understand and review their treatment, and allowing them to be more active in their self-care.

4. Your supervisors, who use the record to evaluate and guide your clinical development. Insofar as the record is an accurate account of what you observed, concluded, and did for the patient, it is one measure of your clinical performance. Similarly, record audits have been used to evaluate the quality of care, though their usefulness has been limited by discrepancies between what is recorded and what is actually done.

5. Clinical investigators use records for research.

6. Administrators for whom the document contains data for assessing disability, mental competency, and eligibility for insurance billing, while also being used in utilization review and lawsuits.

The value of a carefully prepared medical record deserves emphasis. Clearly, the record is a memory aid, preventing loss of important information about patients and about the clinical acts of doctors and other health professionals. It can be used to provide reminders to oneself, for example, to do tests and examinations (e.g., "check the potassium at the next visit," "do an annual pelvic") or to provide services (e.g., "give annual flu shot").

Standards for good records also structure what information is collected and thus promote self-teaching and self-critique of clinical work. For instance, the standard format for a write-up helps you remember what data to collect (e.g., do a family history and a stool guaiac). The format for the assessment and plan should help you ask the following sorts of questions: What problems have been identified? What is the significance of each finding? What other information has been collected (or should have been collected) that bears on this finding? What do I make of each problem? What do I intend to do to clarify my diagnosis? What treatment will I undertake for each problem? How has the patient been educated?

The Problem-Oriented Medical Record (POMR), as described and promoted by Lawrence Weed, represents a useful attempt to systematize the recording and processing of clinical information. Many aspects of this approach have been widely adopted. Rational, orderly clinical action is facilitated by the POMR requirement of defining a list of clinical problems, identifying the data base relevant to each problem, and providing an assessment and a plan—diagnostic, therapeutic, and educational—for each. Examples of problem-oriented notes are included in Part I of this book and in the case example in the Appendix.

Writing for Other Readers

While the vast bulk of medical records are used only by the person who prepares them and perhaps by a few others, the writer must be aware of other audiences. In writing for colleagues, basic goals should be legibility, grammatical construction, correct spelling, brevity, clarity, and a familiar standard format that allows readers readily to find specific data. Only commonly recognized abbreviations should be employed.

In deciding what to report and how to record it (discussed further in the section on confidentiality, which concludes this chapter), remember that medical records are occasionally read by patients and are often available to persons not directly responsible for patient care—for example, secretaries, orderlies, laboratory personnel, and record librarians. Access to some clinical data, even by an office secretary or nurse, may be considered an intrusion on privacy by patients. Moreover, lawyers, insurance companies, and government agencies may obtain access to records. Patients do not need to approve of or agree with all your comments in the record, but you want to present data objectively (e.g., separate out what the patient said, what others reported, and what you have observed yourself) and clearly identify opinion or conjecture. Avoid presenting materials irrelevant to the process of care, especially prejudicial comments or personal reactions that appear in the guise of objective observations.

In deciding what personal information to record, the clinician's goal is not simply to protect the patient. For instance, a diagnosis of hypertension or myocardial infarction may compromise a patient's ability to obtain insurance or employment, but the physician would be acting dishonestly by omitting such information. On the other hand, certain data, regardless of the physician's attitude, when read by others, may constitute a social stigma (e.g., description of sexual fantasies or practices) or an invasion of privacy (e.g., a description of an extramarital affair). As long as the physician does not have a legal obligation to report a behavior (e.g., child abuse, intention to commit personal injury), such matters should be handled discreetly. For instance, when a patient is worried about exposure to a venereal disease, but would not want any notation about it in the record, you might note "concern about an infectious disease," and you could submit the laboratory test under a pseudonym for the patient; a negative test for gonorrhea and syphilis would not need to be included in the record, but a positive test would be reported. Finally, when the inclusion of sensitive personal information is essential for the medical record, take special care about its objectivity and accuracy. (See "Confidentiality: What to Include in the Record" later in this chapter.)

Good clinical manners also dictate that the record not be used for carrying out arguments with consultants or other persons involved in the case, except insofar as major differences in opinion might eventually deserve objective documentation.

Master Problem List

The master problem list is an index or table of contents that provides an outline or overview of all the patient's problems (see Fig. 17-1 and the case examples at the end of this chapter and in Appendix B). At the beginning of a visit, a brief glance at the list reminds the clinician about the major issues in a patient's ongoing care. Such a synopsis becomes particularly valuable when the patient has multiple problems that are delineated in a ponderously long and intricate record. An accurately chosen title for each problem gives the reader an indication of how thoroughly the problem has been characterized (e.g., "fatigue" vs. "psychogenic fatigue" vs. "depression," or "chest pain" vs. "angina" vs. "angina secondary to aortic stenosis [no significant coronary artery disease]"). Over time, one problem may become an element of another (e.g., "right upper extremity weakness" is later subsumed under "multiple sclerosis"). A skin lesion of uncertain significance is a problem, but after being diagnosed as a benign seborrheic keratosis, it becomes a finding that does not require management and thus need not be included on the list, except perhaps as a reminder of the diagnosis. Resolved problems become "inactive."

The master problem list guides the clinician's response to new symptoms and signs, which must be defined either as elements of preexisting

INTERNAL MEDICINE ASSOCIATES
MASTER PROBLEM LIST
1997
Rocco Matasar, M.D.

Ann TYLER
321 22 63

Consultants: Daniels (Thyroid)
Advance directives: None

Problem Number	Date Onset	ACTIVE PROBLEM	RESOLVED

1		HEALTH MAINTENANCE
		    G2P2
		    FH early CAD	

2	1975	Smoking 1 1/2 PPD	
3	1988	Multinodular goiter Euthyroid	
4	1994	Microcytic anemia Guaiac negative Rx iron	3/95
5	1995	Dysmenorrhea Enlarged uterus on ultrasound ?fibroids	
6	1996	Inadequate housing	

Date	Temporary, Old, and Inactive Problems
1971	Appendectomy
1993	Arthralgias hands, resolved

Allergies, Adverse Reactions

Penicillin (pruritic rash)
Ibuprofen (GI upset)

Fig. 17-1 Sample problem list.

problems or as new problems. The list also reminds the conscientious clinician at each visit to consider dealing with every active problem. Thus the problem list serves as a worksheet for patient care, identifying well-characterized chronic problems that require ongoing management as well as new or temporary clinical concerns (e.g., fever, hypokalemia) that also demand attention. The addition of minor problems to the list helps assure that they are not forgotten on subsequent encounters. A special place on the problem list is sometimes reserved for allergies and other reactions to medications about which the clinician needs frequent reminders and a ready source of reference.

The master problem list should be located conspicuously in the record, usually on the inside cover or the first or last page, so that it can be referred to easily. A useful device in office care is to make a master list of established problems and a separate temporary list (e.g. "cystitis," "bronchitis," "hypokalemia, on diuretics"). For instance, a questionable laboratory test may be placed on the temporary problem list until it resolves or is recognized as part of an established problem. Temporary problems that resolve are crossed out; those that persist are transferred to the master problem list (e.g., serial bouts of "cystitis" become "recurrent urinary tract infections").

It is also helpful to have a "s/p" (status post or no longer active) problem list for major medical and psychosocial events that might bear on future clinical decisions but do not need current management (e.g., "s/p appendectomy" limits the possible diagnoses for pain in the right lower quadrant; "s/p hysterectomy" indicates no need for Papanicolaou smears).

In a strict Weed POMR system, each problem is assigned a number that is thereafter always associated with the problem. In common usage, however, problems may be numbered erratically and their titles may not be strictly identical from one usage to the next. The problem list may be re-ordered according to the changing importance of various conditions and the desirability of "splitting" or "lumping" problems. No problem, however, should be lost unintentionally. Assign a resolved or inactive problem to the s/p list when possible, but delete it with caution.

Weed also suggests that problem lists include the date of onset for each problem, when it was recorded, and when it resolved. Some semblance of this system is frequently adopted but requires either a rather conscientious clinician or a very cooperative team of colleagues.

Finally, a problem list that is not kept up to date is a problem itself.

A related form of record-keeping is the pack of 3 × 5 cards that house officers and students often prepare to summarize findings and plans on their inpatients and that sometimes are used for outpatient work. In ambulatory care, these cards usually contain the patient's name, telephone number, unit number, problem list, medication list, and perhaps some other reminders for future visits. Such cards may be more readily and reliably available than the full medical record and can be carried when answering calls away from the office or hospital.

Preparing a Problem List

The preparation of a useful problem list is inseparable from the process of thoughtfully evaluating a patient (see Quick Tips: Preparing a Problem List).

QUICK TIPS

Preparing a Problem List

- Express problems as concise, relatively objective summaries of clinical matters that need attention
- Choose a problem title that represents your most refined understanding of that problem
- Modify descriptions of problems as they evolve
- When two findings may be part of the same problem, treat them as distinct items rather than lumping them together
- When secondary diagnoses require separate management strategies, either cite two problems or include both primary and secondary diagnoses
- Prioritize problems
- Do not include data for which you intend to take no action

The following are a few general rules:

1. Problems need not be diagnoses but should be concise, relatively objective summaries of physical and psychosocial symptoms or complaints, clusters of isolated physical findings or laboratory abnormalities, syndromes, pathophysiological states, health risks, socioeconomic concerns, and other clinical matters that need attention. For example:

   Dysuria
   Petechiae
   Confusion
   Possible abnormal chest x-ray—nodule vs. artifact
   Incomplete standard data base—? allergies
   Health maintenance and disease prevention
   Family history of colonic carcinoma
   Job stress
   Diabetes mellitus
   No health insurance

   Any chronic medical problem belongs on the problem list.

2. Your problem title should represent your most refined understanding for that problem. Do not list a diagnosis unless you are fairly certain it is correct. On the other hand, listing "dyspnea" as a problem is inappropriate when you could have provided the diagnosis of "congestive heart failure."

3. Problems evolve as they are defined. Thus "fatigue" becomes "anemia," which later becomes "iron-deficiency" and "GI bleeding." The latter problem may eventually become "duodenal ulcer, painless, bleeding."

4. When in doubt about whether two findings are part of the same problem, "split" rather than "lump" (e.g., separate "unexplained chest pain" from "unexplained dyspnea"). An initial splitting of problems is favored for medical students who are relatively inexperienced in differential diagnosis. Each problem can be considered separately and then perhaps later lumped into a syndrome or illness (e.g., "nausea," "bradycardia," and "abnormal EKG" become "acute inferior myocardial infarction"; "dysuria" and "vaginal discharge" become "*Trichomonas vaginitis*").

   Also, review of a well-constructed problem list will sometimes suggest further diagnoses (e.g., "hypertension [poorly controlled]" and "elevated mean corpuscular volume; normal serum folate and B12" suggest alcohol abuse).

5. When separate management strategies are needed for secondary diagnoses, either cite two problems or include both primary and secondary diagnoses (e.g., indicate both "diabetes mellitus" and "diabetic retinopathy"; list "carcinoma of the colon," "metastases to the liver," and symptoms resulting from spread of the cancer to the liver, such as "hepatic pain," "nausea," and "pruritus").

6. When constructing or revising a problem list, prioritize problems. In ambulatory care, put health promotion first so that you do not forget it, but the next problem, like the first problem in a hospitalized patient's list, should be the most serious and urgent.

7. Problems require diagnostic evaluation or management. You may choose to retain old problems (s/p problems) on some portion of your master problem list as reminders, but generally do not include data for which you intend no action (e.g., birthmark, right shin).

Flow Sheets

Flow sheets (Fig. 17-2) have several uses:

1. Management guides. Flow sheets aid in following clinical parameters over time (e.g., changes in fasting blood sugar levels with weight and insulin dose or the serial measurements of blood pressure in response to multiple antihypertensive medications) or in organizing even relatively uncomplicated data that are collected over long periods (e.g., periodic serum levels of digoxin). Graphic presentations of data are frequently used for monitoring anticoagulant treatment (medication dose vs. prothrombin time), management of congestive heart failure (weight, pulse, blood pressure, symptoms and signs, and select laboratory values as related to various

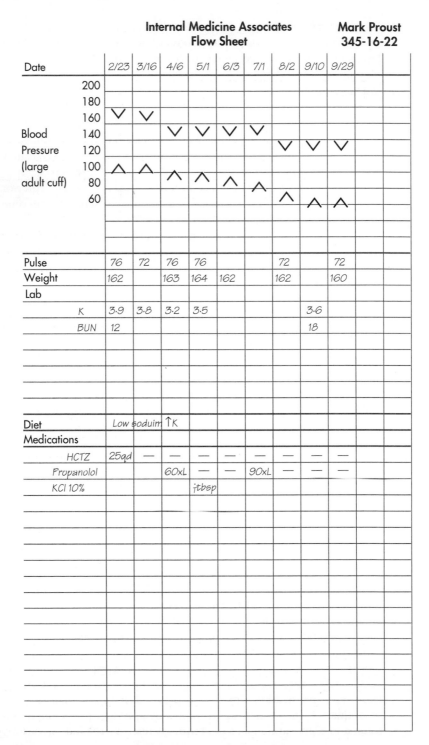

**Internal Medicine Associates
Flow Sheet**

**Mark Proust
345-16-22**

Date		2/23	3/16	4/6	5/1	6/3	7/1	8/2	9/10	9/29		
Blood Pressure (large adult cuff)	200											
	180											
	160	V	V									
	140			V	V	V	V					
	120							V	V	V		
	100	Λ	Λ									
	80			Λ	Λ	Λ	Λ					
	60							Λ	Λ	Λ		
Pulse		76	72	76	76			72		72		
Weight		162		163	164	162		162		160		
Lab												
	K	3.9	3.8	3.2	3.5				3.6			
	BUN	12							18			
Diet		Low soduim ↑K										
Medications												
	HCTZ	25qd	—	—	—	—	—	—	—	—		
	Propanolol			60xL	—	—	90xL	—	—	—		
	KCl 10%				ⅉtbsp							

Fig. 17-2 Sample flow sheet.

Internal Medicine Associates
Preventive Services Checklist

Year	1990							
History and Physical								
Physical Examination	2/90							
Rectal	2/90							
Breast/Testicular exam	2/90							
Pelvic, Pap (+/− chlamydia)								
Tests								
Mammogram								
Stool guaiac	2/90							
Lipids	2/90							
Sigmoidoscopy								
Counseling								
Tobacco	✔							
Alcohol, recreational drugs	✔							
Exercise	✔							
Diet	✔							
Contraception	✔							
Injury prevention	✔							
Seat belts	✔							
Guns	✔							
Violence/abuse	✔							
Advance directives								
Immunizations								
Tetanus/diphtheria	1989							
Flu Shot								
Pneumococcus								
MMR/Polio	1972							

Fig. 17-2—cont'd

medications), and gold treatment for rheumatoid arthritis (requiring frequent monitoring of complete blood counts and urinalysis).

2. Health promotion guides. Flow sheets are useful for keeping track of periodic health promotion and disease prevention efforts: reviewing alcohol and tobacco use, exercise, dental care, and breast self examination; doing a complete or limited physical examination, such as checking weight, blood pressure, breast examination, rectal

examination, Papanicolaou smear, or tonometry; ordering laboratory tests such as the stool guaiac, complete blood count, serum cholesterol, or mammogram; and obtaining special tests for patients with unusual risks (e.g., Vietnamese refugees get skin tests for tuberculosis and stool checks for ova and parasites).

3. Evaluation guides. Flow sheets can also be useful for guiding the evaluation and chronic management of common medical problems. For example, a standard form for new hypertensive patients lists key historical data, physical findings, and laboratory data. Another form on dementia ensures that a complete workup for reversible causes has been performed, reminds the clinician of community resources that should be periodically considered for patient management, while also providing a system for monitoring the progress of the disease in terms of mental function, ability to carry on daily activities, and reliance on family and other supports. A sample evaluation guide is shown in Figure 17-3.

Medication Lists

A sample medication list is included in Figure 17-2. Medication lists should be kept on all long-term patients, either by periodically recording all medications in the chart (usually at the beginning of an office note) or on separate flow sheets that can be readily found in the chart and updated. When other clinicians are involved in the care of a patient, they will appreciate being able to review an accurate, up-to-date medication list. Lists also help the clinician review what drugs were previously used (Which nonsteroidal anti-inflammatory drugs have I tried? What cough syrup worked so well the last time he had a bad cold?) and for preventing adverse drug interactions (Do any of these medications interfere with the drug I want to begin now? Could drug interaction explain the unexpected serum level of this medication?). Medication regimens are frequently confused by patients and clinicians, and need to be reviewed frequently.

What is the name of the medication you are taking?

What strength?

How often are you actually taking them?

When do you take them?

Patients should periodically bring their entire store of pill containers for review. Remember: the container label may neither correctly identify the pills inside nor reflect what the patient is actually taking. In the hospital, where large numbers of medications are being given and are frequently adjusted, a list of medications may be entered daily into the patient's record. This ensures that the health care team is aware of all drug treatments and reviews their usefulness. The most accurate record of what is actually being given in the hospital is the nurses' medication sheet. This sheet is particularly useful

LIPID SCREENING, EVALUATION, AND MANAGEMENT

SCREENING   Every 5 years if no CHD risk factors and total cholesterol
GUIDELINES: <200 mg/dl or LDL <130 mg/dl
               Preferred screening: 12-14 hour fasting total cholesterol,
               HDL, triglycerides; then calculate
               LDL = Total cholesterol − (HDL + triglycerides/5)
               [Cost: Total cholesterol $3.20; full lipid profile additional $23.00]

CORONARY HEART DISEASE RISK PROFILE

___ Family history premature CHD   ___ Myocardial infarction, angina
___ Smoking   ___ Arteriosclerotic cerebrovascular
___ Obesity (≥30% above ideal)   or peripheral vascular disease
___ Hypertension   ___ HDL ≤35 mg/dl
___ Diabetes mellitus

RISK STRATIFICATION AND TREATMENT STRATEGY

LOW RISK: LDL <130—give dietary and risk reduction advice; screen q5yr
MODERATE RISK: LDL 130-160 for male with no risk factors or female with 0-1 risk
                 factors—lipid-lowering diet and q6-12 mos follow-up
HIGH RISK: LDL >160 or LDL 130-160 plus ⊕ CAD *or* Male with 1 risk factor
                 or Female with 2 risk factors—institute lipid-lowering diet;
                 consider drug treatment if remains high risk; follow q1-3 mos
                 until risk reduced; if LDL >190, ⊕ CAD, consider drugs
                 immediately

ADDITIONAL CONSIDERATIONS BASED ON HDL:
Increased risk if CHOLESTEROL/HDL ≥4.5 (unless cholesterol <150)
High risk if CHOLESTEROL/HDL >9.5   Low risk if HDL >70

GENERAL RECOMMENDATIONS FOR DOCUMENTED HYPERLIPIDEMIA
(2 cholesterol determinations):

1. RULE OUT SECONDARY CAUSES (mandatory only before beginning
   drug treatment) [ ]

   HYPERCHOLESTEROLEMIA:
   Hypothyroidism   TFT   ___
   Liver disease   Alk Phos   ___
   Nephrotic syndrome   Urine protein   ___
   Oral contraceptives   ___
            (Cushing's, acute porphyria, dysproteinemia)

   HYPERTRIGLYCERIDEMIA:
   Diabetes mellitus   FBS ___   Drugs: Estrogens   ___
   Obesity   ___   Beta blockers   ___
   Alcohol (1-3 oz/day)   ___   Thiazides   ___

2. SCREEN RELATIVES [ ]

3. DIETARY COUNSELLING [ ]
   Stepped reduction of saturated fatty acids, cholesterol; weight reduction; nutrition
      referral for patients not responding to initial counselling
   Patient education brochure ___   Counselling by nurse/M.D. ___
   Refer to Dietician ___   Refer to Group ___

4. MODIFY RISK FACTORS [ ]
   Exercise ___   Smoking ___   Obesity ___   Blood Pressure ___

5. CONSIDER DRUG TREATMENT IF REMAINS IN HIGH RISK CATEGORY
   especially if LDL >190 *or* >160 with ⊕ CAD or ⊕ risk factors (1 for men, 2
   for women)

Fig. 17-3   Sample evaluation guide.

TARGET LDL-CHOLESTEROL: < 130 mg/dl for patients with ⊕ CAD or ⊕ risk factors (1 for male, 2 for female)
< 160 mg/dl if no CAD, males with no risk factors, females with 0-1 risk factors

LIPID MANAGEMENT FLOW CHART

DATE															
Weight															
Blood pressure															
Cholesterol															
Triglycerides															
HDL															
LDL*															
MEDICATIONS															

*Calculated LDL = Total cholesterol − (HDL + triglycerides/5)

CHOICE OF DRUGS

I. Proven efficacy in reducing CHD risk (for males under 60 yrs old), lowers LDL 15-30%, may increase triglycerides, safe, often difficult to take, inexpensive:

BILE ACID SEQUESTRANTS—monitor GI effects and beware coadministration other drugs [costs ~$550/yr]:
Cholestyramine—Begin 4 g bid with water or juice, increase to 24 g/d in 2-3 doses [available in 9 g packets = 4 g cholestyramine plus 5 g orange-flavored filler or cheaper 378 g cans]
Colestipol—Begin 5 g bid with water or juice, increase to 30 g/d in 2-3 doses [available in 5 g packets or 500 g bottles]

NICOTINIC ACID/NIACIN—least expensive [~$50/yr]; preferable to bile acid sequestrants if hypertriglyceridemia present; monitor flushing and/or pretreatment with aspirin; monitor UGI side-effects, liver toxicity, hyperuricemia, hyperglycemia:
—Begin 100-250 mg qd after dinner; increase dose every 4-7 days, usually to bid pc, then tid pc, then increase each dose by 100-250 mg with meals, but eventually, if needed, up to 3 g/d (rarely 6 g/d)
[available in 50-, 100-, 500-mg tablets. Avoid long-acting preparations.

II. Proven efficacy in reducing CHD risk, lowers LDL 24% to 45%, long-term safety appears good, very easy to take, expensive:
STATINS (various agents)—also modestly reduces triglycerides [cost varies significantly among brands, beginning at $400 to $700/yr]:
Begin 10-20 mg qd with largest meal, then increase *prn* to 20-40 mg qd in one or two doses with meals; monitor GI symptoms, rash, myalgia, CPK, LFTs.

III. Additional medications (can be added to above agents or used if patient does not tolerate above agents)
GEMFIBROZIL (Lopid)—for hypertriglyceridemia; modest lowering LDL and may even increase IDL. Use very causiously with Statins due to problems with myositis.

Fig. 17-3—cont'd

to consult when one wants to know how often a *prn* ("as needed") medication was actually administered.

ABBREVIATED NOTES

In general, very comprehensive write-ups have a pedagogic value early in your training. Even if a full workup has already been entered in the patient's chart, your preparation of a detailed case presentation gives you practice in organizing the data you collected from the patient and in attending to the fine points of the history and physical examination. You develop habits of thoroughness. You also learn to find the right words to convey what the patient reported and to describe what you found on examination. A "complete" history and physical examination eventually becomes second nature to you, even under the stressful conditions of inpatient training. We put "complete" in quotation marks, because no write-up can be an absolutely exhaustive account of the narrative of the patient's life and illness. Moreover, thorough histories are not obtained unfailingly in one encounter. Students, residents, and senior staff frequently find themselves needing to go back to talk with and examine a patient when reflection indicates that more information is needed.

As your proficiency in performing a complete workup increases, and as your familiarity with the clinical method deepens, condensation and conciseness become goals in your written case presentations. You can begin to cut corners, depending on the clinical setting and the wishes of your supervisors. You no longer need to write out a full review of systems to remind yourself about these standard questions, nor to assure your supervisor that you asked. You do a thorough male rectal examination, which, when normal, can often be reported simply as "prostate normal, stool guaiac negative"; yet, when appropriate, you know to write down "no external hemorrhoids," "rectal tone normal," "no masses or tenderness" "prostate smooth, nontender, not enlarged," or "stool soft, brown." Similarly, you become confident of your ability to estimate diaphragmatic excursions upon examination of the chest or to detect venous pulsations on fundoscopy, but you no longer need to practice these skills and you realize that you do not need to check for or report such findings on every patient. In clinical practice, as you become more involved with the exigencies of caring for patients, time pressures will lead you to greater conciseness in obtaining and recording of the history and physical examination. Moreover, you do not bother to report information that is already in the chart or that is unlikely to be useful for patient care. At times, you may abandon prose in favor of a concise, telegraphic recording style.

One word of caution. Shortcuts in recording should not mean shortcuts in patient care. If you write, "review of systems unremarkable," you should be able to look back at the note later and feel confident that you asked a standard set of questions for that portion of the history. While other readers will not know what to make of such a note, you, at least, should know what you ask routinely. Similarly, if you write "Lungs—clear" or "sensation normal," it should indicate to you that you have performed a set physical examination sequence that is standard for yourself in a particular clinical setting. Thus abbreviated records provide less information to others than a comprehensive note, but can represent, in shorthand interpretable by yourself, the full data base that you routinely collect.

As examples of abbreviated write-ups, we include below: (1) a relatively complete description of a present illness accompanied by an abbreviated standard data base, and (2) a brief SOAP note for a short initial visit for a minor illness.

Example 1: An Abbreviated Write-Up

MATTHEW ARNOLD
MGH #113 1986

15 December 1986
This 27-year-old male high school teacher presents with a 5-day history of sore throat, fever, malaise, cough, and ear pain.

#1 Respiratory tract symptoms and #2 otalgia and hearing loss
The patient enjoyed generally excellent health until about 5 days ago, when he developed a sore throat, headache, fever, and malaise. He continued to work until 3 days ago when he developed a nonproductive cough that has interfered with his sleep. Yesterday, he began producing small amounts of phlegm, which was mostly clear but occasionally blood-tinged. He measured his temperature at 101.5° po. Last night he also noted pain and difficulty hearing in the left ear. No medication was taken. The patient is concerned about the significance of his hearing loss and about infecting his child. See #3, Smoking.

#3 Smoking
The patient has smoked two packs per day of cigarettes since age 16. He finds the habit relaxing, particularly at school, which is "like a zoo." He smokes less on weekends, but regularly has a few cigarettes before going to bed and immediately upon arising. He would like to stop, being concerned that he will get emphysema like his father, who has been incapacitated by chronic lung disease since age 54. He is also concerned about the effects of smoke on his 2-year-old daughter, and about encouraging her to smoke. He quit twice in the past few years, but developed severe irritability and fatigue over the first week, and returned to his habit in order to feel calm. His wife has been pressuring him to quit, and he is considering trying to stop on their anniversary, 15 March.

Past medical history
    Hospitalization: None
    Serious illnesses: None
    Medications: None
    Allergies: TETRACYCLINE (rash, stomach upset)
    Habits: EtOH—rare. CAGE test 0/4
        Tobacco—see #3 SMOKING
    Health maintenance:
      Exercise: Plays basketball at least twice a week for an hour, and walks at
          least 1.5 miles to work

Diet: Daily eggs, toast, and bacon or sausage for breakfast; fast-food lunch
(usually hamburger); balanced evening meal
Contraception: Wife uses diaphragm
Seat belts: +
Dental care: +

Social history

Born and raised in Brookline. Taught high school English since graduating college and likes his work, though he notes high pressure. Married 5 years. Wife also a teacher but now caring for their 2-year-old daughter. Describes himself as happy, economically comfortable.

Family history

Father, age 59, smoker with severe emphysema, disabled 5 years
Mother and 2 sibs alive and well

Review of systems

Not obtained

Physical examination

P 92; BP 120/70; R18; T100.8° po
GENERAL: Well-appearing young man with hacking, dry cough
SKIN: Clear
HEENT:
  Eyes: Conjunctivae clear. EOM full. PERRLA.
  Ears: Canals clear. Right TM normal. Left TM erythematous with bulla. Hears
    watch tick right at 6 cm; left at 1 cm. Weber lateralizes left. Air greater
    than bone right; reverse on left.
  Nose: No discharge. Sinuses nontender.
  Mouth: Mild pharyngeal erythema; no enanthem, tonsillar exudate.
  Neck: Supple.
NODES: None palpable
COR: PMI 5th ICS, MCL
  Normal S1. S2 physiologically split with A2>P2
  No murmur, rub, gallop
LUNGS: Unlabored
  Normal vocal fremitus
  Symmetrical resonance
  Few fine scattered bibasilar inspiratory crackles; no tubular breathing,
  wheezing, rub
  No sputum
ABDOMEN: Soft, nontender with active bowel sounds. No mass, L,S,K.
EXTREMITIES: No cyanosis, clubbing, edema

Laboratory

WBC 9,800
CXR—patchy perihilar lower lobe infiltrates

Assessment and plan

#1 PNEUMONITIS, probably *Mycoplasma* pneumonia
  The clinical presentation, association with bullous myringitis, and radiographic
  picture are consistent with "atypical pneumonia" due to *Mycoplasma*.
  Plan:
  Dx—None

Rx—Erythromycin 250 mg po qid for 10 days
  —Terpin hydrate with codeine 5-10 ml q4h as needed, ½ pint, no refill
Pt ed—Review diagnosis, medication, expected course
  —Discuss antibiotics, side effects, previous allergies
  —Suggest measures for protecting daughter
  —Call in case of not responding to Rx, problems with meds

#2 OTALGIA, HEARING LOSS
Bullous myringitis from *Mycoplasma* pneumonia
Plan:
  Dx and Rx—See #1
  Pt ed—reassure about hearing loss

#3 SMOKING
Patient seems well aware of hazards of smoking for himself and his family, and seems well motivated to quit. Nicotine withdrawal seems a significant barrier to quitting.
Plan:
  Dx—None
  Rx—Nicorette gum 1 box Refill × 6 mo
  Pt ed—Set quit date for 15 March; will send reminder letter
    —Given stop-smoking literature
    —Consider relaxation exercises
    —Follow-up in office in mid-April

#4 HEALTH PROMOTION
Further evaluation and discussion planned at next visit.
Dx—Serum cholesterol
Rx—None
Pt ed—Discuss at next visit. Invited to bring wife.

#5 ALLERGIC TETRACYCLINE

OLLIE HOLMES, HMS 1

Example 2: A Brief SOAP Note on a Minor Illness

FRANK KAFKA
Unit #073-1883

33-year-old recently engaged white male, disability claims inspector

Problem #1: URI × 3 days
S: Coryza, myalgia, malaise, temp. 101 po; no otalgia, cough, sputum.
Treated with fluids, acetaminophen. Concerned about TB, needs excuse from work.
O: NAD 98.8 po 122/72 80
  Ears—TMs clear
  Nose—Swollen mucosa, clear discharge; sinuses nontender
  Mouth—No pharyngitis, exudate
  Nodes—Negative
  Chest—Clear to P + A; no sputum
A: URI
P: DX—None

RX—Fluids, rest, acetaminophen
   —Ornade one tab po bid prn #12 NR
   —Letter to work
Pt ed—Discuss diagnosis
     —Reassure about TB; offer chest x-ray and tuberculin skin test later.
     —Return prn persistent symptoms

Problem #2: health maintenance

Problem #3: incomplete data base

S: Patient receiving no ongoing medical care
A: Incomplete data base
P: Dx—CBC, fasting lipids
   Rx—None
   Pt ed—Discuss routine care, premarital counseling
     —RTC 4 weeks for further history, discussion of health maintenance
     (especially family planning) and for routine physical

H. Cushing
HMS 2

MANAGED CARE ORGANIZATION: DEFINING RECORD KEEPING AND CLINICAL QUESTIONS

Because managed care organizations (MCOs) integrate the financing and the provision of care by physicians and hospitals, they may strongly influence professional work by controlling its payment. The care and treatment of patients may now be monitored, standardized by protocols, and restricted by MCOs. Indeed, for physicians to receive payment for services, the content of the medical record must meet the documentation standards of MCOs, in particular, documentation for purposes of billing the insurer. For example, decisions to operate or to do costly diagnostic testing may need MCO approval in advance. Thus before approval of elective operations (hysterectomy, tonsillectomy, cholecystectomy, and so on) and tests (MRI), physicians must ask specified questions, (e.g., "Commonly Asked Questions for Carpal Tunnel Surgery"). In effect, the record and the interview today are influenced by economic demands outside of those communication standards set by the profession itself for patient care and for the interprofessional work of practitioners. If the practice organization for your clinical instruction does not rigidly comply with MCO criteria, your interview or record keeping, of course, can continue to follow the standards of professional organizations, hospitals, and group practices.

CONFIDENTIALITY: WHAT TO INCLUDE IN THE RECORD

A physician receives a telephone call from a patient's spouse or child. What information about the patient's condition can be shared? Might some details be withheld? What if a distant relative calls? An employer? An insurance agent?

A young married man presents with rectal bleeding, and the physician takes an appropriate sexual history. Should relevant matters, such as homosexual relationships, be noted in the record? Should the patient be able to decide what the physician records?

A third patient is endangering the public—spreading an infectious disease [or, alternatively, committing crimes or driving with a poorly controlled seizure disorder]. What steps should the physician take?

▲

Confidentiality and the Doctor-Patient Relationship

Traditionally, all transactions within the clinical encounter are regarded as strictly confidential. The Hippocratic oath states,

> And whatsoever I shall see or hear in the course of my profession, as well as outside my profession in my intercourse with men, if it be what should not be published abroad, I will never divulge, holding such things to be holy secrets.

Without the patient's consent, none of the information arising from the encounter is shared by the physician with outsiders. The rule of "privileged information" applies to facts about diagnosis and treatment, as well as all other matters disclosed by the patient in the clinical interview, regardless of whether they are divulged intentionally or are related to patient care. Moreover, when the physician has permission to talk with others about a patient, communications are limited to topics relevant to the patient's care.

This traditional viewpoint, when applied with common sense rather than with an extremely legalistic mind, serves as a useful guide for clinical practice. For instance, interviews should be carried out in private, and patients should be consulted before any information about their care is shared with relatives, friends, employees, or other third parties. Doctors should conduct patient-related discussions in private and should not chat about patients, use their names, or even describe any of their characteristics in hallways, elevators, and cafeterias where conversations may be overheard. Similarly, avoid criticisms of other health care providers or derogatory remarks about patients or families in public places. In reports to third parties (which should only transpire with the explicit permission of the patient), omit all information the patient prefers not to divulge and avoid reporting irrelevant matters.

Similarly, when the physician consults with other health care workers (who implicitly have a contract with the patient), the scope of communication should be appropriate to the clinical task. Irrelevant personal matters should not be introduced in case presentations. Conversely, personal matters that are germane to diagnosis and treatment are properly discussed among colleagues participating in the patient's care. Whenever a case is publicly discussed among persons not involved in a person's care (e.g., in a teaching session), the anonymity of the patient should be preserved. In discussing a case with a classmate, spouse, or friend, one should also preserve privacy by not using the patient's name or giving other data likely to identify the patient. If you have doubts that privacy will be preserved, no conversation should take place.

However, the physician is free to negotiate with the patient about confidentiality. For instance, one might offer privacy to a minor seeking contraception but also encourage the patient to confide with his or her parents and perhaps even arrange to take part in such a discussion. Similarly, the physician can urge a patient to divulge confidential facts (e.g., alcoholism and drug use) to persons who should share this information, and may seek permission to inform them.

Exceptions to the Rule of Confidentiality

The goal of confidentiality may conflict with other ethical principles. Current medical ethics and practice recognize definite exceptions to the rule of privileged communication in the doctor-patient relationship (see Quick Tips: Exceptions to the Rule of Confidentiality).

QUICK TIPS

Exceptions to the Rule of Confidentiality

- The physician must at all times act ethically and honestly when preparing a medical record for a third party. The patient cannot expect the doctor to withhold information selectively with an intent to deceive.
- Situations may arise in which the interests of society are more highly valued than confidentiality.
- The physician's ethical obligations to various constituencies may require precise definition of how information will be shared.

First, the physician must at all times act ethically and honestly. The patient cannot expect the physician to withhold information selectively with an intent to deceive. For instance, having obtained a patient's permission to prepare a medical report for a third party (e.g., an employer or insurance company), either the physician would complete the form accurately or would indicate that the patient requested that some relevant information not be divulged.

Second, situations arise in which the interests of society are more highly valued than confidentiality. For instance, the physician is obliged to transmit information that assures appropriate management of certain communicable diseases, violent behaviors, and suicidal or homicidal potential. State laws will sanction some abridgements of confidentiality, though legal and ethical principles may not provide clear guidance or, on rare occasion, may even suggest divergent courses.

Third, physicians may have ethical obligations to various constituencies, and the interests of one may conflict with those of another. Physicians who contract with groups (a couple, family, sports team, school, or employer) rather than with individuals may need to define how information will be shared. For instance, the right of adolescent minors to maintain confidentiality from their parents often needs to be negotiated rather than decided on by absolute principles, since both parties have claims on the physician. Similarly, physicians employed by a school, business, or government agency should make explicit their responsibilities to the patient and to the organization.

Confidentiality and the Medical Record

Since its introduction in the early 1900s, the patient's hospital record has been a common document for the institution's medical staff. In the hospital setting and in the private practitioner's office, personal information useful to the collaborative care of the patient can be recorded and ideally is available only to a restricted professional circle. While the record is the property of the hospital or practitioner, access to it should be determined by the patient. Thus the patient may view his or her record, as may professionals who treat the patient and who have an implicit contract to maintain confidentiality. Only with the patient's written permission may others read or copy the record.

Despite these desired norms, access to records inside of medical practices—hospitals, clinics, health maintenance organizations, group practices—is widespread. No longer restricted, the staff that writes in or reads the record includes nurses and aides, technicians in various diagnostic services, nutritionists, social workers, secretaries, medical librarians, employees in the transport service, admitting officers, utilization review and billing personnel, and a host of other members of the hospital bureaucracy. Strict privacy may not be regularly respected. Confidentiality is particularly problematic in small communities where the staff and patients are part of the same network, when the patient is a hospital staff member, or when the person being treated is a public figure or celebrity.

Moreover, through a variety of common and usually legitimate procedures, the record is readily accessed by persons outside of medical practices, including representatives of insurance companies, welfare agencies, utilization review organizations, courts, and compensation boards. The entire record may be divulged, regardless of the purpose of the outside review. Similarly, computerized records, including clinical notes, laboratory tests, or simply charges for procedures, may be obtained by a variety of people.

Therefore the physician has little control over the dispersion of information once it is recorded in the record. Indeed, the physician should warn certain patients (e.g., those undergoing testing for the HIV virus) of their potential lack of privacy. Remember: the record is public.

An Ethical Perspective on Confidentiality and the Record

Given this diffusion of medical records, what information should be recorded and what is considered confidential? The first and basic ethical principle is to serve the well-being of the patient or, stated negatively, to do no harm. A second principle is to follow the will of the patient (assuming he or she is competent). Third, the physician should adhere to fundamental professional standards, such as being honest and providing good care. Conflicts commonly arise when the physician's notion of good care differs from the patient's sense of what is desirable. For instance, physicians-in-training may want to demonstrate their thoroughness in a write-up, thus including information (e.g., about sexual practices) that the patient considers confidential. A physician may record pejorative judgments (e.g., that the patient is feigning illness) because such opinions seem important to share with colleagues. Similarly, in response to concerns about malpractice or utilization review, a clinician may feel that the recording of confidential matters is necessary to document that proper care was provided. The abridgement of patient privacy in deference to professional interests deserves ethical reflection.

A first step in deciding about the recording of personal information is to decide whether it is important for the patient's care. Does it need to be stated explicitly? For instance, would it be sufficient to educate the patient about his or her responsibility of transmitting the information to practitioners providing care?

If recording of personal information is judged valuable or essential, is it potentially damaging to the patient? If so, has the patient consented to the inclusion of such material in the record? If not, what are the physician's legal and ethical obligations? Can professional responsibilities be carried out without divulging potentially damaging information?

The recording of detailed facts about many private matters is generally of no benefit to patients and serves little use to other practitioners who care for the patient. Some brief, perhaps slightly elliptical, mention of these topics may be considered helpful, but should be handled cautiously. For instance, the details of the patient's sexual practices and concerns need not be included in the record, but the physician may simply indicate that a sexual history has been taken ("Discussed patient's sexual concerns and behaviors"), thus underscoring the topic's importance while allowing the next practitioner to take his or her own history. In the case of identifying sexual orientation, a first step is usually to ask the patient how he or she feels about including this data in the record, as well as educating the patient to the importance of physicians' awareness of this information. Recognized psychiatric disorders generally deserve recording in the form of standard diagnoses, but stigmatized occupations and other deviant behaviors generally need not be mentioned. Again, the inclusion of information about stigmatized matters, when useful to the clinical process, should generally be negotiated with the patient, and patients may be educated about providing such information when relevant.

Extreme care in documentation is required when the medical record is likely to serve legal purposes (e.g., caring for a victim of a crime or accident, reporting child abuse, explaining the basis for involuntary psychiatric hospitalization). In these circumstances, when describing uncertain facts that have been obtained from the patient, neutral language is preferred: "The patient reportedly was hit by a stranger."

What is Confidential?

Would you be comfortable reading the record to the patient? Private topics usually include:

- Sexual history, practices, and concerns
- Stigmatized conditions, such as mental illness, suicide in the family, and venereal diseases
- Deviant or illegal activities, such as drug use, prostitution, or crime
- Delinquency, arrests, and prison sentences

Just as some of the topics listed above are not universally considered confidential matters, many patients will view other information as private. There is no rule for defining what will be considered confidential by a patient, but one reflection may give some guidance about whether to write down the personal stories and facts volunteered to you or gleaned from patients who so often are strangers to you: Would I want this information recorded about myself or my family? At the same time, be aware that the use of your personal standards may not coincide with the patient's. Beware of any behavior, feelings, or thoughts that the patient considers "secret" or private—facts never communicated to casual acquaintances, close friends, or relatives. If you have any serious doubt, you should omit the information from the record or check with the patient about its inclusion.

SUGGESTED READINGS

An Introduction to Records

Bjorn JC, Cross HD: *The problem-oriented private practice of medicine: a system for comprehensive health care*, Chicago, 1970, Modern Hospital Press.

Physician's Current Procedural Terminology, Chicago, 1997, American Medical Association.

Reiser SJ: The clinical record in medicine. II: Reforming content and purpose, *Ann Intern Med* 114:980, 1991.

Shenkin BN, Warner DC: Giving the patient his medical record: a proposal to improve the system, *N Engl J Med* 289:688, 1973.

Weed LL: *Medical records, medical education, and patient care: the problem-oriented record as a basic tool*, Chicago, 1971, Mosby.

Confidentiality

Marsh P: The "deeper meaning" of confidentiality within the physician-patient relationship, *Ethics Sci Med* 6:131, 1979.

Siegler M: Confidentiality in medicine—a decrepit concept, *N Engl J Med* 307:1518, 1982.

Ubel PA, Zell MM, Miller DJ, et al: Elevator talk: observational study of inappropriate comments in public space, *Am J Med* 99:190, 1995.

Computerized Records

Slack WV: *Cybermedicine: how computing empowers doctors and patients for better health care*, Los Angeles, 1997, Jossey-Bass.

CHAPTER 18

ORAL CASE PRESENTATIONS

It is one thing for a man to understand a matter for himself and for his own use, and another thing to understand and explain it for the use of others.

PETER MERE LATHMAN

The oral case presentation is the primary means by which clinicians convey information about patients to each other. For students, the presentation is also the major means for demonstrating their clinical competence to peers and supervisors. In practicing clear, carefully organized, and terse presentations and in having them critiqued, the student acquires a basic skill for interprofessional communication.

Excellence of oral presentation in the theater of ward rounds reflects your basic grasp of the patient's condition and your capacity to reduce complex data to readily understandable form. In learning to present well, you develop skills in obtaining, organizing, and conveying clinical information, in diagnostic reasoning, and in therapeutics.

SIMILARITIES AND DIFFERENCES BETWEEN WRITTEN AND ORAL PRESENTATIONS

Formal oral presentations and case write-ups share many features:
- An orderly, familiar organizational format
- A full characterization of symptoms
- Reconstruction of the patient's narrative into a coherent description of an illness, not merely a recitation of isolated facts
- Presentation within the description of the present illness of whatever past medical history, social and family history, and review of systems are relevant to the differential diagnosis
- Separation of "subjective" data (derived from inquiry of the patient or other sources) and "objective" (physician-observed) data and of impressions and plans (though this rule may be breached selectively for the sake of brevity)

However, oral case presentations and case write-ups serve distinct functions. The "complete" history of the medical record is a repository of information, a detailed documentation of clinical acts and the course of an illness. It includes data that may be of peripheral or uncertain significance in the immediate care of the patient. The oral presentation, however, gives a concise, compressed account of only the most essential facts. Moreover, the content of oral presentations varies markedly, depending on their purpose, such as quickly providing an overview for colleagues on rounds, opening an extended discussion about a disease for a teaching conference, or obtaining consultation on a troublesome feature of a case.

In oral presentations, the student should bear in mind the limitations of a listener. A reader reviews a medical record alone, adjusting the speed at which new information is encountered, allowing time for thought, skimming over unnecessary detail, or returning to portions of a write-up that were not appreciated at first glance. A listener, however, has but a single hearing to register all the important details of a case and to think about the information while listening. To help the listener with this difficult task, the oral presentation needs to be especially clear, uncluttered, and easily grasped. The listener should be guided through a reasoning process that helps him or her consider a differential diagnosis—beginning with a few broad strokes that give an overall picture of the patient and the patient's problem, followed by data that focus attention on key matters, then by more detailed information that clarifies and answers further questions and elaborates on the uncertainties of the case. The organization of the oral presentation is similar to that used in newspaper articles: begin with headlines, follow with lead sentences, and progress to more detailed descriptions of matters that are not of central importance but that become of interest when the broader issues have been appreciated.

You help your listener grasp the data by maintaining the familiar, recognizable order of the written case report. Beware of jumping back and forth between descriptions of separate problems, between active problems and the standard data base, or between history and physical findings. When the information being presented is out of the expected order or does not bear on the listener's problem-solving process of the moment, it is perceived as distracting, confusing, and even irritating.

A final point to bear in mind is that listeners, much more than readers, are influenced by your style of presentation. A monotonous droner can make Shakespeare sound dull; a lively raconteur can entertain you, at least briefly, with a recitation of the phone book. Every student has conversational skills that allow him or her to tell a story well—not by drably recalling facts, but by creating a vivid picture, leading the listener through the tale, and focusing on interesting and pertinent aspects. Such universal skills need not be discarded in deference to somber clinical goals. Use your manner of presentation and your selection of data to enliven the story. Engage your listeners and maintain their attention.

LENGTH

Oral presentations may vary enormously in their length. The student must gauge the amount of time and detail appropriate to presentations in different settings with different persons. Ask your preceptors for guidance. In some settings, a few seconds are sufficient.

[To a colleague:] You might get a call this weekend from Mrs. Sherman. She's a healthy young woman with her first urinary tract infection, presenting with fever, dysuria, and mild flank discomfort. Cultures are pending. She seems to be responding on her second day of trimethoprim-sulfa. She's a bit worried, and I encouraged her to call if she spikes a fever or starts feeling worse.

[To an attending physician:] Mrs. Miller is a very active 68-year-old woman who is followed here regularly for her blood pressure and routine checkups. She just wants a flu shot. She's had them before without problems. Her blood pressure is fine today, and I'd just like to give her the shot.

In other circumstances, presentations may last 5 minutes or more and will recapitulate much of the medical record.

In teaching settings, oral presentations generally fall into two categories: the "bullet" or "capsule," often lasting less than a minute, typically given either in stand-up ward rounds, in the office hallway, or over the telephone; and "formal case presentations," lasting 5 to 7 minutes, usually given to supervisors and colleagues at the bedside or in a sit-down conference. "Complete case presentations," which recapitulate the bulk of the written record and might last 10 minutes, are sometimes required of beginning students. Most of the comments that follow are directed toward formal case presentations, but the advice can be applied to presentations of any length.

FORMAT

The order of the presentation should parallel that of the write-up: a headline sentence that includes identifying data and the reason for visit, followed by the history, physical examination, laboratory examination and procedures, assessment, and plan. Within each of these sections you should follow the familiar organization of the case record. The history begins with the present illness and may be followed by a brief past medical history, including its usual subsections, which in turn may be followed by an abridged social and family history and review of systems. The physical examination begins with a statement about appearance and vital signs and then generally proceeds from head to toe, concluding with the neurological examination. The laboratory data begin with common tests (blood counts, basic chemistries, urinalysis, chest x-ray, electrocardiogram, and microbiological studies), followed by relatively more complex and unusual data (arterial blood gases, rheumatoid factor, joint fluid examination, and computed tomography scan). The assessment may begin with a brief summary, address the most severe, acute, or central clinical problem, proceed to important but secondary or less urgent matters, and then finish with peripheral matters. The plan starts with diagnostic measures, then proposed treatments, followed by patient education. Deviations from this conventional sequence jar the listener and may also lead you to repeat yourself. If you omit any topics, your audience will assume that you consider them irrelevant.

A summary statement is sometimes expected at the end of a long formal presentation.

> In summary, then, this 52-year-old single seamstress presents with classic symptoms of stable, mild angina and no identified risk factors or further evidence of cardiovascular disease. Her examination is unremarkable. I would like to obtain some basic studies, including fasting blood sugar, lipids, electrocardiogram, and chest x-ray, and teach her to use nitroglycerin.

CONTENT

Here are a few general suggestions about the content of an oral presentation (see Quick Tips: Oral Presentation Content).

QUICK TIPS

Oral Presentation Content

- Begin with an opening statement—broad overview of the patient, reason for the visit, duration of complaint
- The body of your presentation should focus on one or more major problems in the history of the present illness
- Include all significant abnormal *and* any normal findings from physical examination and laboratory data that contribute to answering what is wrong with the patient

---

Opening Statement

The opening statement should give a broad overview of the patient (the "identifying data" and past illnesses of major significance), the reason for the visit, and the duration of the complaint. These are the headlines that orient your listener to the remainder of the presentation, including key components of the "prior probabilities" on which clinical problem-solving will be based.

Begin with the patient's age and sex. If relevant, include marital status, race, ethnicity, or occupation. If the patient has a history of a major medical problem that bears strongly on the understanding of the present illness—such as a recent heart attack, cancer, diabetes, alcoholism, manic depressive illness—mention it in a few words.

Next, give the reason for the visit. It need not be a verbatim report of the patient's complaint; it should be a few words that set the stage for more detailed consideration of the patient's problem, as viewed by the presenter, perhaps already hinting at the leading diagnosis or diagnoses. You may want to give the patient's reason for the visit as well as the major problem that you have identified. Make sure you also give the duration of the symptoms.

> Mrs. O'Connor is a 56-year-old widowed telephone operator with long-standing insulin-dependent diabetes who now complains of weekly dizzy spells over the past 2 months.

> Mr. Lucas is a 42-year-old jogging journalist who presents with knee problems for 3 months and was found for the first time to be hypertensive.

Body of the Report

The bulk of the presentation focuses on one or more major problems in the history of the present illness. Present the most important problem first, along with all the relevant information—relevant historical findings and standard data base, including "pertinent negatives." Cover all data about one problem or organ or physiological system before going on to another. Beware of skipping back and forth, unless there are critical relationships between different problems or systems. Within the first few sentences, you should lay out a map for your listener, allowing him or her to grasp the general issues at hand and to begin sorting out the details that affirm or refute various hypotheses. If a patient complains of fatigue, but has anemia and bloody stools, you may want immediately to let your listener know that this is a case of gastrointestinal bleeding, rather than waiting to get to the presentation of the stool examination or laboratory data. Two patients who complain of weight loss (one who has lung cancer, the other hyperthyroidism) are presented as follows:

> Gabriel Humphrey is a 55-year-old married fireman—a long-time smoker and chronic lunger—who presents with fatigue, a 20-pound weight loss, and worsened chronic cough.

> Susan Dale, a 55-year-old recently widowed housewife, presents with a few months of excessive nervousness, heat intolerance, and a 20-pound weight loss despite a good appetite.

What To Include?

Do not suffer the illusion that a good presentation merely requires a recital of all relevant facts. You need to select the essential information and organize it into a coherent story that can be told in a limited time. The inclusion of any data should be justifiable in terms of its usefulness in figuring out the patient's problems. Thus, in deciding what data to present, you ideally should have a firm grasp on the differential diagnosis and management issues. You may also recognize the idiosyncrasies of the listener (who, for instance, may either demand or be irritated by a presentation of basic social history, independent of your assessment of the importance of this data in appreciating a particular patient).

Consider two patients with similar stories of fatigue and painless jaundice. For the first patient, who you think has alcoholic liver disease, you say,

"This 58-year-old separated white male, unemployed printer, and chronic alcoholic, presents with painless jaundice and fatigue." You then go on to describe the patient's drinking, other complications of alcoholism, the onset of symptoms, and a few pertinent facts that indicate that it is unlikely that the patient has another cause for jaundice, such as gallstones blocking the common duct. For the second patient, who you think has metastatic cancer, you begin, "This 58-year-old white male, retired postal worker, who underwent resection of a colonic carcinoma 2 years ago, presents with fatigue and painless jaundice." You then describe the presentation of the malignancy, the interval course of the cancer, the onset of new symptoms, and the absence of evidence to support other diagnoses, such as hepatitis or gall bladder disease.

Your presentation does not have to answer every question. In briefer presentations, you need only sketch out key facts; the listener's inquiries will guide you to offering further details. In longer presentations, the listener should also be expected to ask questions afterward, but feel that you offered the important facts of the case. A supervisor is usually most pleased to have the major questions answered, yet to be allowed to ask a few clarifying points. Of course, you try to be prepared to answer every question that might arise.

Do not be surprised if you are asked to repeat details that you already included: listening is imperfect. Also, in some settings, interruptions are permitted for questioning the presenter, and you will need to adjust your delivery to the immediate demands of the audience.

Present the Patient and the Illness

In general, present the "bare bones" of the case, but flesh them out in such a way as to make your report engaging and to allow the listener a feeling for the patient as a person. Sometimes, quoting the patient will give the audience a sense of what kind of person is being presented.

> Even when he appeared in no distress, he said the discomfort is the worst thing he ever felt and kept saying, "you've got to help me" or "you've got to believe me."
>
> After a few weeks of this constant pain, inability to sleep, and oozing from the wound, he said to his son, "I think we maybe better show this to the doctor, if it keeps up."

Little or No Standard Data Base

Focus on the present illness. All data relevant to understanding the patient's major problems are presented in conjunction with those problems. The standard data base is otherwise generally omitted or severely abbreviated.

> The remainder of the history is only notable for a recurrent low back pain with sciatica on the right and a 30 pack-year smoking history.

More specifically, the past medical history that bears directly on current problems is mentioned in conjunction with the present illness; other matters—substantial but resolved, remote in time, or irrelevant—are mentioned in a very brief summary or are omitted. Similarly, the social history and family history are noted in a few sentences or omitted. Essentially items from the review of systems that are unrelated to the present problems may be mentioned in passing. Avoid presenting any information as part of the standard data base that has already been described under the present illness.

The Compressed Physical Examination

The presentation of the physical examination begins with a few broad comments, allowing your audience to conjure up a picture of the patient's general appearance and condition. You will select or omit data in the physical examination, using principles similar to those described for the present illness. At times, only abnormal findings are mentioned. For instance, in a bullet presentation, a person with angina might be described as follows: "The patient is normotensive, and the physical examination is entirely unremarkable." In a lengthier formal presentation on the same patient, you might describe the vital signs, the appearance of the blood vessels on ophthalmoscopic examination, the carotid and jugular venous pulses, a detailed cardiac examination, and the peripheral pulses. If time allowed, you might also note the presence or absence of chest wall tenderness or the cutaneous stigmata of hyperlipidemia. In longer presentations, every organ system (e.g., heart, lungs) or major region of the physical examination (HEENT, abdomen, extremities) would be mentioned, including either a description of relevant findings or a statement that the examination was normal. As a general rule, include all significant abnormal findings and any normal findings that contribute to the process of figuring out what is wrong with the patient; omit insignificant or irrelevant abnormalities and other normal findings.

Laboratory Data

Laboratory findings are often best appreciated when written on a blackboard or in handouts, especially when these facts need to be presented in detail. Radiographs and ECG printouts should be available for review and may be shown to the audience before you give your own interpretation.

Shortcuts

Good presentations often resort to a number of shortcuts. In bullets, extreme condensation is expected by the listener; anything not mentioned is assumed to be normal or irrelevant. For the sake of brevity, you may, at times, offer summative, integrative, and interpretive statements rather than simply presenting data. For instance, you may specify that certain parts of the history, physical or laboratory examinations were done but did not provide any information pertinent to a better understanding of the patient's major problems.

> The past medical history, social history, family history, and review of systems were otherwise noncontributory.

> The remainder of the history is remarkable only for a tubal ligation 3 years ago, a strong family history of diabetes, and occasional premenstrual cramps.

> Other minor problems include long-standing tension headaches, hemorrhoids, and psoriasis.

The physical examination and laboratory data may also be condensed.

> There were no stigmata of chronic liver disease. The examination of the heart, lungs, and abdomen was within normal limits; no right upper quadrant tenderness could be elicited.

> The CBC, blood sugar, electrolytes, BUN, and liver function tests were within normal limits.

Common Omissions in Outpatient Presentations

Students frequently omit the following data in ambulatory case presentations:
1. A full description of the dimensions of the symptom, such as duration, frequency, and severity
2. The patient's perspective, including attributions, requests, and the trigger for the visit
3. Medications, including name, dose, frequency, and appraisal of compliance

FURTHER ORGANIZATIONAL SUGGESTIONS

As mentioned in Chapter 6, Consulting With Your Preceptor, three organizational approaches are commonly used to describe the present illness and may be used in various parts of the same presentation. First, in "symptom characterization," a key symptom is identified and its "dimensions" are presented in a thorough, orderly fashion. Second, in a "chronological report," the crucial events are described as they evolved over time (e.g., for a patient with peritonitis from ambulatory peritoneal dialysis, you note the history of exposure to nephrotoxins, the early diagnosis of renal failure and development of end-stage renal disease, the course of peritoneal dialysis, and, finally, the development of the current episode of peritonitis). Third, usually in conjunction with one of the previous two methods, "hypothesis testing" or "problem solving" serves as the logic for presenting data. Here, one of the diagnoses under consideration becomes the focus of the presentation, and information is provided that tends to confirm or disconfirm this diagnosis. For example, the presence or absence of diabetes or hypertension is mentioned in a patient with possible angina. Similarly, for a patient with suspected gonorrhea, give a history of venereal disease and sexual encounters. All three organizational formats may be used in the same presentation.

If two or more major and unrelated problems are evident, you can help your audience follow a complicated presentation by starting with a list of major problems or by introducing all problems in the headline sentence.

> This 76-year-old widowed, retired plumber, who has not seen a physician since his transurethral prostatectomy 8 years ago, now presents with progressive haziness of vision in his left eye, stiffness of the left shoulder, and recurrent difficulty in voiding.

In this case, you might present three "present problems" (beginning with the most important one), followed by one brief standard data base and a physical examination that focuses on the three acute problems. At other times, you may want to use a format similar to that of the SOAP note, presenting together the history, physical examination, and laboratory work relevant to each separate problem.

PRESENTING UPDATES

When presenting a progress report (a description of new data that have been collected since an initial case discussion), you generally will want to jog your listeners' memories by beginning with a sentence or two that recapitulates the major features of the case.

> Mrs. Henry, the 23-year-old house painter with anxiety attacks, who we thought was probably not thyrotoxic, had normal thyroid function tests. We started her 2 weeks ago on alprazolam 0.25 mg tid, and she's back today, saying she had only two mild attacks. She's also talking more about how she feels about leaving her family.

PREPARATION AND REVIEW

The basis for preparing an oral case presentation is a thorough patient evaluation, selected reading, and completion of a comprehensive write-up. Ideally, you should be prepared to discuss the etiology, pathophysiology, diagnosis, complications, differential diagnosis, treatment, and course of any conditions under consideration. You should also be familiar with the use of any diagnostic tests, medications, or other treatments relevant to the case. In presenting cases before you have had time to digest the facts or read about the patient's problems, you aspire to a similar background fund of information, but are only expected to organize your thoughts in a manner appropriate to your stage of training.

Good presentations take practice. Talk about your case to anyone who will listen! Before a formal case discussion, practice your presentation at least a few times. Prepare an outline or use notes, but do not read your presentation. Time yourself and make sure your formal presentations last no longer than 5 to 7 minutes. Rehearse bullets too. Audiotape your trials or actual presentations and review them on your own or with your colleagues and preceptors. Listen for excessive "uhs and ahs," pauses, and repetition. After your presentations, ask for guidance and feedback.

CONCLUSION

The content and organization of an oral case presentation reflect your fundamental appreciation of the patient and his or her problem. Students and physicians develop their own styles of presenting, and no single format is right for every patient, setting, listener, or presenter. The two most common problems with student presentations are excess length and poor organization. Review your presentation with the following points in mind.

Guideliness for Oral Presentation

1. Paint a broad picture and then follow with logically organized details that the listener needs for understanding the case. Put yourself in the listener's shoes and make sure he or she will have the information necessary to obtain an accurate view of the patient and the illness.
2. Beware of simply reciting facts. A presentation should give a fair, undistorted report of the data, yet its organization and manner of delivery should also advocate for a clinical conclusion. Construct a cogent argument in favor of a diagnosis or, at least, of a limited differential diagnosis. For a return visit or follow-up on a hospitalized patient, the presentation might focus more on management than on diagnosis and thus might point to a need for new diagnostic studies, a change in medication, or a referral to a specialist.
3. Present the patient and the illness. Even in a bullet, a few words or nuances can give your listeners a sense of the person you are presenting.
4. Make the format appropriate to the setting. Be familiar with the interests and expectations of your listeners, their time constraints, and their educational and patient-care goals.
5. Be brief and lucid. Consider whether anything can be condensed, distilled, clarified, or omitted. Try not to repeat yourself.
6. Don't feel that you have to answer every anticipated question. Expect your listeners to ask for elaboration and clarification.
7. Speak crisply and clearly. Give an energetic, enthusiastic, animated account. Remember: your patient has the most fascinating case of athlete's foot that anyone has ever encountered.
8. Engage your listeners. Be a raconteur. Part of the challenge of presenting well is to make the case come alive, helping the listener to care about both the diagnostic questions and the personal plight of the patient. How would you vividly describe the patient to a friend? If the patient has ever been a tightrope walker, beauty contest winner, or center fielder in the minor leagues, this information belongs in the presentation. What makes this case special? A few well-chosen words that suggest how this person and this problem are interesting can help you get more attention as a learner, as well as inciting enthusiasm toward your patients, thus helping them get better care.

ADDENDUM: DISCUSSING CASES WITH THE PATIENT PRESENT

We strongly endorse the inclusion, insofar as is practical, of direct patient contact (and, at times, contact with families) in clinical supervision and teaching exercises. A favorite method for case review begins not with a case presentation but with a patient interview, focusing on the immediate physician-patient interaction and the collection and processing of raw clinical data.

Case presentations and discussions with the patient present, however, do pose problems, especially in time-pressured clinical settings. Many patients will misunderstand the purpose and meaning of portions of the presentation and may want to interrupt with rebuttal, clarification, or questioning. The presenter will rightly be hesitant to mention worrisome diagnostic possibilities or to include information that would not normally be disclosed by the patient in public. A more convenient format may be to present away from the patient, then to go to the patient, saying, for instance:

> We've had a little time to discuss your health problems, but now I would like to hear a bit directly from you.

As you leave the patient, you might say:

> Okay, we're going to sit down together and go over this some more, and then I'll come back to discuss our conclusions with you. Is there anything you would like to add or ask about now?

Insofar as some or all of a case presentation or discussion occurs in the patient's presence, consider the following:

- Introduce the process to the patient, preferably before any case discussion. Let the patient know beforehand who will be seeing him or her, why, when, for how long, what will have been discussed ahead of time, what will be expected of the patient (e.g., should he or she clarify points in the presentation? should questions be asked?), what will be done afterward, and how the process will be of use to the patient. Address concerns about confidentiality.
- Insofar as is reasonable, introduce the patient to everyone present and to their roles.
- When in the patient's presence, be prepared to give all your attention to the patient. If the health care team is going to use technical language or talk among themselves without intending to include the patient, excuse yourselves: "Now we're going to engage in some doctor-talk."
- Eye contact with the patient or a few gestures that acknowledge his or her presence will help prevent the process from becoming dehumanizing. Alter the standard format of the presentation appropriately, speaking of "Mrs. Smith" or "she" rather than "the patient." In the patient's presence, you should not give data that are obvious (e.g., sex, race, general appearance).

- Say goodbye, assuring the patient that you will come back later for more discussion. In general, a few words of thanks are appropriate, as well as a statement, ideally an optimistic one, about how the group will work on helping the patient.
- At a later time, review with the patient his or her impressions of the exercise and any questions about what was said. Summarize any discussion from which the patient was excluded.

Conversely, if the patient is presented but not present, your colleagues and supervisors should consider arranging some time to see the patient, exchange a few words, develop a rudimentary relationship, and let the patient know of their involvement in the care process. Ideally, supervisors will review portions of the interview with the patient, check physical findings, offer an opinion, and give the patient and family an opportunity to ask questions.

SUGGESTED READING
Yurchak P: A guide to medical case presentations, *Resident Staff Physician* 27:109, 1981.

CHAPTER 19

COLLABORATIVE CARE

The treatment of the disease may be entirely impersonal; the care of the patient must be completely personal.

FRANCIS WELD PEABODY

REFERRAL AND CONSULTATION

Making a Referral

Consultations serve essential functions in the care of patients and in the physician's continuing professional education. A few important principles in the referral process deserve attention.

Clarify Your Purpose (and the Patient's) in Making the Referral

What do you want the consultant to do? Like all personal interactions, the referral is likely to be most effective when both parties hold similar expectations or goals. What are your uncertainties, concerns, and requests? For instance, do you want the consultant to give an opinion about a confusing problem, advise you about the current drug of choice, do a procedure, assume responsibility for ongoing management of a problem, review the case to ensure that the best possible care was provided, endorse what you have done, or transfer the patient to his or her care? Did you suggest the consultation or was it requested by the patient or a family member? Be specific about what you and the patient want—what aspects of the patient's care to review, what clinical findings to evaluate, what diagnostic steps and therapies to address, what procedures you want considered, and how to communicate consultation findings with the patient and family. If timeliness is an issue, make sure you indicate when you want the consultation done.

Examples of clearly stated requests include:

[A note in the record:]
   Consult: Dr. Bigby.
   Is the mole on his right shoulder malignant? Please biopsy it, if indicated. I have discussed the likelihood of needing a biopsy with the patient. Both the patient and I would prefer that I present her with the results of the biopsy.
   Thank you,
   Chester Jones, M.D.

[A note in the record to a nurse-practitioner:]
   To Ms. Janeco:
   Kindly see this gentleman every 2 months to check his blood pressure, monitor for signs of congestive heart failure, and encourage compliance with

medications and diet. He should also have a flu shot in the fall and be referred back to me for an annual checkup in a year. Thanks.
M. Querner, M.D.

[A referral note to a social worker:]
Thank you for seeing this unfortunate 62-year-old widow who has metastatic breast cancer and lacks close friends or relatives. She is very unhappy with her housing and is having difficulty paying for medications, getting to appointments with her oncologist, and caring for herself at home. I think she would benefit from some practical help, such as referral for elderly housing and transportation, assistance submitting her medical bills to her insurance company, and a homemaker, but will also appreciate your ongoing support and availability should further problems arise.

[A telephone call:]
Bill, I need your help but I don't think you need to see this patient. She's 37 and has had recurrent UTIs, roughly one yearly for about 8 years, and now presents with another episode. Her IVP was normal a few years ago. Now her urine has gram-negative rods and lots of white cells; the culture is pending. She also has multiple drug allergies—penicillin, cephalosporins, and sulfa, and a history of nephrotoxicity with aminoglycosides. How do you think I should proceed?

[A letter:]
Dear Dr. Smith:
Mrs. Percy would like a second opinion about the need for a cholecystectomy. Enclosed is a summary of her clinical evaluation, including laboratory and radiological studies. We have recommended the operation.
Sincerely yours,
James Jackson, M.D.

[A record note:]
Consult: Dr. Peabody:
I believe this patient should be transferred to your service for further management. Please accept, if you agree.
Thank you,
John Ware, M.D.

Attend to Common Courtesies

Engage the consultant on a personal level, rather than strictly through formal channels. A personal call to the consultant will be appreciated and will promote collaborative care. Personal information about the patient and delicate issues are best handled by direct contact rather than in writing. A few words about the patient's personality, including his or her expectations about the consultation, can be helpful. A call should often be followed by a written note, especially in complicated cases and when you want to make sure important points are remembered. When the consultation is straightforward and you already have an ongoing relationship with the consultant, a brief written note can be satisfactory. Afterward, consider entering a note of thanks in the record or personally communicating gratitude to the consultant.

In clinics, large group practices, and academic units where referral is made to "the service" rather than to an individual clinician and where the senior consultant may be assisted by a clinical fellow or resident, you will often want to identify who the consultant will be and then contact him or her so that you can make the process more personal. You might leave a note: "Please call me at extension 3745 before seeing the patient."

Have All Relevant Data Available

Present the consultant with the material he or she needs to do the kind of consultation you want. You may want to write a note that summarizes the relevant history, physical examination, or laboratory data. You can also refer to a note in the record or merely make the chart, radiographs, and other previous studies available.

Prepare the Patient

The patient should consent to the consultation, of course, but also be prepared for it. What is the consultation for? How will it help? How will it be carried out? What are the costs? What about discomforts, especially if a procedure is anticipated? What kind of questions should the patient ask the consultant, and what kind of explanations can be expected? Is this a one-time visit or the beginning of a long-term relationship?

Give Your Consultants Follow-up

Let them know when you (and the patient) found a consultation useful and what the outcome was. Also review conflicts. For instance, if the consultant made arrangements for care without discussing them with you, then mutual review is needed to resolve interprofessional differences and establish a suitable collaborative plan. Such communications may be difficult, especially as specialists and generalists compete for patients.

Providing Consultation

A similar set of rules applies to providing a consultation, a job that frequently falls on students when they serve on both inpatient and outpatient subspecialty rotations. Consultation is part of the professional work of many physicians and should provide for the needs of the patient and the educational interests of the referring clinician.

Clarify Why You Are Being Consulted

A personal call to the referring physician may be helpful before you see the patient. Recognize a broad range of reasons for seeking consultation, some of which may not be made explicit: wanting assistance with an entire case that is confusing, advice on a rather circumscribed aspect of patient care, desire to transfer primary caretaking responsibility, desire for reassurance that everything is being done well, specific requests for a special service (e.g., a biopsy procedure), advice sought by the patient, wanting help (or relief) when the doctor-patient relationship is distressed or there are conflicts among the health care team, and so on. Consultations may be attended by considerable discomfort on the part of the clinician—uncertainty, guilt, feeling distrusted by the patient or pressured by the nurses or a patient's relative—and may be complicated by the referring physician's reluctance to admit uncertainty or to cede clinical authority to other specialists. You can provide a more satisfying and successful consultation for both the patient and the referring physician when you recognize these issues.

How urgent is the consultation? Are you asked to make general suggestions or specific recommendations (e.g., dosage of a drug), provide an academic discussion of the problems posed by the patient, or assume overall responsibility for care? Will follow-up be expected and appreciated, or will it be considered meddling? How are you asked to relate to the patient? What channels of communication are preferred? Be wary of "taking over" any aspect of the patient's care unless negotiated with the referring physician. Both primary care physicians and specialists are particularly sensitive about (1) consultants who jump ahead with major diagnostic or therapeutic maneuvers or further referrals without involving the referring physician (e.g., scheduling open heart surgery, obtaining an endocrinological consultation for a problem that the primary care physician feels confident to handle), and (2) not returning patients to the referring physician ("I'll follow him for his heart problem now"). Be clear about how soon you will provide your services.

Keep Consultation Notes Brief

Consultation notes should be kept brief to allow selected reading. You may feel compelled to write out a detailed history and physical examination and an exhaustive differential diagnosis, and perhaps to summarize a long chart or to provide elaborate documentation that is not readily available in the record. Separate out these portions of the consultation note so that they are recognized as optional reading. Your note should conclude with a very brief summary, accompanied by a terse impression and specific recommendations, geared to your audience.

In general, you need not support your recommendations in detail but you should briefly indicate what information led you to your diagnosis or recommendations. You may offer a few references but do not expect them to be read. If you believe that a particular reference would be appreciated by your readers, provide a copy.

Disagreement should be handled tactfully. Sarcasm is never appropriate, and criticism should generally be avoided, though it may be implied.

Give Specific Recommendations

Unless you are absolutely sure that your colleagues know how to do a test, prescribe a drug or other treatment, arrange for a procedure, and so on, spell out your recommendations clearly.

Communicate in Person

Communicate your impressions in person as well as through a terse note. The referring physician's further questions are surest to be answered when he or she is given the opportunity to ask about them directly. Subtleties, personal issues, disagreements, and criticisms are best handled person-to-person rather than in writing. Remember that referral is often sought for support and encouragement rather than just for technical knowledge or procedures. Your success as a consultant may hinge on addressing such issues.

Follow-up

For your own education, at least a minimal amount of follow-up is required for each case. By reviewing the chart or getting a hallway progress report from the referring physician, you should ascertain whether the consultation was appreciated and followed, and whether it helped the patient and the doctor. For many other cases, you should remain in contact with the patient or at least leave the door open for further communication.

MENTAL HEALTH REFERRAL

Of patients in medical practice:
- 50% to 80% have psychological distress
- 15% to 20% have a psychiatric disorder
- Of those with a psychiatric disorder, only 50% are diagnosed by medical practitioners
- Of those diagnosed, 25% are referred to psychiatrists or mental health specialists

Referrals to psychiatrists, psychologists, psychiatric social workers, drug and alcohol counselors, and other mental health practitioners pose particular difficulties. Among patients with psychiatric problems, many neither define their illness as psychological, nor even recognize that psychological factors are playing a part. If they do acknowledge that "nerves" or emotions are contributing to their distress, they still may feel these factors are not very important, certainly not something requiring professional help. Moreover, since psychiatric disorders and treatments may be stigmatized, even a person who believes that he or she would benefit from psychological help may not want to consult a mental health specialist: "I'm not crazy, doc!" Thus recommendations for psychiatric referral are often not accepted or, if accepted initially, the patient does not arrange for or keep the appointment or stay in treatment.

Some brief, general guidelines for facilitating referral of reluctant patients are provided in this section.

Negotiating About the Problem and Its Management

When the practitioner believes a patient would benefit from specialized mental health evaluation and treatment, but the patient is reluctant to see a counselor, the referral has often been proposed prematurely. Discussion needs to be reopened about the patient's and physician's definition of the problem. The physician may recognize the necessity for a referral after a few minutes of the interview but may need several follow-up visits to complete a medical workup, understand the patient's view, develop a therapeutic alliance, effectively communicate a psychosocial assessment, and then negotiate a referral (see Quick Tips: Negotiating a Mental Health Referral).

The physician and patient need not have an identical view of the meaning of the illness. Patients may agree to referrals based on their own definition of the problem: for "nervousness" rather than hallucinations; for help

---

QUICK TIPS

Negotiating a Mental Health Referral Management

- Patients may accept a referral based on their own definition of the problem.
- Recommend a treatment to address the patient's immediate discomfort.
- Deal with the patient's resistance by exploring with him or her the reasons, practical concerns, and apparent excuses.
- If possible, offer the patient a taste of the psychotherapeutic process; then point out the benefits of continuing with a trained counselor.

---

with transportation and medical bills rather than for emotional support; for being "sensitive and upset" rather than for unrealistic fears; for "insomnia and fatigue" rather than depression; for getting a spouse to behave rather than for examining a marital relationship; or for helping one's children rather than oneself. Referrals are also most acceptable when the recommended treatment promises to address the patient's immediate discomfort.

If the patient is reluctant, address the "resistance"—patients' stated opposition to referral and those behaviors (e.g., missing an appointment) that may indirectly signal reluctance. Explore their reasons, noting both practical concerns (the inevitable "realistic" barriers to getting psychological help) and a host of apparent excuses (reflecting, for instance, inadequate motivation to change or reluctance to engage in an intimate helping relationship).

Some "realistic" resistances are issues of time, place, money, privacy, and, especially for patients who have never had counseling, the unfamiliar process of psychotherapy. These issues can often be addressed directly through explanation, discussion, and practical problem-solving (e.g., finding a nearby consultant, getting an evening appointment, requesting reduced fees, describing the evaluation procedure). Sometimes it helps to acknowledge barriers and to either credit patients for overcoming them or to encourage them to do so.

Less realistic resistances are often harder to tease out, and sometimes are brought forth only with coaxing. What kind of ideas does the patient have about the evaluation process and psychiatric treatment? For instance, if the patient says "I'm not crazy," you might ask, "What makes you think that we think you're off your rocker if you go to a shrink?" Other patients will suggest that they will be humiliated, taken advantage of sexually, "pried into," "seen through," or criticized. Take these responses as useful bits of information about how the patient views the world. Common issues that may underlie a patient's resistance (and that need to be addressed in making referrals) include abandonment by the primary physician, the stigma of mental health problems, illness as a personal weakness or failing, fear of an unknown process, what to do if one dislikes the therapist, whether talk is useless or stirs up too many disagreeable feelings, and previous bad experiences with counseling.

"Doing the First Session"

When resistance is strong, the best path is often to avoid confrontation. For patients who are good candidates for psychotherapy, a successful tactic is to "do the first session" oneself. In other words, even though the physician has enough information to make an intelligent referral, the patient needs to understand and experience the value of psychotherapy. This is accomplished by offering the patient a taste of the psychotherapeutic process—one or more long visits for further exploration of emotional problems and enjoyment of a nonjudgmental, accepting relationship. Referral then offers more of the same but better:

> It seems that you find this kind of session useful. I wonder whether you wouldn't benefit from seeing a counselor who is better trained in these matters than I and who might see you more regularly and give you more time?

The Clinician's Resistance

A final bit of resistance that needs to be addressed is your own. Asking for help from a psychiatrist or other consultant can be a blow to one's self-esteem, suggesting failure or incompetence, especially if one feels harshly scrutinized by the consultant. Referral may seem like losing a patient or losing control of the case. The referring physician's negative attitude toward mental health practitioners, however, should not be communicated to or projected upon the patient.

SUGGESTED READING

Bursztajn H, Barsky AJ: Facilitating patient acceptance of a psychiatric referral, *Arch Intern Med* 145:73, 1985.

AFTERWORD: A HISTORY OF HISTORY-TAKING*

You have now read about and practiced the medical interview. As a newly informed reader and beginning practitioner, we offer you a few final words about the history of interviewing and its place in the clinical method. We hope this brief account gives you a wider perspective on your lifetime practice of this clinical skill.

THE CLINICAL METHOD

The clinical method that is central to "doctoring" is not solely medical science. It combines, as you may have observed, both a technical and a communicative method. The technical, of course, is science-based, most evident in the new technologies for diagnosis and treatment that are derived from basic and clinical research. The communicative method—the questioning, listening, and talking of the interview—focuses on biographical knowledge of the patient and is derived from a behavioral science perspective on interpersonal relations. Both the technical and communicative methods are concerned with information from patients. The subjective, historical information emerges from the medical interview; the objective facts come from physical examination and special laboratory examinations of the body. Both kinds of information are essential for diagnosis and treatment. Thus, typically, in arriving at a diagnosis, the interview reveals the patient's complaints and suggests one or more likely causes, while examination and tests of the patient confirm or disconfirm the diagnostic hypotheses raised by the subjective report. For treatment, the interview reveals the patient's needs and perspectives, which are essential information in the choice of appropriate medical therapies, while communication about diagnosis and management makes the clinician's scientific expertise available to and usable by patients.

THE EVOLUTION OF THE MEDICAL INTERVIEW

A brief account of the history of the interview in this century illustrates that the communicative method in medicine is not a fixed, ancient, unalterable art. It has undergone profound changes analogous to the more familiar,

*This section is an abbreviated version of a longer essay of the same title: Stoeckle JD, Billings JA: A history of history-taking: The medical interview, *J Gen Intern Med* 2:119, 1987; used with permission.

publicized changes in medical technologies. In the following discussion, the evolution of history-taking is traced through medical records and modes of clinical instruction, and explicated as a reflection of the contributions of clinical and behavioral sciences and social forces to clinical practice.

The Interview as Revealed in Medical Records

To learn about doctor-patient communication, even as recently as 1900, is difficult. Only suggestive clues about the dialogue are found in old office records. Medical records, as we conceive of them today, were seldom kept, being considered unnecessary by the solo practitioner who knew and had no trouble remembering the patient, family, and illness. For the most part, the office record was a list of visits and charges contained in account ledgers or on a filing card that might also indicate the complaint, results of the physical examination, and prescriptions. Dr. William Hammock Goodson, wrote of a 1933 visit,

> Mrs. VP 9/2/33 Dislocation of right elbow in fall to floor while dancing. Reduced under Ethyl Chloride, and put in sling. X-ray made and showed no break of any bones in arm. Services $15.00 Rec'd on account $1.00.

These office notes of doctors reveal little of what the conversation may have been.

Fortunately, hospital records contained a more detailed recording. Throughout the nineteenth century, institutional records consisted of two parts—the history of illness and the physical examination—two basic components of medical diagnosis. The history described the present illness, focusing on bodily complaints, but it also contained at the least a one-line personal identification, noting the patient's occupation, sometimes a report of habits, (smoking or drinking), and then a note on sickness and death in the family. These were the first elements of a brief biography. Illustrating this clinical method, a history and physical examination from Richard C. Cabot's *Case Teaching in Medicine* (1906) reads:

> The patient is a married woman, age 34, large and fat in person. She has had two children and three miscarriages, the last 6 weeks ago. Otherwise, she says her health has always been good, until within 3 or 4 months; has been in the habit of drinking beer freely, but has not been intemperate. For 2 weeks there has been pronounced jaundice, anorexia, and bilious vomiting soon after eating; dizziness, flatulence, occasional diarrhea with pain at epigastrum; slight edema of feet and ankles. These symptoms have been increasing. There has been no headache and no hemorrhages or chills. The tongue was clean, the pulse 80, temperature 97.8. The heart and lungs were normal. The liver much enlarged and smooth. The spleen was felt below the ribs. There was no ascites. The urine had a sp. gr. of 1017, was of a deep yellow color, and contained a trace of albumin and much bile; sediment normal. The blood was negative.

From this hospital record, the interview appears to have consisted of a brief personal inquiry and an interrogation about bodily complaints. For diagnosis, the history of physical complaints was most important. In those early decades of the 1900s, diagnosis was based on the logic of internal consistency rather than on today's confirmation by "lab tests" with their sensitivities and specificities. Thus the history of bodily distress and the physical examination provided the essential data (clues) from which the doctor, like a medical sleuth, could clinically reason (deduce) the diagnosis of the patient's disease, comparing its symptoms and signs for their consistency with previously known cases.

Eventually, history-taking was expected to provide more personal and social information in addition to bodily complaints. As Physician to Out-Patients around the turn of this century, Cabot expanded the inquiry, arguing for inclusion of detailed facts about the patient's background. The additional information would assure more accurate—indeed more scientific—diagnosis, since illness, as in the Hippocratic view, developed out of the entire life of the individual and therefore was always social-psychological, certainly not medical alone. To accommodate the personal and social information, the recorded history was gradually standardized into those topics familiar today as chief complaint, history of present illness, past medical history, family history, and social history. These five items constituted the "complete history"— complete because it contained more than the medical facts alone. The wide adoption of the case method of teaching made these topical divisions a common format for recording.

This recording format for the hospital chart remained essentially unchanged until the 1970s, when Lawrence Weed argued for a reordering of information by *problems,* the separation of "subjective" and "objective" components, and the reframing of the diagnosis and treatment as "assessment" and "plan." Such a revision would make the record (and presumably the clinical process) more scientific and accountable. Moreover, ordering information into problems would ensure that unexplained complaints and test results were registered for continuing evaluation.

Instruction as Demonstration-Supervision, 1900 to 1940s

Despite longtime pedagogical praise of the value of careful history-taking, instructional texts were not written on how to do it. Teaching in the first four decades of this century was an oral exercise, a demonstration, and later, a supervision. History-taking was first shown at the bedside by senior clinicians who "took the patient's story," and was then imitated (or not) by students as they "worked-up" patients alone on the hospital wards and in outpatient clinics. In the language of educational theory, the students learned from role models.

As today, instruction also included the student's bedside presentation of a summarized history to senior staff who might then quiz the student about the particulars of the account and, in turn, question the patient again in the student's presence, verifying the consistency of the report and perhaps eliciting more or different facts. In effect, such presentation and review provided supervision of history-taking, a pedagogical method that was indirect because the student was never observed eliciting the patient's story. Direct supervision by viewing and listening to the student's history-taking at the bedside or in the clinic office was rare, presumably so as not to intrude on the privacy of the student-patient relationship. The student was learning how to take a history but also how to form an alliance and how to begin exercising therapeutic responsibility, both of which might be impaired by the presence of the older instructor, a "real," and often "private," doctor, whom the patient might prefer and seek for continuing care outside the teaching clinic.

Even though clinicians during this period did not publish how-to-do texts on history-taking, suggestions on what questions to ask did appear in three sources. First, in texts on physical diagnosis, an outline of the history might be appended, making up 5 to 10 pages of a 400-page volume. Such texts listed topics for interrogation on the several anatomical organ systems. Second, history questions also appeared in instructional manuals for students in courses on the clinical method. While such manuals did not list questions, they noted topics to explore about illnesses and bodily functions. They included a family and social history, thus indicating that an interview should produce facts that might explain sources of emotional distress and the hereditary basis of medical disorders, while also providing information about the patient as a person. As today, the assumption was that "learning what the patient is like" would facilitate personal care; the doctor who "knows the patient" could tailor treatment to the individual. A third source for learning what to ask was the textbook of medicine. Since these publications described the characteristic symptoms and signs of medical disorders, they could, of course, be implicit guides to useful questions.

While these three types of publications were early guides to questions, they did not address *process* skills: how to ask questions and evoke responses, or how to listen, talk, and explain. Eventually, of course, texts and articles on the process of history-taking did appear, stimulated by the following influences: fresh ideas out of psychiatry; the social, behavioral, and communication sciences; information derived from audio and video recording of doctor-patient encounters; and by pressure on the doctor-patient relationship from social changes exterior to the profession. The contributions from psychiatry and the emerging social science disciplines added new content and new modes of questioning and responding, while modern recording technology brought modern pedagogical tactics.

Psychiatry: History-Taking as Interviewing, 1940s

In the 1940s the first systematic instruction in how to do history-taking began as psychiatrists were invited to join the staffs of general hospitals. The invitation came after psychiatrists successfully collaborated with medical colleagues during World War II. Psychiatrists brought their wartime experience with soldiers under stress and their skills in office psychotherapy to the care of medical patients and to the instruction of students. Moreover, these clinicians used audiotaped interviews to analyze the process of history-taking, and they described how best to question, comment, and listen. For example, after reviewing the transcribed interviews of psychiatric residents, Felix Deutch and William F. Murphy wrote their classic text, *The Clinical Interview* (1954).

They noted:

> If the examiner allows him [the patient] to talk without asking leading questions . . . the patient will usually give a detailed account of his complaints and ideas about his illness.

They suggested:

> The examiner waits until he feels that the patient will not continue spontaneously, and he repeats one of the points in the patient's last sentence in interrogative form . . . The patient then as a rule gives new information centering around his symptoms and is stimulated to further associations.

This method of "associative exploration," which stimulates self-disclosure about emotional factors, was soon taught to medical students and residents. Even earlier, Jacob Finesinger and Florence Powdermaker had developed instructional films for the Veterans Administration to teach "psychotherapeutic interviewing," which included recognition of nonverbal behaviors. The doctor was advised to be "minimally active" by using open-ended questioning, similar to the associative format of Deutch and Murphy. In effect, the psychoanalytical technique of encouraging free association was transferred to the medical inquiry.

Films of office psychiatry, new equivalents of bedside teaching demonstrations, could be shown to audiences distant from the actual encounter. More significant, history-taking was transformed. No longer a rote interrogation, history-taking became a recognized clinical skill—medical interviewing—whereby it was acknowledged that the doctor and the patient engage in a complex interpersonal process involving a variety of communication techniques and behaviors.

In redefining history taking as medical interviewing, psychiatrists were eager to demonstrate that psychological factors invariably accompanied physical disease. The adoption of nondirective questioning would not only elicit bodily complaints and biographies but also reveal psychological components of illness, namely details about the patient's personality (such as defenses), relationships (such as conflicts), and emotional reactions (such as depression, grief, shame, guilt, anger) that might influence the course of disease, if not bring it on. The medical practitioner was now expected to obtain information for both psychological diagnosis and psychological treatment; the encounter, in turn, was expected to be psychotherapeutic.

Social Science: Interviewing by Questionnaire, 1950s

At the same time that psychiatrists were teaching about interviewing, social scientists, working outside of medical practice, studied how to question the public about its opinions. In their survey research in the field, social scientists sampled the public and then wrote "how-to-do-it" books, for example, *Interviewing, Its Forms and Functions* by Richardson, Dohrenwend, and Klein, and *The Art of Asking Questions* by Payne. These texts noted that only slightly different wording and construction of questions could produce different answers, anticipating recent clinical-decision studies on the same theme. In trying to make the interview a valid scientific "instrument" for measurement, social scientists searched for and observed interview bias in their field workers, similar to the way psychiatrists noted transference and countertransference in the office encounter. Increasing sophistication in surveying by telephone, questionnaire, and field interviews had little direct influence on teaching medical students how to do face-to-face interrogation in the office. Yet today's use of patient-administered history questionnaires, which are presumed to save the doctor time, may have been influenced by four decades of opinion surveys. The public became readily accustomed to filling out forms, such as a checklist medical history—a set of silent, unattended questions, self-administered in the waiting room, that might make the unobserved patient less ashamed of self-disclosure, while giving the doctor shortcuts for the interview. Later, detailed history questionnaires were also administered by computers. On initial use, patients found the computer encounter as acceptable as (or even preferable to) talking with a real doctor; however, the printout overloaded the doctor with details that did not require medical attention.

Behavioral Sciences: Learning Interpersonal Skills away from the Office and Bedside, 1970s

Under a new rubric the social sciences eventually did directly influence interview instruction. Since the 1970s, clinical and social psychologists, who were now referred to as behavioral scientists, along with new communication specialists, were brought into teaching medical clinics and family practice centers to instruct on the conduct of the interview and on counseling techniques. These behavioral science teachers aimed to improve the student's counseling skills and appreciation of interpersonal and linguistic processes in the doctor-patient discourse. Thus instruction was not only about questioning for diagnosis but, once again, explicitly included elements of psychotherapy that had been previously researched by psychologists in educational settings. "Unconditional regard," "empathy," and "genuineness" were now to be *learned* as essential interpersonal communicative behaviors in medical settings.

Moreover, the interview was to be more cooperative and the patient's role more participatory. Behavioral scientists were influenced by the social psychologist Kurt Lewin, who had argued that democratic relations in groups were valuable to the individual. He also had observed in studies of working groups that decisions were more effective when achieved with participation. More recent writers have concluded that information transmittal enhances patient involvement, thus fostering a doctor-patient relationship of mutual participation that is particularly useful in the management of chronic illness.

The behavioral scientists also transformed and relocated the instruction itself. Interpersonal skills, such as empathy, were taught in classrooms away from the office and bedside. Students now role-played patient or doctor, or interviewed "simulated" or "standardized" patients (e.g., actresses and actors with specific scripts about an illness). In simulated encounters, students could rehearse communication skills while being directly observed or videotaped; later they could review and explain their performances in small peer groups with instructors. Classroom interview training was distinct from the demonstration-supervision with patients on the wards and in the clinics. These distanced methods permitted the student's lines and poses to be acted out, observed, prompted, and critiqued by the student and instructor safely away from the stress of a real performance in the "theater" of the medical office.

Supervision was also considerably enhanced. Previously, medical students had reported their encounters with patients from memory, notes, and case records. The analysis of the interaction, based on students' own self-reports and self-appraisals—an "interpersonal process recall"—helped them learn about themselves and about the patient too. Recall became distinctive when a videotape replay of the actual discourse and the behaviors of both doctor and patient were used to stimulate self- and group-reflection. Videotape replay displayed textual facts about what the patient, the doctor, and the illness, taken together, were like. The recording could be a "text" for teaching behavioral sciences in medicine, where, for example, manifestations of ethnicity and social class could be heard, observed, and discussed. Moreover, the nonverbal behaviors of doctor and patient, previously described by linguists, were also readily recognized on videotape in the 1980s. These behaviors could be studied to better understand the patient, the interviewer, or the dynamics of the encounter itself, adding still another instructional dimension.

Communication Sciences: From Medical Advice to Patient Education, 1980s

As previously noted, instruction traditionally focused only on medical information-gathering, but later included psychological diagnosis and treatment. Today, instruction has expanded still further to include the communication of information about illness, namely patient *education,* a function previously taken for granted as *medical advice.*

The segment of the clinical encounter that typically comes after the physical examination—the communication about diagnosis, treatment, prognosis, and prevention—became a new pedagogical focus. Information transmittal was now defined as patient education, a concept that alters the dynamics of the doctor-patient exchange. Education requires "feedback" from patients on the nature and quality of their understanding, a reciprocity quite unlike the one-way, authoritarian direction often expected by doctors and patients in the past. In the particular instance of "informed consent," the doctor is required not only to inform but also to discuss risks and benefits—information that was previously transmitted according to practitioners' judgments of patients' need to know.

Secular Changes

In recent years a number of new topics have been introduced into the routine history, while old interview topics, particularly sexuality and substance abuse, have been both reemphasized and reframed. Sexuality is explored more often for a variety of reasons: increased openness about sex on the part of patients and doctors, changing sexual behaviors and new patterns of sexually transmitted disease, wider recognition of sexual dissatisfaction in the everyday psychological distress presented to the doctor, and a greater concern about sexual performance and satisfaction of the disabled as they strive for normalization in society. Similarly, drug and alcohol abuse are increasingly recognized as producing serious medical and psychological disorders, and systematic inquiry about these behaviors is promoted with the hope of improving problem recognition and treatment.

Like sexuality and substance abuse, other topics are more readily disclosed now than in the past, though still are not easily confronted by students and physicians. Talking about "death and dying," for instance, has become less taboo, especially as the profession and the public have recognized that physical comfort and psychosocial support for the terminally ill and the bereaved require such discussion. More recently, attention to patients' preferences with regard to resuscitation—the Do Not Resuscitate (DNR) status—has opened new discussions about the usefulness of various interventions for persons facing life-threatening illness. Attention to patients' choices in lifesaving treatment has become a regular feature of the clinical interview at the bedside and office.

In addition to the elicitation of information about drinking, drugs, sex, and now dying, old mundane inquiries about eating, exercise, and smoking—topics that had long been a part of the history of personal habits—have acquired new importance as behavioral risk factors for cardiovascular disease and cancer. Preventive medicine and techniques for motivating patients to care better for themselves have increasingly become a part of the physician's practice. The doctor's traditional medical or moral advice about healthy lifestyles has been transformed into behavioral counseling.

THE INTERVIEW AND THE IDEOLOGY OF TODAY'S RELATIONSHIP

The medical interview has been gradually transformed by reforms from within and outside the profession. These many changes in the medical interview (as taught, if not practiced) also transmit an ideology of what today's doctor-patient relationship should be, not unlike our notions of the proper care of children or the right conduct of everyday human relations. Such beliefs about the proper doctor-patient relation may not be explicitly addressed but are evident in the material of current interviewing texts and in the behaviors of clinical instructors, medical students, and practitioners. While textbooks may claim only to instruct about clinical skills, astute readers will recognize that they also contain unstated notions which define what the doctor-patient relationship should be like. Similarly, clinical instructors address the relationship inadvertently, for example, as they demonstrate respect for patients regardless of class, race, gender, age, ethnicity, or how "undesirable" the patient seems. Likewise, students and practitioners are defining the proper relationship insofar as they attend to the patient's perspective and attempt to tailor care to the individual. When relationships of all kinds—between students and teachers, women and men, clients and professionals, consumers and institutions—have been criticized for their unequal exchange, the inequality between patients and doctors is also addressed by instructors, medical students, and practitioners who promote (while laypersons seek) more patient participation in the politics of the relationship and more autonomy in decision-making.

Looking ahead, technology is changing our communication with patients. Our attention in this text has been on face-to-face encounters, in the hospital with those sick in bed, in the office with those seeking and returning for medical help. These traditional face-to-face encounters remain, but other options for listening and talking are coming: (1) e-mail between patient and doctor, (2) then, beyond the telephone, televideo for monitoring the home-based disabled (or even for neighborhood residents for seeking advice), (3) computerized transmittal of laboratory results by phone, and of course, (4) Internet where, on questioning, advice can come from doctor to patients on what is known and what to do.

Today's ideology for the doctor-patient relationship can be characterized as follows:

An Ideal Doctor-Patient Relationship

- Make the relationship more democratic by giving patients choices in decisions about the scope of diagnosis and the alternatives of treatment
- Develop patient participation in the relationship by transmitting appropriate information about illness and treatment, enabling patients to make choices
- Negotiate with patients about their requests and choices; similarly, acknowledge and negotiate conflict, even if in the relationship itself
- Attend to patients' feelings about illnesses and treatment and respond to their feelings with positive regard, genuine concern, and empathy

- Provide helping actions by eliciting, acknowledging, and responding to patients' own perspectives on their illness and care
- Convey respect to patients without regard to their class, gender, sexual orientation, race, ethnicity, or age
- Promote health education, self-help, and preventive behaviors by communicating information about diagnosis, treatment, health maintenance, and prevention and by helping with behavioral change
- Be self-reflective in the acts of questioning, listening, and talking to learn from one's personal responses, and, in turn, to modulate one's own feelings and prejudices in responding to patients

These several behaviors define today's doctor-patient relationship, reflecting old and new values that are social, psychological, ethical, and even religious. While such guidelines suggest how today's doctors and patients should behave, either person may diverge from these prescriptive ideals or find that one ideal conflicts with another. For instance, the doctor who responds vigorously to a conviction about the importance of patient education is at risk of either transmitting so much information that the patient is overwhelmed or of providing information different from what the patient desires. Similarly, the doctor who seeks to encourage patient autonomy in decision-making will encounter patients who do not want to participate and who would rather have the physician decide. Respectful treatment might require that the practitioner take charge without exploring further the patient's feelings or values. In these and other instances, the good relationship, as in the past and in the future, means accommodation by both the doctor and the patient.

SUGGESTED READING
Lipkin M, Quill TE, Napodano RJ: The medical interview: a core curriculum for residencies in internal medicine, *Ann Intern Med* 100:277, 1984.

COMPLETE CASE WRITE-UP

Early in your clinical training, you will be required to prepare "complete write-ups." These detailed case presentations are intended as pedagogical exercises rather than as models for notes in the patient's chart. They help you to become familiar with the entire history and physical findings and with the phrases that describe normal as well as abnormal findings. Also, your preparation of an elaborate note on the present illness assists you in learning differential diagnosis.

In actual clinical practice, conciseness and brevity are highly valued in both oral and written presentations. You will learn how portions of a detailed and exhaustive history and physical findings can be condensed, abbreviated, or omitted. The following example, however, is meant to show you a relatively "complete" write-up.

Mark Proust
MGH #345-16-22
4 April 1992

This 46-year-old white, male, married accountant presents for a "complete checkup" after being told he had high blood pressure at a worksite screening program last week.

HPI

#1 Hypertension

In the past 10 years, during office visits for colds, the patient has been told that he had slightly elevated blood pressure. Since he was feeling well, he never sought follow-up care. Blood pressure of 160/100 was noted 8 years ago at the employee health service. Records from the worksite screening program on 1 April 1992 indicate blood pressure of 150/110 and 168/100.

His father, age 69, has angina and hypertension. His brother, age 39, was recently begun on a "water pill" for hypertension, and his sister, age 36, is said to have had high blood pressure during her last pregnancy.

The patient has enjoyed generally excellent health and recalls no complete checkups since discharge from the army 22 years ago. He has no history of nephritis, kidney disease or infection, or protein in the urine, nor does he note polyuria, nocturia, or polydipsia. He denies palpitations, paroxysmal, headaches, postural dizziness, or excess perspiration. He reports no weight gain, easy bruising, fatigue, muscle weakness, or emotional lability. He does not drink alcohol regularly or drink caffeinated beverages.

He denies any history to suggest angina, CHF, CVA, or intermittent claudication. There is no family history of diabetes, hyperlipidemia, or early cardiovascular disease. He has never been obese, nor has he smoked cigarettes. He plays tennis at least once a week and has never had a sedentary life-style.

PMH

Hospitalizations: 1955 T&A, Wellesley Hospital

1959 Appendectomy, Wellesley Hospital

Illnesses: Usual childhood diseases; no rheumatic fever.

Hay fever, Asthma—Notes mild wheezing, rhinorrhea, and itchy eyes during spring and early summer since age 9. Some years, he has mild tightness in his chest with nonproductive cough, wheezing, and mild DOE. He never obtained medical attention such as emergency ward visits, prescription medication, or allergy testing. He denies paroxysmal attacks or interference with or precipitation by exercise. He uses various over-the-counter preparations—pills but not sprays or inhalants. No nasal polyps, aspirin sensitivity. No sinusitis, bronchitis, chronic cough, pleurisy, pneumonia, hemoptysis, TB. Family history ⊕ for asthma (mother, son) and eczema (son).

No heart problems, cancer, diabetes, ulcer.

Medications: Seasonal use of over-the-counter pills for asthma, hay fever; occasional Tylenol; multivitamin 1 qd.

Allergies: None known to food or medications, but see Hay fever, Asthma in PMH.

Habits: Cigarettes—never smoked.

EtOH—two to three beers or glasses of wine only at occasional parties.

CAGE test negative.

Recreational drugs—none.

Exposures: None known to toxic chemicals, dusts, radiation.

Travel: None outside Massachusetts.

Diet: See #1 Hypertension. No attention to cholesterol, salt, or weight maintenance.

Health maintenance: No routine medical, dental care.

Full childhood immunizations and recent tetanus booster;

No Pneumovax or flu vaccine.

Uses smoke detectors, no seat belts.

Exercise: see #1 Hypertension.

Family planning—wife had tubal ligation.

SH

Mr. Proust grew up in Wellesley, where he completed high school. He served in the Army for 2 years and then attended junior college and became an accountant. He initially worked for a large Boston firm, but now shares a private office with two partners in Allston. He is happy with his work and his associates and is satisfied with his financial security. He describes himself as competitive, impatient, and harassed by a sense of time urgency.

He has been married for 18 years and has two sons. His wife is a homemaker and part-time secretary. She and the children enjoy good health. He describes his family life as satisfying, though his oldest son has recently done poorly in high school and bickers excessively with his mother. Otherwise, he denies recent unusual stresses.

He and his wife enjoy dancing and tennis in their free time. Vacations are spent traveling by car and camping out.

Insurance: BC/BS Master Medical.

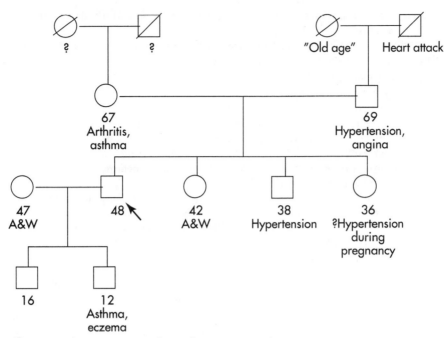

⊕ Angina, hypertension, asthma, degenerative arthritis

⊖ DM

ROS

Constitutional —Good general health, energy
—No fevers, sweats, weight change, fatigue.
Skin—No rash, pruritus, bruising, change in hair or nails
—Notes no change in "mole" on his forearm.
Head—Rare headaches; no dizziness, trauma.
Eyes—No irritation, change in vision, diplopia, other visual disturbances.
—Wears glasses for driving × 10 years; no change in prescription from optometry check last year.
Ears—Acuity good; no tinnitus, pain, discharge.
Nose—No epistaxis; see Hay fever.
Mouth—No sores, dental problems, difficulty swallowing, sore throat, hoarseness;
Teeth in good repair; sees dentist annually.
Resp—See Asthma in PMH.
CVS—No history murmur, palpitations, PND, orthopnea, edema, calf pain on exertion.
GI—No anorexia, N, V, indigestion, gas, heartburn, food intolerance, pain, jaundice, hepatitis, change in color or frequency of stool, melena, hemorrhoids, rectal bleeding.
GU—No dysuria, hematuria, stones, polyuria, nocturia, penile sores, VD, sexual difficulties, testicular pain or swelling, hernia.
Extremities—No pain or stiffness, swelling, deformity; no phlebitis, varicosities.

Neuro—Normal smell, taste, speech, strength, sensation; no paresthesias, fainting, seizures.

Mental status—No nervousness, depression, difficulty sleeping, change in memory.

Endocrine—No heat or cold intolerance.

Physical examination

p 76 reg; R 18, unlabored; Weight 162, no shoes

BP	small cuff	L arm 178/115	R arm 176/112	sitting
	large cuff	L arm 165/104	R arm 168/102	lying
	large cuff	L arm 168/106	R arm 170/104	standing
	thigh cuff		R arm 176/106	sitting

General appearance—Healthy-looking, muscular man, appearing stated age.

Skin—Clear except for R forearm:

1.1-cm irregularly pigmented (brown, tan, blue, black) flat lesion; smooth borders except slight irregularity at inferior aspect

No other unusual moles, rash. Hair distribution and texture normal.

Nails normal. No striae, ecchymoses.

Head—Normocephalic, atraumatic.

No moon facies.

Eyes—Conjunctivae clear, anicteric; no proptosis, lid-lag; PERRLA, EOM full, no nystagmus. No arcus. Reads near card 20/30 R & L with glasses. Fields full to confrontation. Fundi: media clear; A:V ratio 1:2, minimal AV nicking; no hemorrhages, exudates, arteriolar thickening. Discs flat.

Ears—No tophi. Canal clear, TMs normal light reflex. Hears watch tick at 2 inches.

Nose—Septum midline, intact. Membranes normal; no polyps, discharge, sinus tenderness.

Mouth—Lips and membranes unremarkable. Teeth in good repair. Tongue well papillated. Pharynx benign, no tonsils.

Neck—Supple, full ROM. Thyroid palpable, smooth, small.

Trachea midline.

No buffalo hump.

Nodes—No palpable cervical, supraclavicular, axillary, inguinal nodes.

Cor—JVP 5 cm Carotids 2+, normal upstroke, no bruit.

PMI 5th intercostal space, midclavicular line, well localized; no heave, thrust, S1 normal intensity. A2 > P2, split physiologically. Quiet S4 at lower left sternal border.

No S3, click, murmur, rub.

Breasts—No gynecomastia, tenderness.

Lungs—Thorax symmetrical; no increased AP diameter or use of accessory muscles. 4- to 5-cm diaphragmatic excursions bilaterally.

Normal to percussion.

Clear to auscultation—no rales, rhonchi, rubs. Forced expiration produces no wheezing.

Abd—Flat, soft, nontender with active bowel sounds in four quadrants. Liver percusses 10 cm in midclavicular line; no hepatosplenomegaly, mass, CVA tenderness, ascites. No widened aorta. No bruits, including both CVA.

GU—Normal male genitalia, circumcised. No scrotal mass, inguinal hernia.

Rectal—No hemorrhoids, fissure. Normal rectal tone. Prostate small; no mass. Stool soft, brown, guaiac negative.

Ext—Pulses   R   L

	R	L
Fem	2+	2+ no radiofemoral delay
DP	2+	2+
PT	2+	2+
Cap filling	5 to 6 sec	5 sec

No cyanosis, clubbing, edema, varicosities, cords.

Neuro—CNS

I not tested.

II acuity, fields—see Eyes

III, IV, VI EOM intact.

V facial sensation and corneal reflex intact, jaw strength good.

VII symmetrical expression.

VIII see Ears.

IX, X uvula midline; gag, phonation normal.

XI shrug good.

XII tongue midline.

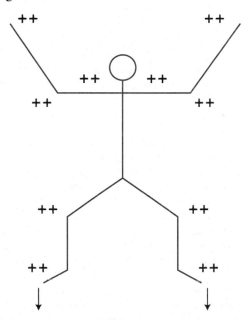

DTRs

Strength: grasp, shoulder strength good; walks on heels and toes.

Sensation: position, vibration, sharp-dull in lower extremities intact.

Coord: FTN, HTS, alternating hand motion intact.

Gait unremarkable. Romberg not tested.

Tremor, asterixis negative.

Mental status—alert, oriented, appropriate, normal affect. Higher cognitive functions not tested.

Lab

Pending

Assessment and plan

#1 Hypertension, essential

There are no symptoms or signs to suggest a primary illness producing hypertension (e.g., renal disease, pheochromocytoma, Cushing's, aldosteronism). The positive family history and evidence of long-standing, mild blood pressure elevation also favor the diagnosis of essential hypertension. There is no evidence of end-organ damage, though the S4 and mild AV nicking are noteworthy. No co-risk factors for cardiovascular disease are identified, though he may be "Type A."

A few tests to screen for renal or adrenal corticosteroid abnormalities will be suggested, as well as an ECG and chest x-ray to assess cardiac disease, and fasting blood studies for hyperglycemia and hyperlipidemia. We will also measure his calcium and uric acid before diuretic therapy.

Plan

Dx—CBC, FBS, cholesterol, HDL, triglycerides (12-hr fasting), lytes, calcium, uric acid, BUN

—Urinalysis

—ECG

—CXR PA/lat

—Set aside time at next visit for further evaluation of possible Type A personality.

Rx—To Nutritionist to evaluate salt intake, instruct on moderate salt restriction (5 gm) and potassium supplementation, and counsel on reduction in dietary cholesterol. Will be seen with wife, who does most of the cooking.

—Pending lab work, begin hydrochlorothiazide 50 mg po qam (with orange juice or banana) #60 Refill × 5.

Pt ed—Discuss asymptomatic nature of hypertension, its dangers

—Review medication regimen, side effects

—Review need for long-term follow-up and treatment

—Advised not to discontinue Rx without discussing with M.D.

—Advise hypertension screening for relatives

—Advise continuing routine aerobic exercise

—We will want to monitor his blood pressure during allergy season (see #2), since over-the-counter medications may affect it

—Follow-up appointment, 3 weeks, with physician assistant, Ms. Matthews.

#2 Hay fever, Asthma—seasonal, mild

The patient is satisfied with his sporadic use of over-the-counter preparations and seems to have no significant disability from his condition.

Plan

Rx—Nonprescription preparations per patient.

Pt ed—Discuss avoidance of allergens and lung irritants, and possible usefulness of medical attention and prescription drugs if symptoms are troublesome or if he develops purulent bronchitis.

#3 Pigmented lesion, right forearm

Probable benign nevus, but has a few disturbing features: slightly irregular coloration and borders.

Plan

Dx—To Dermatology.

Pt ed—Advise on probable benign nature but need for definitive diagnosis, possible biopsy.

#4 Health maintenance

The patient is advised, per #1, on diet and exercise, and will obtain some screening tests. His regular visits for blood pressure checks will be supplemented periodically with further health assessment, physical examination, stool guaiac cards, and reminder to use seat belts.

Plan

Dx—see #1.

Pt ed—Discuss routine care.

Walter Cannon

HMS 2

SAMPLE PROBLEM LIST

INTERNAL MEDICINE ASSOCIATES
MASTER PROBLEM LIST
1992

| Mark PROUST |
| #345 16 22 |

Consultants:
Advance directives:

Problem Number	Date Onset	ACTIVE PROBLEM	RESOLVED
1		HEALTH MAINTENANCE	
2	1982	Hypertension, essential +FH	
	1992	Begin treatment	
3	1955	Seasonal rhinitis Asthma, mild, intermittent	

Date	Temporary, Old, and Inactive Problems
1955	T&A
1959	Appendectomy
4/92	Mole right forearm

Allergies, Adverse Reactions

Basic Outpatient Medical History Form

PATIENT PROFILE AND REASON FOR VISIT

HISTORY OF PRESENT ILLNESS

PAST MEDICAL HISTORY

Hospitalizations, Operations, Injuries
Pregnancies
Serious Illnesses
Medications
Allergies
Habits   Tobacco   Alcohol   Recreational drugs (IVDA)
Exposures (including occupational, family violence/abuse, and travel)

HEALTH MAINTENANCE

Physical examination	Dental care	Vision	Hearing
Pelvic/Pap	Mammogram	BSE/TSE	DES (1938-71)
Diet	Cholesterol		Guaiac/sigmoidoscopy
Exercise			
Immunizations	Last Td	Pneumovax	Annual flu shot
Seat belts	Guns in house	Other injury prevention	
Family planning			
STD	AIDS risk		
Ca++ supplementation		Hormone replacement	
Advanced Directives		Health care proxy	

SOCIAL HISTORY

FAMILY HISTORY

REVIEW OF SYSTEMS

Criteria for Case Write-ups*

1. STANDARD FORMAT

The "complete" write-up† consists of the following:

Patient demographic data (name, hospital number)

Date and Title (identifying writer)

Headline Sentence

    Patient profile (age, sex, marital status, occupation, and major medical conditions)

    Reason for the visit or chief complaint (usually includes the duration of the complaint)

Source (if other than patient) **and Reliability** (if questionable)

History of Present Illness (HPI)

The Standard Data Base

  Past Medical History (PMH)

    Hospitalizations, Operations, Injuries

    Pregnancies

    Serious Illnesses

    Medications

    Allergies, Adverse Reactions

    Habits (alcohol, tobacco, recreational drugs)

    Exposures (including occupational, family violence, and travel)

    Health Maintenance

      Routine medical/dental care, including Pap smear

      Mammogram, breast self-exam; menopausal hormones and calcium

      Diet, lipids, exercise

      Immunizations, including childhood immunizations, tetanus, influenza vaccine, and pneumonia vaccine

      Risks for injury, including use of seat belts, guns in house

      Family planning, STD counseling, HIV prevention

      Advance care planning

    Social History (SH)

    Family History (FH)

    Review of Systems (ROS)

---

*Many clinicians and educators at Harvard Medical School contributed to this section, but particularly LuAnn Wilkerson and Elizabeth Armstrong.

†The requirements for "completeness" change over the course of training, so the student and preceptor must continually redefine the scope of the write-up.

Physical Examination (PE)
Hospital Course
Assessment, including Problem List
Plan
   Diagnostic
   Therapeutic
   Patient Education
Signature, Printed Name, Year in medical school

The HPI and SH are generally written in prose, whereas the PMH and FH are usually presented in a tabular format with headings, subheadings, and so on. The FH may also be presented as a genogram. A problem-oriented format is desirable in the history of the present illness and the assessment. *A number of alternative formats are acceptable, but they should include the above information and be used consistently.*

---

2. CLARITY OF WRITING

- The case presentation is legible, grammatical, and correctly spelled.
- The writing is lucid and succinct.
- The layout mirrors the organizational outline of the write-up, facilitating reading or scanning.
  - *OWRAAU (only widely recognized abbreviations are used).*
  - *Medicines are noted with their chemical or generic names; brand names may be included in parentheses. Look up the correct spelling of unfamiliar drugs.*
  - *Events are dated in terms that are meaningful to future readers (e.g., "4 days before admission" rather than "last Thursday").*
  - *Descriptive terms are meaningful and fresh (e.g., "thin, stooped, frail"); hackneyed phrases (e.g., "well-nourished, well-developed") are avoided.*

---

3. DATA ACQUISITION: ACCURACY, PRECISION, COMPLETENESS

- The write-up accurately reflects the data acquired in the interview.
- Data acquired from persons other than the patient or from the medical record are properly attributed.
- Acknowledgement of an interpreter's assistance is noted.
- Each category and subcategory of the standard history and physical examination is addressed.
  - *The constraints of time and setting may justify an abbreviated work-up in which less essential data are omitted. When necessary, set priorities for what information must be collected now and what may be acquired later.*

- Symptoms, signs, and other historical data are completely and clearly characterized (see, for example, the sections on clarification, precision, and characterizing the symptom).
  - *All the relevant "dimensions" of a symptom are reported.*
  - *Terms reported by patients or others are not taken at face value. Vague descriptions are clarified. When patients use medical vocabulary or previous diagnoses, appropriate clinical data are elicited to justify applying such terms. Don't say a patient has "angina"; describe the symptom.*
  - *Rather than writing, "No other significant health problems" or "otherwise in good health," indicate specifically what you inquired about. Include pertinent "negatives": "No chest pain or shortness of breath."*
  - *Medications are fully and accurately recorded: dose, timing, route, other directions.*
  - *Omissions in data acquisition are acknowledged.*

---

4. PRESENTATION OF DATA: ORGANIZATION AND CLINICAL REASONING

- The history of the present illness provides a thorough, coherent, and logical story of the illness.
- The following criteria are met:
  - *Symptoms are described fully, precisely, and logically.*
  - *The chronology of events is clear.*
  - *All data germane to understanding the patient's problem are noted, including "pertinent negatives" and relevant portions of the standard data base. You do not need to include information the patient thinks is relevant if you find it irrelevant. Parts of the SH, FH, or ROS may be included in the HPI and either duplicated in the later section or acknowledged in the later section with "See HPI."*
  - *The organization reflects an appreciation of how clinical data are used to solve the problem posed by the patient and thus reveals thought and study about the case.*
  - *The history of the present illness addresses not only the patient's major problem, but also other active problems.*
  - *Similarly, the presentation of the physical examination reveals extra attention to positive and negative findings relevant to the differential diagnosis.*
  - *Each section and subsection of the history, physical, assessment, and plan includes only the information appropriate to that part of the write-up.*
  - *In the history and physical examination, data are presented in a precise, objective manner, allowing the reader to arrive at his or her own conclusion about the significance of findings. The clinician's*

impressions—inferences about the data—are presented in the assessment.

---

5. PATIENT AS A PERSON

- The write-up provides a sense of the patient as a person and reflects an awareness of pertinent psychosocial issues. *Make the patient come alive.*
- Psychosocial data may be presented in the headline, history of present illness, social history, mental status, or other portions of the write-up. The history of the present illness generally includes the patient's perspective (e.g., attributions, requests), disability or functional status (how the symptoms have affected the patient's life), how the patient has responded emotionally, and pertinent social history.

---

6. ASSESSMENT

- The Problem List identifies all major issues in patient care (though discussion may be limited to a few major problems).
- The Problem List demonstrates:
  - *An appreciation of priorities*
  - *Interrelationship of problems*
  - *Responsiveness to preventive health issues*
- The discussion addresses the clinical significance of major problems.
  - *The assessment generally includes an identification of the major historical and physical findings.*
  - *A summary statement is often useful.*
  - *As students become more familiar with pathophysiology, the write-up demonstrates awareness of basic disease mechanisms and of clinical approaches to diagnosis and management.*
  - *The assessment does not merely reflect what the student should have known immediately after obtaining supervision from his or her preceptor; it reflects both thought about the case and further study.*
  - *References to relevant sections of clinical texts or journals are desirable.*

---

7. FORMULATION OF A PLAN

- Plans include diagnostic efforts, therapy, and patient education. Where indicated, attention is directed to preventive medicine and follow-up.
  - *Students at early stages of training are not expected to formulate an assessment or a detailed, appropriate plan. However, at a minimum, any plans decided upon by the preceptor are recorded accurately, and the student attempts to outline an approach for major problems.*

- *Since students regularly omit important data from their history and physical examinations but are only aware of the omission after further study and preparation of the write-up, this section includes an indication of what further basic information would ideally have been collected.*

8. PROMPTNESS

- Write-ups should be submitted within 48 hours after the patient is evaluated. In many clinical settings the case presentation should be placed in the record within a few hours of the clinical encounter.

INDEX